**Book**

# INFRASOUND
# AND
# LOW FREQUENCY
# VIBRATION

# Infrasound
# and
# Low Frequency
# Vibration

*edited by*

## W. TEMPEST

*Department of Electrical Engineering*
*University of Salford*
*England*

1976

## ACADEMIC PRESS

### LONDON   NEW YORK   SAN FRANCISCO

*A Subsidiary of Harcourt Brace Jovanovich, Publishers*

ACADEMIC PRESS INC. (LONDON) LTD.
24/28 Oval Road,
London NW1

*United States Edition published by*
ACADEMIC PRESS INC.
111 Fifth Avenue
New York, New York 10003

Library of Congress Catalog Card Number: 76 016989
ISBN: 0 12 085450 5

0 12 6854505

*Printed in Great Britain by*
JOHN WRIGHT & SONS LTD., AT THE STONEBRIDGE PRESS, BRISTOL

# LIST OF CONTRIBUTORS

C. ASHLEY, *U.O.P. Bostrom (UK) Ltd., Northampton, NN5 5AB, England*

M. E. BRYAN, *Department of Electrical Engineering, University of Salford, M5 4WT, England*

DORIS M. COWLEY, *British Standards Institution, London, W1A 2BS, England*

MARGARET J. EVANS, *University of Manchester, Manchester, M13 9Q, England*

H. E. VON GIERKE, *Wright-Patterson Air Force Base, Ohio 45433, USA*

M. J. GRIFFIN, *Institute of Sound and Vibration Research, University of Southampton, SO9 5NH, England*

K. KYRIAKIDES, *Sandy Brown Associates, London, W1P 5HP, England*

H. G. LEVENTHALL, *Chelsea College, Pulton Place, London, SW6 5PR, England*

E. J. LOVESEY, *Royal Aircraft Establishment, Farnborough, GU14 6TD, England*

C. W. NIXON, *Wright-Patterson Air Force Base, Ohio 45433, USA*

D. E. PARKER, *Department of Psychology, Miami University, Ohio 45056, USA*

B. K. N. RAO, *Department of Mechanical Engineering, University of Birmingham, B15 2TT, England*

J. T. REASON, *Department of Psychology, University of Leicester, Leicester, LE1 7RH, England*

W. TEMPEST, *Department of Electrical Engineering, University of Salford, M5 4WT, England*

N. S. YEOWART, *Department of Electrical Engineering, University of Salford, M5 4WT, England*

# PREFACE

This book is concerned with what might well be termed the "environmental" aspects of infrasound and low frequency vibration. In this context "environmental" refers to the relationship between the human being and the infrasound and/or vibration environment in which he finds himself.

Infrasound is here defined as airborne sound in the frequency range below 20 Hz, and until the early 1960's it had only been the subject of a very few, rather academic, studies. At about that time the development of new noise sources, particularly larger jet engines and rocket motors, led to the (incidental) generation of high levels of infrasound. It became quickly apparent that this new noise hazard could be perceived, could cause annoyance, interfere with task performance, and, it was suspected, cause biological damage. Now, after a decade of research, mainly in Britain and the United States, some answers are beginning to emerge to the questions posed ten years earlier. This book aims to bring together contributions from some of the leading workers in the field and to set out the current "state of the art". The reader will find that only some of the effects originally attributed to infrasound have been verified. Annoyance can certainly occur, and at the other end of the scale there is very little evidence of biological damage. Between these extremes, there is the area of task performance, and general well-being, where, at the moment, there are real differences of opinion between workers. This book does not attempt to reconcile these differing views. To do so at this stage would be arbitrary, and premature, but both sides describe their research and draw their conclusions. It is hoped that further interest may be stimulated, and the disagreement finally reconciled. Although not directly concerned with the human reaction to infrasound, animal studies in this field allow many investigations which could not possibly be performed on humans. This work is discussed in Chapter 7, and throws some light on the physiological processes involved. It seems possible that, in the long term, work with laboratory animals will contribute as much to understanding infrasound as will human studies.

The final four chapters are concerned with vibration at low frequencies and its effect on the human organism; a field closely related to, but very different from, infrasound. The parallels lie in the frequency range involved, the fact that in both vibration and infrasound the inner ear is an important receptor, that vibration and infrasound occur together in many environments and in the similarity of many of the effects demonstrated or postulated. Historically, however, the subjects have developed quite differently. A glance at the long lists of references to the chapters on vibration show that here is a problem that has been known for several decades, and to which many workers have made contributions. The effects of vibration can be broadly considered in two frequency ranges: a low range, where the main consequence of exposure is motion sickness, and the interest is concentrated largely on the nervous system; in the higher range the body is "shaken about" and one thinks of the effects mainly in anatomical and physiological terms. In both areas of frequency this book tries to present the current view on the effect of vibration on the human subject.

Finally, the editor would like to take this opportunity to thank all the authors for their contributions, the staff of the Academic Press for their very skilful assistance in the preparation of the book, and his wife Brenda, for her help as assistant editor, proof-reader, secretary and typist throughout the whole period of collecting and finalizing the manuscript.

Salford                                                             W. TEMPEST
August 1976

# CONTENTS

LIST OF CONTRIBUTORS . . . . . . . . v

PREFACE . . . . . . . . . . . vii


## 1. ENVIRONMENTAL INFRASOUND: ITS OCCURRENCE AND MEASUREMENT

   I Introduction . . . . . . . . . 1
  II Detection of Infrasound . . . . . . . 1
 III Recording of Infrasound . . . . . . . 4
 IV Analysis of Infrasound . . . . . . . 6
  V Typical Sources of Infrasound . . . . . . 6
 VI Impulsive Noise . . . . . . . . . 13
VII Long Term Monitoring and Analysis of Infrasound . . . 15


## 2. INFRASOUND IN TRANSPORTATION

   I Introduction . . . . . . . . . 19
  II Measurement Techniques . . . . . . . 20
 III Infrasound in Passenger Cars . . . . . . 21
 IV Infrasound in Commercial Vehicles . . . . . 26
  V Infrasound in Other Forms of Transport . . . 30
 VI Infrasound in Surface Transportation—Summary . . . 31
VII Infrasound in Helicopters and Ships . . . . . 33
VIII Effects of Infrasound in Transportation . . . . 33
 IX Conclusions . . . . . . . . . 35


## 3. THRESHOLDS OF HEARING AND LOUDNESS FOR VERY LOW FREQUENCIES

   I Introduction . . . . . . . . . 37
  II The Threshold of Hearing for very low Frequencies . . 38
 III Comparison of Recent Binaural Threshold Data . . . 57
 IV Low Frequency Equal Loudness Relationships . . . 59
  V Low Frequency Equal Annoyance Relationships . . . 61
 VI Summary of Low Frequency Equal Loudness and Equal
     Annoyance Contours . . . . . . . 63

## 4. Low Frequency Noise Annoyance

    I Annoyance, Loudness and Noisiness  .    .    .    .    .    65
   II Low Frequency Annoyance .    .    .    .    .    .    66
  III Low Frequency Noise Sources   .    .    .    .    .    67
  IV Annoyance in Transportation   .    .    .    .    .    68
    V Annoyance due to Low Frequency Noise in the Work Environment  .    .    .    .    .    .    .    81
  VI Annoyance due to Low Frequency Noise in the Home Environment  .    .    .    .    .    .    .    85
 VII Discussion .    .    .    .    .    .    .    .    91

## 5. Physiological and Psychological Effects of Infrasound at Moderate Intensities

    I Introduction    .    .    .    .    .    .    .    97
   II Physiological Effects .    .    .    .    .    .    97
  III Psychological Effects .    .    .    .    .    109

## 6. Effects of Intense Infrasound on Man

    I Introduction    .    .    .    .    .    .    .    115
   II Sources of Infrasound .    .    .    .    .    .    116
  III Investigative Methods .    .    .    .    .    118
  IV Physiological and Performance Effects .    .    125
    V Whole Body Effects   .    .    .    .    .    136
  VI Preliminary Tolerance Levels   .    .    .    144
 VII Summary .    .    .    .    .    .    .    147

## 7. Effects of Sound on The Vestibular System

    I Introduction    .    .    .    .    .    .    .    151
   II Vestibular Responses to Acoustical Stimulation   .    .    158
  III Discussion .    .    .    .    .    .    175
  IV Summary and Conclusions   .    .    .    .    182

## 8. Subjective Effects of Vibration

    I Introduction    .    .    .    .    .    .    .    187
   II The Sensations of Vibration .    .    .    .    187
  III Types of Motion .    .    .    .    .    194

IV Effects of Directional Vibration on Performance . . . 199
V Vibration of Specific Parts of Body and Effects of Posture . 203
VI Physiological Effects of Vibration . . . . . . 211
VII Ride Indices and Vibration in Transport . . . . 218
VIII Measurement Techniques . . . . . . . 225
IX Conclusions . . . . . . . . . 228

## 9. The Occurrence and Effects Upon Performance of Low Frequency Vibration

I Introduction . . . . . . . . . 235
II Performance Effects . . . . . . . . 240
III The Occurrence of Vibrations in Vehicles . . . . 257

## 10. Vibration and Visual Acuity

I Introduction . . . . . . . . . 263
II The Mechanism for Seeing . . . . . . . 264
III Object Vibration . . . . . . . . 269
IV Subject Vibration . . . . . . . . 280
V Object and Subject Vibration . . . . . . 293
VI General Conclusions . . . . . . . . 294

## 11. Motion Sickness and Associated Phenomena

I Introduction . . . . . . . . . 299
II The Nature of the Phenomenon . . . . . . 301
III The Role of the Vestibular System . . . . . 305
IV The Otolith Overstimulation Theory . . . . . 306
V The Sensory Conflict Theory. . . . . . . 309
VI Quantitative Studies of Oscillatory Stimulation . . . 321
VII Factors Influencing Susceptibility . . . . . . 326
VIII The Prevention of Motion Sickness . . . . . 336
IX Conclusion . . . . . . . . . . 342

Appendix: International Standards in the Vibration Field . 349

Index . . . . . . . . . . 359

# 1. Environmental Infrasound: its Occurrence and Measurement

*H. G. Leventhall* and *K. Kyriakides*

## I. Introduction

This chapter considers infrasound in city and industrial environments, produced mainly by human activity, e.g. industrial processes, transport etc., but excluding nuclear explosions and rockets. Many processes which produce infrasound also give continuous energy into the lower audio-frequency range so that a sharp division of interest at about 20 Hz is not desirable. Methods for the detection, recording and analysis of infrasound are discussed first and this is followed by a description of typical sources and spectra.

## II. Detection of Infrasound

The detection of infrasound presented difficulties to early workers since commercial equipment was not available and a number of special microphone systems capable of responding to pressure fluctuations in the infrasonic region were developed. The stimulus for these came initially from the interest in naturally occurring infrasound, but the subsequent need to detect sonic booms led to the commercial development of low frequency microphones which were of direct use for infrasound. There have also been commercial designs specifically for infrasound.

The earlier microphones had limitations on overall frequency response and dynamic range and were often quite bulky. Their principles of operation were as follows.:

a. *Condenser microphone* (Baird and Barwell, 1940). The microphone diaphragm was enclosed in a cavity and external pressure fluctuations were passed through a needle valve which gave a controlled leakage rate into the cavity. A second needle valve to the rear of the diaphragm controlled the pressure equalisation rate. In this way the microphone could be used to select a band of frequencies. For example, Baird and Barwell adjusted the front leak so that frequencies less than about 1 Hz were passed without attenuation whilst the pressure equalisation leakage was much slower, to permit the detection of frequencies below 1 Hz, but to give equalisation for atmospheric pressure changes.

b. *Moving coil microphone* (Vakhitov, 1964). An acoustic resonator was incorporated into the microphone in order to raise the low frequency response. The resonator consisted of a hole drilled through the centre magnet pole, along the axis of the coil, communicating with an auxiliary cavity. The lower frequency limit depends on the dimensions of the hole and volume of the cavity, but the response of the microphone was typically from about 6 Hz to 100 Hz.

c. *Optical detector* (Gavreau *et al.*, 1966). A large cylinder (volume 120 litres) was closed at one end with a rubber diaphragm which had a small mirror attached at the centre. Movement of the diaphragm was detected by a light reflected from the mirror through a screen of opacity dependent on its length and falling on to a photocell. The useful range was from about 0.1 Hz to 40 Hz.

d. *Solion infrasonic microphone* (Collins *et al.*, 1964). The solion is an electro-chemical device, its name being derived from "ions in solution". The electrolytic solution is contained by flexible diaphragms and differential pressure fluctuations cause flow of the electrolyte which, in the system used (the redox system), is converted to a fluctuating electrical output. The frequency range is from 0.0001 Hz to 30 Hz.

e. *Thermistor microphone* (Fehr, 1970). Air flow over a thermistor bead carrying a steady current causes cooling of the bead and a change in resistance which may be detected by connecting the thermistor in a bridge circuit. The output of the bridge due to unbalance depends on the resistance change. Rectification was avoided by using a second thermistor adjacent to the first so that it was warmed by the heat lost from the first one, thus ensuring that the bridge output changed polarity as the air flow direction changed. The frequency range is from about 0.001 Hz to 22 Hz.

The microphones described above are representative of those specially developed for infrasonic work. They are not all suitable for the full range, from about 1 Hz to 100 Hz, which might be of interest in studying environmental low frequency noise in towns and industry, and some of them are not easily portable. However, alternative smaller microphones which are useful for field work are also available. These are described next.

*Piezo-electric microphones*. The low frequency limit of a microphone employing a diaphragm depends on the pressure equalisation hole connecting the rear of the diaphragm to the atmosphere. If this hole is blocked or omitted, and the capsule sealed, the diaphragm will, ideally, respond to static pressure changes. The diaphragm deflection is transmitted to the sensing element which may not be able to maintain its response down to very low frequencies because of charge leakage through external resistance (or, in the limiting case, through the leakage resistance of the element itself) during the fluctuation of the exciting pressure. A piezo-electric microphone has been adapted to operate down to 0.1 Hz (Hood and Leventhall, 1971). A B and K 4117 microphone, which normally has a lower limit of 3 Hz, was modified by blocking the equalisation hole and using a high input impedance amplifier in the first stage of signal amplification. Residual air leakage limited the acoustic low frequency cut-off to 0.1 Hz. The electrical low frequency cut-off, $f$, was obtained from the microphone capacitance (4000 pF) and amplifier input resistance ($10^9$ $\Omega$) using $2\pi f RC = 1$. Hence

$$f = \frac{1}{2\pi RC} = 0.04 \text{ Hz}$$

giving the frequency at which the electrical response of the system is 3 dB down. The Pons type MIF70 is a piezo-electric microphone specially designed for infrasound. It has a diameter of 330 mm and an upper frequency limit of 20 Hz.

*Condenser microphones*. The condenser microphone may be used in a similar manner to the piezo-electric microphone described above. However, since the capacitance of a condenser microphone is much lower than that of the piezo-electric (say, 60 pF compared with 4000 pF), the lower frequency limit might be determined electrically rather than acoustically. For example, a microphone of capacitance 60 pF used with an amplifier having input resistance of $10^9$ $\Omega$ has a lower limit of about 2.5 Hz due to the time constant of the electrical system, even though the microphone acoustic cut-off frequency may be lower.

A condenser microphone also lends itself to use in a high frequency tuned circuit, or balanced bridge system, operating in the megahertz region. Diaphragm movement in the tuned circuit causes a frequency modulation which is subsequently demodulated to regain the low frequency. Diaphragm movement in the balanced bridge causes an amplitude variation of the high frequency which is detected to give the original waveform.

Commercial frequency modulation systems are available, e.g. the B and K Type 2631 carrier system with either one inch or half inch microphones, and the Sennheiser MKH-110-1. These microphones respond over the audio as well as the infrasonic region. If interest is only in infrasound, it may be advantageous to limit the high frequency response. This may be done with a "front leak" obtained by enclosing the capsule in a chamber with a small opening which is of too high impedance to transmit high frequencies, thus combining low pass filtering of airborne acoustic waves with wind shielding.

## MICROPHONE CALIBRATION

An infrasonic microphone should be calibrated at low frequencies. A simple method is the pistonphone which uses constant peak displacement of a diaphragm to produce constant pressure changes. However, difficulties arise at low frequencies when heat loss to the walls of the pistonphone causes a reduction in pressure during the period of the diaphragm displacement. This occurs when the pressure changes are turning from adiabatic to isothermal and can cause an error of up to 3 dB (Beranek, 1949). The effect is minimised by using a large volume compared with the surface area of the pistonphone cavity. For example, a cylindrical cavity of 5 cm diameter, 10 cm long has less than 0.5 dB error at 0.2 Hz.

An alternative method of calibration is to use constant force, instead of constant displacement excitation of the pistonphone, by employing an electromagnetic vibrator fed with constant current to drive the diaphragm. The pistonphone volume should be small to ensure that the stiffness of the system is due to the enclosed air, rather than to the vibrator suspension, and then, when the pressure tends to drop due to heat conduction, the deficit is made up by the constant force of the vibrator.

## III. Recording of Infrasound

The location of an infrasonic noise source is often in a place where analysis on site is not possible. A recording is therefore necessary. Ultraviolet recorders give a graphic trace of the waveform but it may not be easy to determine the frequency components and amplitudes from inspection of the trace. Magnetic tape recording, permitting subsequent analogue or digital analysis of the noise, is preferable, but a conventional tape recorder cannot be used at very low frequencies. A modulation system is required for the recording. Frequency modulation is the most widely used method but, although multi-channel portable

F.M. tape recorders are available commercially, they are expensive. However, it is a simple matter to build an F.M. adapter to use with an existing conventional tape recorder, and at least one commercial version is available. The unmodulated recording frequency is placed towards the upper end of the tape recorder range and the input to the modulator causes a variation of frequency which follows the low frequency input. The frequency-modulated high frequency is recorded on the tape and subsequently replayed through detector circuits which

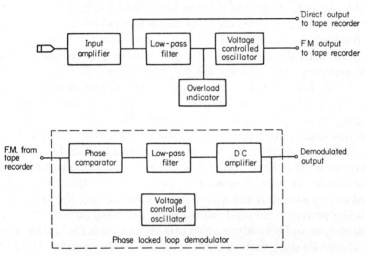

*Fig.* 1 Block diagram of tape-recording system.

restore the low frequency information. The recording system at present being used by the authors is based on an integrated circuit voltage controlled oscillator in which the unmodulated frequency is set to 10 kHz. Figure 1 illustrates the recording system. The high input impedance amplifier following the microphone ensures a good low frequency response. The low pass filter removes higher frequencies, which are not required in the recording and may cause overloading. The modulator output consists of frequency-modulated rectangular waves which are recorded. Demodulation is carried out with a phase locked loop. In the integrated circuit form the phase locked loop is a simple and inexpensive solution in areas where it was previously too complex and expensive.

The response of the F.M. channel is 3 dB down at about 450 Hz. When the F.M. unit is used with a two-channel (stereo) tape recorder there is wide overlap with the normal audio channel permitting recording from low infrasonic frequencies through the audio frequency range.

## IV. Analysis of Infrasound

Commercial analysers are now available down into the infrasonic range, e.g. the B and K range extends down to 2 Hz. Vibration analysers operating down to low frequencies have been produced for some time and most major manufacturers supply equipment suitable for infrasonic work.

Active filters based on operational amplifiers may be constructed very easily to operate in the infrasonic region and it is possible to assemble an octave or one-third octave filter bank. However, a one-third octave filter centred on 2 Hz has a bandwidth of about 0.46 Hz. Slow fluctuations in output level will result from the analysis of wide-band noise with this filter and a long averaging time will be required to ensure accuracy. The relation $e = 1/\sqrt{(BT)}$, where $e$ is the relative error, $B$ the bandwidth and $T$ the averaging time, shows that an averaging time of over 200 seconds is required for a relative error of 1 dB. The averaging time is correspondingly greater for narrower band analysis at this frequency. For example, a 1% bandwidth analysis at 2 Hz would require an averaging time of nearly one and a half hours for 1 dB relative error. It is clear that some analogue instrumentation becomes impracticable at low frequencies. However, analysis may also be carried out by sampling the waveform and computing the spectrum and this is the preferred method for the very low frequencies.

Heterodyne and homodyne analysers are available for low frequencies. They should be used with caution towards the lower end of their ranges since the sum and difference components produced by the internal mixing process are separated by only twice the tuning frequency. This is normally of no consequence in the audio-frequency range since a narrow analysing filter can reject the unwanted component. The rejection is adequate if the ratio of the filter bandwidth to the tuning frequency is very small, a condition which is not satisfied in all instruments at their lowest frequencies.

## V. Typical Sources of Infrasound

Sources of infrasound are basically the same as those of audio-frequency noise, including turbulence, resonance, pulsating and reciprocating processes. Infrasound occurs in a wide variety of locations some of which will now be described.

### A. INFRASOUND IN TRANSPORT

Several measurements of infrasonic noise in vehicles have been reported (Hood and Leventhall, 1971; Stephens, 1971; Tempest and

Bryan, 1972; Anastassiades *et al.*, 1973). The infrasonic noise inside a saloon car travelling at 100 km/h with a front quarter-light window open is shown in Fig. 2. Turbulence contributes to the high level at low frequencies. When only a rear window is open there is a peak at about 16 Hz resulting from a suspected Helmholtz resonance within

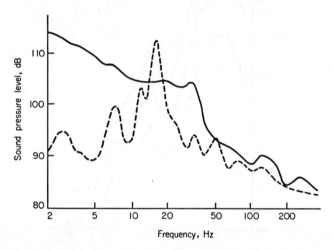

*Fig.* 2 Noise in saloon car at 100 km/h. —— quarter-light windows open; – – – – rear window open (5% bandwidth analysis).

the car body. The rise at low frequencies is typical of noise in cars produced by turbulence, whilst we have found that a peak in the infrasonic region is consistently produced by an open rear window. Infrasonic levels in vehicles are discussed in more detail in Chapter 2.

Low frequency noise generated by wind turbulence is illustrated in Fig. 3, which is the statistical analysis of noise recorded inside a small commercial vehicle when standing stationary in a high wind. The peaks are associated with vehicle body panel resonances.

Single vehicles and streams of traffic produce low frequency noise in the vicinity of roads. Figure 4 shows the noise measured in the room of a house when a 30 ton lorry accelerated past at a distance of 27 m from the window. The peaks at 16 Hz and 64 Hz can be related to the firing rate of the engine.

The overall noise produced by a stream of vehicles must be analysed statistically. Traffic noise on a large busy motorway junction is shown in Fig. 5. The peak at 63 Hz is caused by slow-moving heavy vehicles. This peak normally changes to 125 Hz for rapid traffic flow.

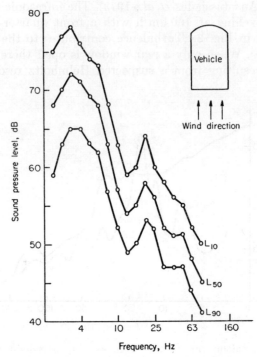

*Fig.* 3 Wind turbulence effects in small commercial vehicle (one-third octave bandwidth analysis).

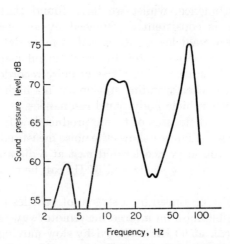

*Fig.* 4 Noise in a house due to single heavy vehicle (5% bandwidth analysis).

The noise both outside and inside a double-glazed house on a busy road is given in Fig. 6. The peak is at 63 Hz and the attenuation of the double glazing at low frequencies is as indicated.

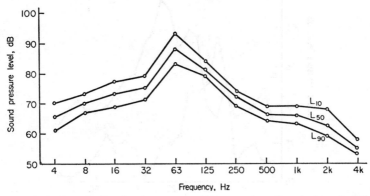

*Fig.* 5 Statistical analysis of noise near a motorway junction (octave bandwidth analysis).

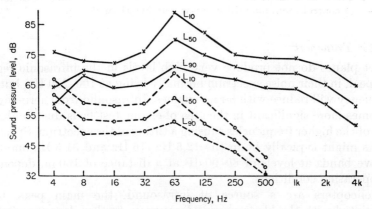

*Fig.* 6 Statistical analysis of noise outside and inside a double-glazed house (octave bandwidth analysis). × — × outside; ○ – – – ○ inside.

### 1. *Infrasonic Noise from Trains*

The noise levels in a diesel train have been reported by Tempest (1973), see also Chapters 2 and 4.

### 2. *Infrasonic Noise in Ships*

The noise levels in the first class lounge and the control room of a cross-channel passenger vessel are given in Fig. 7. Further data on noise in the engine rooms of ships are to be found in Chapter 2.

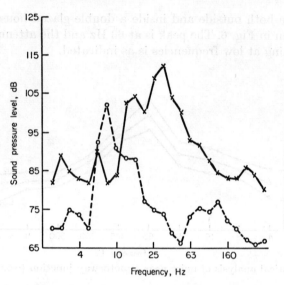

*Fig.* 7 Noise in a cross-channel passenger vessel. × — × first class lounge; ○ – – – ○ control room (one-third octave bandwidth analysis).

## 3. *Air Transport*

Jet planes do not produce very high levels in the infrasonic region, the peak in their noise spectrum normally being at 100–200 Hz, but this frequency will reduce with larger engines. Infrasound from aero-engines becomes more significant in the area of engine test beds due to absorption of the higher frequencies causing a tilting of the spectrum. Spectrum peaks might typically be in the 12.5 Hz, 16 Hz and 31.5 Hz one-third octave bands at levels of 80–90 dB at a distance of 100 m, depending on operating conditions.

Helicopters are a source of infrasound, the main peak being associated with the blade passing frequency, further data are given in Chapter 2.

## B. INFRASONIC NOISE IN INDUSTRY

The noise close to a blast furnace in a steelworks is given in Fig. 8. There is a prominent peak at about 7 Hz which is thought to be due to an acoustic resonance within the structure of the blast furnace.

High levels of low frequency noise have also been measured from a tuyere furnace which produced 123 dB at 25 Hz at the charging platform. Nearby domestic buildings were subjected to uncomfortable noise.

Other sources of high levels at low frequencies include the shaker tables in a foundry knock-out plant, which have produced a level of 120 dB at 25 Hz.

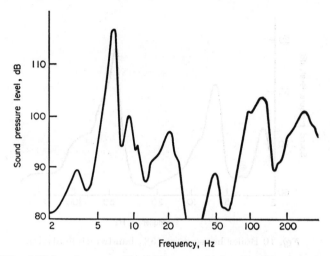

*Fig.* 8 Noise close to a blast furnace (5% bandwidth analysis).

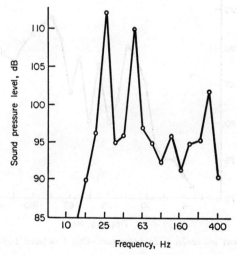

*Fig.* 9 Compressor noise in a factory (one-third octave bandwidth analysis).

The noise from stationary diesel engines or compressors is similar to that in ships. Figure 9 shows a typical spectrum of compressor room noise. Boiler house noise may also contain high levels of infrasound generated by combustion. Figure 10 shows an analysis of the noise in the boiler house of an apartment block. The high level low frequency components are probably caused by resonances within the boiler/flue system. Combustion noise in a factory is given in Fig. 11.

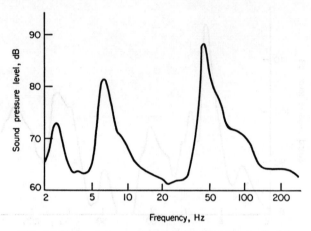

*Fig.* 10 Boiler house noise (5% bandwidth analysis).

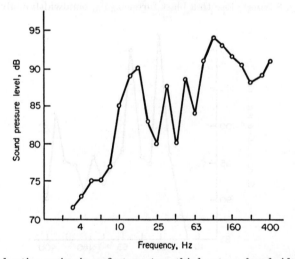

*Fig.* 11 Combustion noise in a factory (one-third octave bandwidth analysis).

## C. VENTILATION SYSTEMS

Interest in infrasound was stimulated partly by experience with disturbing noise from ventilation systems (Gavreau *et al.*, 1966). In large buildings the positioning of outlet grilles in relation to corridors can produce low frequency resonances. Incorrect installation of a suspended ceiling may also result in high levels of low frequency noise due to ceiling vibration. Figure 12 shows the noise levels in a small office in which the hangers for the suspended ceiling were in contact with ventilation ducts in the ceiling void. The result of the faulty installation was that the ceiling panels vibrated, producing the peak

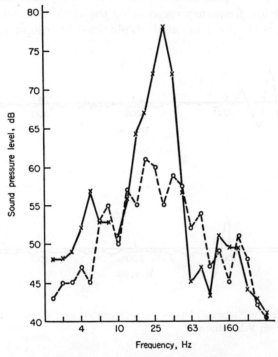

*Fig.* 12 Noise in a small office. ×—× before treatment; ○ ─ ─ ─ ○ after treatment (one-third octave bandwidth analysis).

at about 30 Hz which corresponded with a room mode. Correction of the installation reduced the levels as shown in the lower curve. Other examples of ventilation system noise with high levels at low frequencies are given by Tempest (1973), see also Chapter 4.

## VI. Impulsive Noise

It is well known that sonic booms, blast waves and gun fire contain low frequency components. An illustration of recording and analysing techniques is given by the analysis of the noise of gun fire during a salute on a ceremonial occasion in Hyde Park, London. The terrain in Hyde Park is substantially flat and was free from obstacles in the vicinity of the guns so it was possible to consider only the initial impulse and exclude reflections. The noise was recorded at a distance of 250 m from the source on both the infrasonic and audio-frequency channels of the tape-recording system described above, and replayed into a digitising system which gave a record on punched tape. Figure 13 shows a computer plot of the waveforms from both channels. The effect of poor low frequency response on the audio channel is apparent. Figure 14 gives the spectrum analysis obtained by computation and also

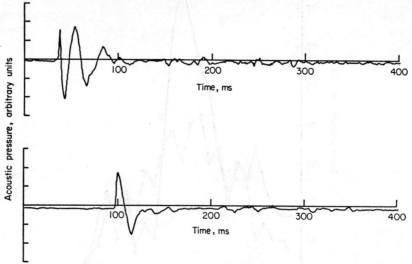

*Fig.* 13 Gun fire waveforms. Upper trace recorded on "direct" channel; lower trace recorded on F.M. channel.

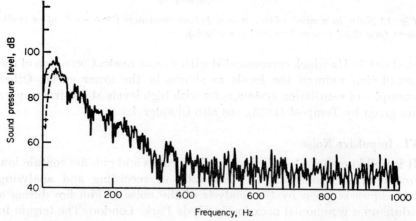

*Fig.* 14 Gun fire spectrum. ——— from F.M. channel; – – – – – from direct channel.

illustrates the effect of inadequate low frequency response. (The spectrum above 500 Hz should be ignored because it exceeds the upper frequency limit of the F.M. system.)

## VII. Long Term Monitoring and Analysis of Infrasound

A system designed and constructed in the authors' laboratory consists of a bank of one-third octave filters from 1.25 Hz to 160 Hz. The incoming signal is amplified and fed simultaneously to all filters. The filter outputs are rectified, averaged and fed through a data logger to a digitiser and punched tape. A clock controls the commencement of the logging scan which is immediately preceded by automatic disconnection

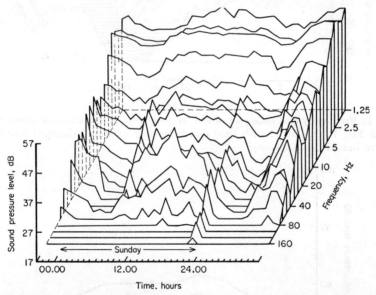

*Fig.* 15 Frequency and time plot of low frequency noise in a small anechoic room. Samples at 1 hour intervals (one-third octave bandwidth analysis).

of the rectifier circuits from the averaging circuits, which contain low leakage capacitors. In this way, the result of scanning the averaging circuits corresponds to integration up to a particular instant of time. Time intervals between scans may be selected to be from 2 minutes to 120 minutes. The time constant of the averaging circuits of the lower frequency filters are about 275 seconds, gradually decreasing with increase of frequency to 10 seconds.

The punched tape output of the data logger contains information on frequency, level and time, permitting three-dimensional computer plots to be produced. Figure 15 shows infrasonic and low frequency

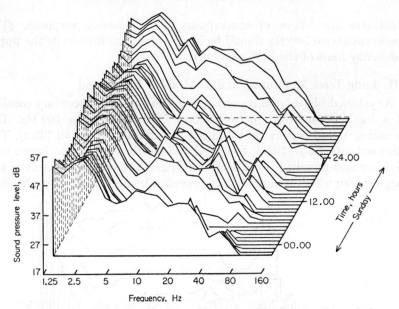

*Fig.* 16 Frequency and time plot of low frequency noise in a small anechoic room (as in Fig. 15) replotted with time and frequency axes interchanged (one-third octave bandwidth analysis).

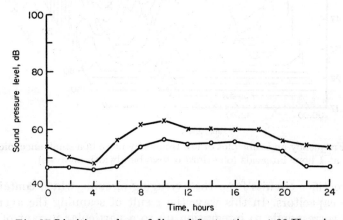

*Fig.* 17 Limiting values of diurnal fluctuations at 20 Hz noise.

noise levels measured in a small anechoic room. Sampling was at 1 hour intervals over a 39 hour period. The same data can be replotted as in Fig. 16 to present the information from a different aspect.

Monitoring over a longer period permits maximum and minimum levels to be extracted from the data. For example, for outdoor measurements Fig. 17 gives the limiting values of the output of the 20 Hz one-third octave filter on any Wednesday over a 10 week period. The general trend of the diurnal fluctuations follows that to be expected from traffic noise. Similar variations over a continuous 1 week period in the 2.5 Hz one-third octave band are shown in Fig. 18. The difference between maximum and minimum levels is greater at 2.5 Hz than at 20 Hz. The levels were generally highest in the middle part of the day,

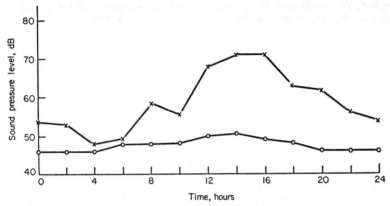

*Fig.* 18 Limiting values of diurnal fluctuations at 2.5 Hz noise.

but the maximum levels shown occurred on one day only and were about 5 dB higher than on any other day. This could have been due to wind effects or to favourable propagation from distant sources. For example, Liszka (1974) used a chain of tripartite arrays in Sweden to monitor infrasound at 2 Hz and was able to identify hydroelectric power plants, industrial plants and oilfields in the North Sea as probable sources.

This chapter has described the occurrence of infrasound and low frequency noise from a variety of man-made sources. The infrasonic content is sometimes a distinct contribution, as for example with resonances or diesel engines, but it is often the lower end of a spectrum which continues to much higher frequencies.

REFERENCES

Anastassiades, A. J., Panayotopoulos, C. J. and Thanassoulas, C. P. (1973). *J. Sound Vib.* **29**, 257–259.
Baird, F. and Barwell, C. J., (1940). *J. Sc. Tech.* **21B**, 314–329.
Beranek, L. L. (1949). "Acoustic Measurements", John Wiley, New York.

Collins, J. L., Richie, W. C. and English, G. E. (1964). *J. Acoust. Soc. Am.* **36**, 1283–1287.

Fehr, U. (1970). *J. Aud. Eng. Soc.* **18**, 128–132.

Gavreau, V., Condat, R. and Saul, H. (1966). *Acustica* **17**, 1–10.

Hood, R. A. and Leventhall, H. G. (1971). *Acustica* **25**, 10–13.

Liszka, L. (1974). *J. Acoust. Soc. Am.* **56**, 1383–1388.

Stephens, R. W. B. (1971). *Revista di Acustica* **11**, 48–55.

Tempest, W. (1973). *Acustica* **29**, 205–209.

Tempest, W. and Bryan, M. E. (1972). *Applied Acoustics* **5**, 133–139.

Vakhitov, Ya. Sh. (1964). *Societ Physics (Acoustics)* **10**, 199–200.

# 2. Infrasound in Transportation

*W. Tempest*

## I. Introduction

Transportation is an important area, perhaps *the* most important area, where the effects of infrasound may impinge on the welfare of the community. However, the extent and significance of the effects of infrasound have not yet been evaluated, and to some degree the discussion must therefore be speculative.

The existing situation can be summed up briefly as follows. High levels of infrasound have been measured in numerous transportation situations, the sources of the infrasound being aerodynamic, road roughness or, in some cases, engine noise; this much has been firmly established.

As regards the effects of infrasound; at the levels involved, the data available are far from unanimous in their conclusions. All the work has been performed in the laboratory and a number of adverse effects on balance and task performance have been recorded, but other workers in different laboratories have failed to reproduce the results. Animal experiments have shown some very interesting data at high intensities, but again have not been easily reproducible. A little work on abnormal humans has suggested that there are some individuals of abnormally high sensitivity, but no systematic study has been reported.

There is another, quite indirect approach to the problem, which derives from studies that have established that intense noise at normal frequencies can effect vigilance. It seems possible that similar effects could occur in the infrasonic range.

This chapter is therefore based on the proposition that infrasound exists in transportation, that there is some laboratory evidence to suggest that it may have adverse effects on people, that there are unexplained phenomena in transportation, and that any possible facts which might help to relate the above should be brought together.

## II. Measurement Techniques

The significance of infrasound has only been recognised in the last decade, progress on the collection of data has been impeded by the absence, for much of this period, of commercially available equipment.

Probably the first investigation of transportation noise to extend below 20 Hz was that of Aspinall (1966), who used a magnetic tape recorder and found that, using a direct (as distinct from a modulation) recording technique, and replaying at four times the recording speed, he could obtain a useful response down to 10 Hz.

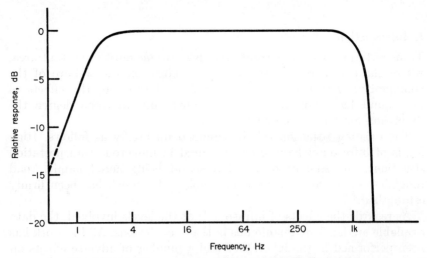

*Fig.* 1 Frequency response of infrasound recording system.

The measurement range was extended downwards by Tempest and Bryan (1972), who fed the output of a sound level meter through a frequency modulation attachment to a battery-driven tape recorder. This system could be used on frequencies down to the octave centred on 2 Hz and the published design (Tempest and Bryan, 1967) has since provided the basis of the equipment used by several other workers in the field.

Figure 1 gives the overall frequency response of the system from the acoustic input of the microphone to the output of the play-back recorder. The replay system was designed to operate at the same tape speed as the recorder, since this permitted continuous monitoring of the system performance during replay, and provided an opportunity to note any obvious faults or malfunctioning of the apparatus. Octave band analysis was normally used, the signal was fed through a band-pass filter to a long time-constant random noise voltmeter, the low frequency band-pass filters were designed specially for this application and have been described elsewhere (Tempest and Yeowart, 1966).

## III. Infrasound in Passenger Cars

The study by Aspinall (1966) already referred to was concerned particularly with the phenomenon of "wind throb" or "wind flutter" which can occur in passenger cars when a major window is open.

His investigation was extensive, and established that, depending on the conditions of the test (i.e. vehicle type, speed and wind direction), there were two distinct types of wind throb which he termed "periodic" and "broad-band".

Periodic wind throb was most commonly obtained when travelling in such a direction that the wind was blowing towards the open window, the actual yaw angle being in the region of 5–10°. At moderate speeds, under this condition, it was found that the sound pressure level measured inside the car had a very large peak in intensity at a single frequency. It is postulated that the sound is generated by a jet-edge mechanism, presumably due to the airstream striking the rear frame of the open window. This generator is coupled to the interior of the car, which, with the same open window as a neck, acts as a Helmholtz resonator to produce a system similar to a musical wind instrument. Direct measurements of the behaviour of the Helmholtz resonator were made using a specially constructed low frequency loudspeaker to excite the vehicle interior via the open window. It was found that while the resonator effect was clearly present, the "Q" was low, typically in the region of five, presumably due to the many departures of a car interior from a simple rigid walled volume. Such departures include leaks through door seals and holes to the engine compartment, interior damping by seats etc.; and, in some cases, coupling to the smaller volume of air in the boot.

Figure 2 shows three examples of the sound pressure level spectra obtained by Aspinall, under conditions which produced periodic wind throb. All three were obtained on the same vehicle and illustrate the points:

(a) Periodic wind throb levels can exceed 120 dB.
(b) The sharpness of the peak is in fact sharper than the "Q" of the vehicle interior itself, indicating some form of positive feedback mechanism.
(c) The behaviour is that of a system with poor frequency stability in that the frequency of maximum energy varies with the speed of the vehicle.

2

Aspinall reported that wind noise of a rather different character was often found when the wind was in a direction away from the window. In this case the "wind throb" was of a broad-band nature, but still

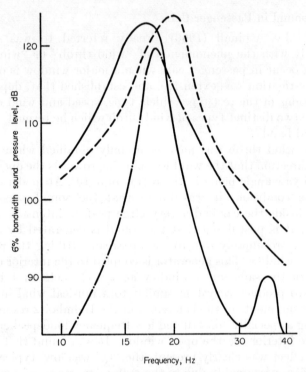

*Fig.* 2 Sound pressure level spectra obtained inside a car with one rear window open under conditions of periodic wind throb. – – – – 113 km/h; ——— 97 km/h; —·—·— 64 km/h. (From Aspinall 1966.)

attained high enough levels to cause passenger discomfort. Figure 3 shows the spectrum measured inside a car under "broad-band wind throb" conditions. This is about 10 dB lower at its maximum than the periodic wind throb levels, and shows evidence of a smaller discrete frequency peak at 12 Hz. It was concluded that the broad-band wind throb was due to the excitation of turbulent flow produced by separation of the airstream passing around the windscreen of the car, the actual spectrum being influenced by resonance of the car interior volume.

Aspinall's work on wind throb was limited to the range of frequencies from 10 Hz upwards, and aimed to provide an understanding of the mechanism of generation with a view to helping vehicle designers reduce the effects. In this he achieved some success, and his report reaches certain conclusions about ways in which "wind throb" can be reduced. More recent work, which has extended the frequency range down to 1.5 Hz, has been mainly concerned with the incidence and human aspects of the problem, rather than the physics of the sound sources.

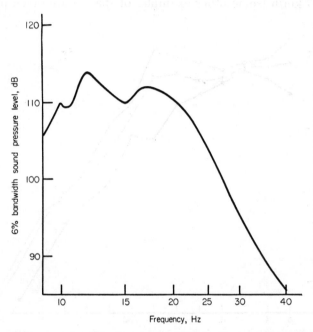

*Fig.* 3 Sound pressure level spectrum obtained inside a car at 97km/h under broad-band wind throb conditions. (From Aspinall 1966.)

Tempest and Bryan (1972) have reported octave band sound pressure level measurements in a variety of cars over the frequency range from 2 Hz to 16 kHz, and over a range of speeds from 64 km/h upwards. The aim of the work was to establish the levels of infrasound to which passengers and drivers were subjected in normal conditions. The measurements were therefore made so as to avoid features which could have rendered the data untypical, such as (a) rough or noisy road surfaces, (b) conditions of high wind and (c) any audible periodic wind throb.

The frequency modulation recording technique has already been mentioned. The sound level meter was normally used in the front passenger seat of the car, with the microphone at a position on a level with the front passenger's head. Infrasound was recorded for a period of approximately 1 minute under steady conditions. Octave bands from 32 Hz upwards were measured directly either just before, or just after, the recordings. A pistonphone was used to calibrate the sound level meters, and to record a reference level on each tape recording.

Figure 4 shows typical overall frequency spectra obtained in three cars at 97 km/h (some other examples of spectra are given in Chapter

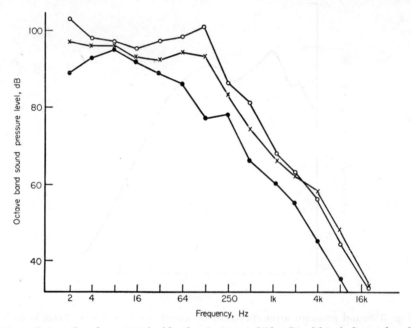

*Fig.* 4 Octave band spectra inside three cars at 97 km/h with windows closed. ○ — ○ small car; × — × large car; ● — ● limousine.

4). The pattern of the results obtained in various cars follows Fig. 4, a substantially flat spectrum for 2–32 Hz followed by progressive reduction in octave band levels at higher frequencies.

The variables which were found to influence the levels of infrasound in a systematic way were vehicle speed, vehicle size and opening windows. The effects of the first two of these are demonstrated in Fig. 5, which shows the mean level of infrasound (defined as the average of the octave bands from 2 Hz to 32 Hz) for four different vehicles at speeds from 64 km/h to 161 km/h; with data at higher speeds for one vehicle. The general pattern of the data is clear, that the level of infrasound increases with increasing speed and decreases with increasing vehicle size. It should be mentioned here that the "small" and "large" vehicles were passenger cars and the "medium" vehicle was an estate car, all of integral steel construction; while the limousine was a coach-built vehicle on a separate chassis. The difference between the largest and smallest vehicles averages 7.1 dB, and the rate of increase of infrasound with speed is 1.8 dB per 16 km/h. This latter figure can now be used to estimate the rate of growth of infrasonic energy with speed and gives the result:

$$P \propto V^{2.7}$$

where $P$ is the power in the range 2–32 Hz and $V$ is the vehicle speed.

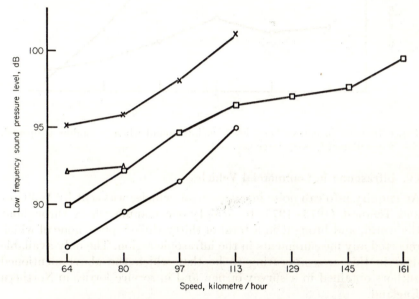

*Fig.* 5 Infrasound level (mean of octave bands 2–32 Hz) measured in four cars at speeds from 64 to 161 km/h. ×—× small car; △—△ medium-sized car; □—□ large car; ○—○ limousine.

The opening of a window (in conditions which did not produce periodic wind throb) invariably increased the level of infrasound considerably. Figure 6 shows the mean effect at 97 km/h and 113 km/h for two cars, the "small" and "large" saloons. In the former case a front sliding window was opened 15 cm and raised the level by about 13 dB to a level of 112 dB at 113 km/h. In the latter case a triangular front quarter-light was opened 40° and increased the level by about 6 dB to 102 dB at 113 km/h.

Other data in cars have been reported by Hood and Leventhall (1971) and by Bruel and Olesen (1973), each of whom published a spectrum for one vehicle. These data are in general agreement with those of Tempest and Bryan (1972).

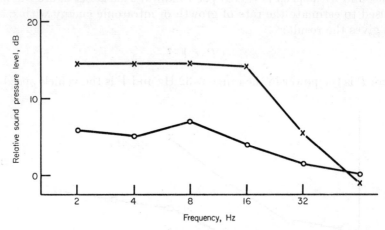

*Fig.* 6 Increase in octave band levels of infrasound when a window is opened. × — × small car; ○ — ○ large car.

## IV. Infrasound in Commercial Vehicles

An enquiry into cab noise in commercial vehicles was sent by Williams and Tempest (1973, 1975) to seventy-one manufacturers throughout the world, and brought in a total of thirty-three replies, none of which reported any measurements in the infrasonic region. The only available data in this area appearing to be that which the above-mentioned authors obtained in a survey of new and in-service lorries in Northern England.

Williams and Tempest obtained data in four types of vehicles: (1) tractor units, (2) tractors and trailers, laden and unladen, (3) rigid chassis box vehicles and (4) rigid chassis low loaders. The speeds normally used were 48 km/h, 64 km/h and 80 km/h and additional parameters investigated were the effects of opening windows, the effect of coasting with the engine switched off and the effect of road surface changes.

Figure 7 shows the spectra obtained in a typical new vehicle, in this case a 32 tonne tractor and trailer unit, measured with the windows closed. Figure 8 shows, for another tractor–trailer unit of similar gross weight, spectra obtained at 48 km/h and 80 km/h with the driver's side-window open and closed. Both figures show the same general pattern as that found in passenger cars; maximum octave band sound pressure levels in the infrasonic region, a steeply falling spectrum at higher frequencies, and a significant increase in infrasound when a window is opened.

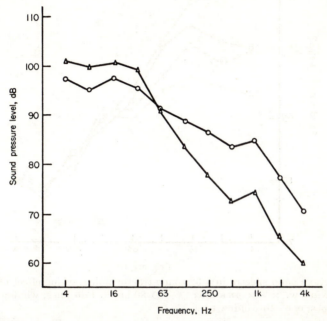

*Fig.* 7 Octave band spectra obtained in cab of a new 32 tonne tractor unit. △ — △ 48 km/h; ○ — ○ 80 km/h.

The effect of vehicle speed on the level of infrasound is shown in Fig. 9 where the 4–32 Hz average octave band levels are plotted for speeds from 48 km/h to 80 km/h. In this case each point represents the mean data for three vehicles of different types.

Two tests were performed to investigate the contribution of engine noise and road noise to the overall level of infrasound. Figure 10 shows the spectra in one new vehicle at 80 km/h in the driving and coasting (engine in neutral) condition. These spectra show a slight decrease in the 63–1000 Hz region in the coasting condition, but the infrasonic levels are unaltered; the conclusion that engine noise does not contribute in the infrasonic bands is to be expected since the calculated frequencies of the engine firing rate and rotational speed all lie in the region above 20 Hz at normal vehicle speeds. This particular vehicle had a well-insulated cab which minimized the contribution of the engine to the cab noise.

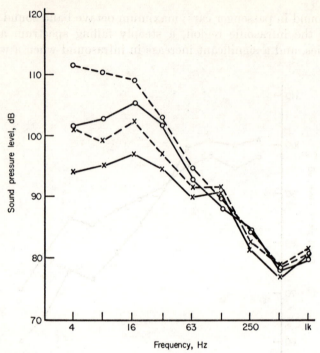

*Fig.* 8 Octave band spectra in a 32 tonne tractor unit showing effect of opening one cab window. × — × 48 km/h; ○ — ○ 80 km/h. Full lines, windows closed; broken lines, one cab window open.

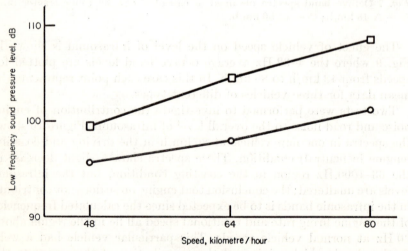

*Fig.* 9 Mean infrasound levels in lorry cabs (4–32 Hz octave bands, three lorries) as a function of speed. □ — □ windows open; ○ — ○ windows closed.

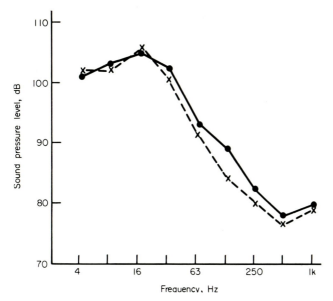

*Fig.* 10 Octave band spectra for driving and coasting conditions in a new lorry at 80 km/h. ● — ● driving; × – – – × coasting.

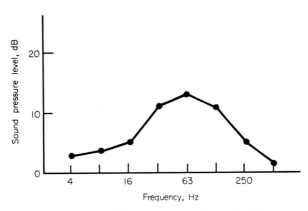

*Fig.* 11 Increase in octave band levels when a lorry is driven over a cobbled surface at 48 km/h.

The effects of a rough road surface were studied by examining the change in octave band levels when a lorry was driven from a smooth to a cobbled road surface at 48 km/h. The result of this test is shown in Fig. 11, which reveals a maximum of 13 dB at 63 Hz, but shows only a small increase of 3–5 dB in the infrasonic region.

3

To give some impression of the range of levels to be found in various lorries, data for a range of heavy vehicles have been combined in Fig. 12 to show the distribution of levels measured. The feature of particular interest in the figure is the convergence of the data into a range of $\pm 16$ dB at 2 kHz. Included in Fig. 12 are data from both new

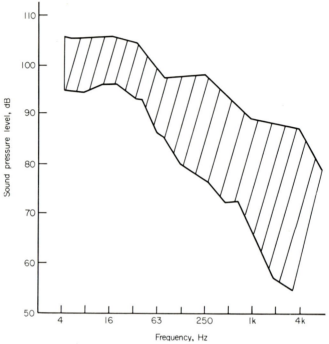

*Fig.* 12 Distribution of spectra obtained over a range of vehicles demonstrating convergence at the lower frequencies.

and used lorries of various types and in this context Fig. 12 supports the hypothesis that audible noise levels are considerably influenced by the age and type of vehicle, but that infrasound in not so affected, hence indicating that the level of infrasound is fundamental to the basic design of the vehicle, and is not influenced by detail differences in design or condition.

## V. Infrasound in Other Forms of Transport

Data on the levels of infrasound in vehicles other than road vehicles are relatively sparse. The only data from rail transport appear to be those quoted elsewhere in this book (Chapter 4) for the levels in motorised and unmotorised diesel multiple-unit passenger trains.

The octave band sound pressure levels and the means of the octave bands are set out in Table I. The train in which these data were obtained consisted of open-type coaches, with some open windows in each coach at the time of testing. Two features of the data deserve comment; the unmotorised coach levels fall in the middle of the range of passenger car figures, and show a very similar rate of increase with vehicle speed.

TABLE I: Infrasonic spectra of diesel multiple-unit passenger train

| | Octave band spl in dB | | | | | |
| Frequency band (Hz) | 2 | 4 | 8 | 16 | 32 | Mean |
|---|---|---|---|---|---|---|
| Unmotored coach 64 km/h | 91 | 91 | 91 | 91 | 92 | 91.2 |
| Unmotored coach 97–103 km/h | 96 | 96 | 95 | 95 | 96 | 95.6 |
| Motored coach[a] 80 km/h | 99 | 99 | 97 | 101 | 101 | 99.4 |
| Motored coach[b] 80 km/h | 94 | 96 | 95 | 105 | 107 | 99.4 |

[a] mean of two runs.
[b] in this condition a loud resonance, presumably between the diesel engine and the coach structure, was audible.

The motorised coach data show evidence of noise from the engine and/or transmission system leading to an increase in the level in the 16 Hz and 32 Hz bands.

## VI. Infrasound in Surface Transportation—Summary

Figure 13 shows the mean infrasonic sound pressure levels obtained in cars, lorries and trains as a function of speed. All the data fall into a fairly narrow range, and show a very similar variation with vehicle speed, thus suggesting that the predominant mode of noise generation is the same in all cases.

Possible sources of infrasound include:

(1) Engine and/or transmission vibration.
(2) Running wheel vibration.
(3) Road (or rail) irregularities.
(4) Aerodynamically generated sound due to the motion of the vehicle through the air.

The role of (1), engine–transmission vibration, would seem to be clear from the train and lorry data. Diesel-engined vehicles have a contribution from this source in the 16 and 32 Hz regions, but not at lower frequencies.

There is no evidence that vibration due to unbalanced running wheels is an important source of infrasound. In one case (the limousine), a severe wheel vibration was noticed at 113 km/h, and a corresponding increase in level in the 16 Hz band (from 92 dB at 97 km/h to 103 dB at 113 km/h) was recorded. However, this subjectively very obvious vibration had no parallel in the other tests carried out. In general the flat spectra obtained in the 2–32 Hz region would argue against major components of noise from this source.

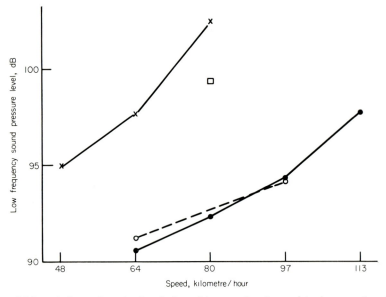

*Fig.* 13 Mean infrasonic noise levels found in cars, lorries and trains as a function of speed. ×——× lorries; ●——● cars; ○ – – – ○ train (unmotored); □ diesel train (motored coach).

The role of running surface irregularities in the generation of infrasound is harder to establish with certainty, but the similar levels found in trains, cars and lorries would argue against this source, since it would be expected that track irregularities would be considerably less than road irregularities.

This leaves aerodynamically generated noise as the predominant source in the infrasonic region, a conclusion that is supported by the work of Aspinall (1966), who found high levels of infrasound in the airstream outside the vehicle.

## VII. Infrasound in Helicopters and Ships

Helicopters and ships present a quite different picture from surface vehicles, since the primary source of infrasound is not a random aerodynamic fluctuation, but arises from the means of propulsion. The only available helicopter data (see Table II) appears to be that of Hood

TABLE II: Noise level peaks in helicopters

| Helicopter type | Speed in knots | Blade frequency (Hz) | Peak levels of noise |
|---|---|---|---|
| 2-seat | 70 | 11·5 | 118 dB at 11·5 Hz |
| 5-seat | 100 | 28 | 120 dB at 28 Hz<br>105 dB at 56 Hz |

and Leventhall (1971), who found, using a narrow band (6–7%) analyser, flat spectra in the 90–100 dB region, with a large peak of about 120 dB at the blade passing repetition frequency.

Available data on noise in diesel-engined ships also come from the work of Hood and Leventhall (1971), who measured engine-room noise in two ferry-boats of 400 and 800 tonnes respectively. Their data are summarised in Table III.

TABLE III: Engine-room noise levels in two ferry-boats

| Vessel | Engine firing (rate/sec) | Infrasonic noise peaks |
|---|---|---|
| 400 tonne ferry | 13 | 133 dB at 13 Hz |
| 800 tonne ferry | 7 | 118 dB at 7 Hz<br>108 dB at 14 Hz<br>111 dB at 21 Hz |

## VIII. Effects of Infrasound in Transportation

Much of this book is devoted to reports on laboratory experiments to measure and evaluate the effects of infrasound on human and animal organisms; however, as far as the author is aware, there are no data available which directly associate infrasound with transportation. For this reason it is only possible to proceed by deduction, and in the current state of knowledge many of the deductions must be quite tentative.

The work on task performance of a type most closely resembling a driving situation is that of Hood *et al.* (1972), who measured both reaction time and performance in a pointer-following task. In the pointer-following task the subject used a steering wheel to drive a pointer with which he attempted to follow a randomly oscillating reference line. The reference line moved over a maximum excursion of ± 25 cm, and was driven by a random noise voltage in the frequency band 0.05–0.4 Hz. An electronic integrator was used to integrate the modulus of the error between the reference and the pointer, the error score being noted every minute, the total test lasting for 10 minutes. This task was performed in levels of 80 dB, 110 dB and 120 dB noise in a band from 2 Hz to 15 Hz.

This experiment showed an increase in error at 110 dB against 80 dB for six out of seven observers, the mean increase being approximately 14%. However, the average performance improved again at 120 dB, the mean increase in error over 80 dB falling to 9%. The same authors' reaction time test showed a similar result, reaction time (seven-subject average) increasing by 9% at 110 dB, but only 8% at 120 dB. These experiments are clearly inconclusive. The samples were small, and while the pattern of first a deterioration in performance, followed by a slight improvement at higher levels, can be explained by the hypothesis of some form of compensation, it would be more satisfactory to repeat the work with larger samples and with some form of multiple task which would test the compensation theory.

The work of Evans and Tempest (1972) is described in detail elsewhere in this book (Chapter 5), but in essence they report evidence of vertical nystagmus in the dark, beginning in normal observers at about 120 dB sound pressure level. This effect is not a large one, for example it does not occur when the eyes are able to "fix" on some visible object, and, in any case, it only begins at the extreme upper end of the range of levels normally found in vehicles. There may be greater significance in some of the other observations noted by these authors, particularly the feelings of lethargy and euphoria, which some observers reported as being similar to slight intoxication. These effects are not easy to quantify, and the evidence remains in the form of subjective reports. However, this effect has an interesting parallel in another field, that of balance disturbance due to motion. It would seem to be widely accepted, on the basis of available experimental data, that if infrasound has any significant effects on normal observers at levels up to 120 dB, then these effects probably arise from stimulation of the organs of equilibrium. It is well established that some forms of rotary motion can cause balance disturbance, but it is also reported (Reason,

Chapter 11) that low level stimulation of the organ of balance, insufficient to cause dizziness or motion sickness, can induce sensations of extreme lethargy.

Evans and Tempest (1972) also report tests on a small number of observers who described themselves as being abnormally sensitive to balance disturbance, and who were found to be highly susceptible to infrasound; these observers reported serious discomfort and balance disturbance at levels which would not significantly affect normal observers. This result is clearly useful evidence that infrasound can affect the sense of equilibrium, and also suggests that it may be a source of real hazard to a minority of the population. There are no data available on the size of this minority.

The work of Hood and Leventhall (1971) has an interesting parallel in the study of industrial noise, where it is reported (for example Broadbent, 1969) that levels of noise over 90 dB cause a deterioration in performance in vigilance tasks. It is hypothesised that this deterioration is due to a form of overload of the perceptive system; whether infrasound can similarly overload an aspect of perception is at present a matter of speculation.

## IX. Conclusions

Data have been presented which show that infrasound up to 120 dB levels is encountered in road and rail transportation, and that even higher levels are to be found in ships' engine rooms and in helicopters.

The literature of laboratory work on the effects of infrasound provides some rather inconclusive reports of performance deterioration and balance disturbance in the range of intensities reported in vehicles. Evidence is also presented of sensations of euphoria and lethargy. Parallels are drawn between the lethargy produced by infrasound and rotary motion, and also the similarity between infrasound and high intensity audible noise in impairing relaxation time and vigilance respectively. It is reported that some individuals who report sensitivity to balance disturbance also show an unusual sensitivity to infrasound.

In total these effects suggest that infrasound may well have an adverse affect on the performance of drivers. In this respect it probably adds to the already known influences of noise, motion, heat and fatigue, and in this way it may be a factor in some accidents. The magnitude of the role of infrasound in relation to the other factors mentioned is, at the moment, quite impossible to evaluate and further research is clearly needed to decide whether it is significant or entirely trivial.

The role of infrasound as a factor in comfort in transportation has been dealt with in Chapter 4.

## REFERENCES

Aspinall, D. T. (1966). "An empirical investigation of low frequency wind noise in motor cars", MIRA Report No. 1966/2.

Broadbent, D. E. (1969). *In* "Experimental Psychology in Industry" (D. H. Holding, ed.), Chap. 22. Penguin Books, Harmondsworth.

Bruel, P. V. and Olesen, H. P. (1973). *Brüel Kjaer tech. Rev.* No. 3, 14–25.

Evans, Margaret J. and Tempest, W. (1972). *J. Sound Vib.* **22**, 19–24.

Hood, R. A. and Leventhall, H. G. (1971). *Acustica* **25**, 10–13.

Hood, R. A., Leventhall, H. G. and Kyriakides, K. (1972). *Proceeedings of the British Acoustical Society* **1**, No. 3, Paper 71–107.

Tempest, W. and Bryan, M. E. (1967). *Electron. Engng* **39**, 87–89.

Tempest, W. and Bryan, M. E. (1972). *Applied Acoustics* **5**, 133–139.

Tempest, W. and Yeowart, N. S. (1966). *Electron. Engng* **38**, 397–399.

Williams, D. and Tempest, W. (1973). *Proceedings of the British Acoustical Society* **2**, No. 3.

Williams, D. and Tempest, W. (1975). *J. Sound Vib.* **43**, 97–107.

# 3. Thresholds of Hearing and Loudness for Very Low Frequencies

*N. S. Yeowart*

## I. Introduction

General textbooks on sound give the impression that the range of human hearing covers a 10-octave region from 20 Hz to 20 kHz. Outside this range the usual auditory and subjective sensations are generally said not to exist. If one neglects the spectacular and artificial case of hearing by bone conduction at frequencies beyond 30 kHz, then normal observers can hear sounds beyond 14 kHz and younger subjects up to 20 kHz. The ability of the person to hear in the upper range is fairly sensitive to his, or her, age. At the other end of the scale, the accepted limit of 20 Hz for the hearing mechanism can be understood in terms of the physical difficulties which arise when one tries to produce a sound frequency this low. Acoustical engineers have generally been satisfied with a narrower frequency range when studying the effects of noise on man. For example, the range of 50 Hz to 10 kHz was found to be sufficient to describe the human response to every-day sounds. In this case, atmospheric attenuation quickly removed the higher frequencies as distance from the source increased, and the sensitivity of the ear was known to be falling rapidly for frequencies below 50 Hz, so little if any contribution to loudness was expected.

In the last decade new noise sources have developed, e.g. air-conditioning systems for large halls, which produce intense sound pressures below 20 Hz. The obvious discomfort of people exposed to this low frequency noise has indicated that human reaction to frequencies below 20 Hz is indeed far from non-existent; in fact, in some cases, it could be realistically described as being violent.

In the following sections the various key experiments in determining the threshold of hearing below about 25 Hz are presented in chronological order. The chronology itself is interesting as it shows the resurgence of interest in the low frequency field over the last decade.

Current means of measuring low frequency loudness are also explained.

## II. The Threshold of Hearing for very low Frequencies

The early work on the threshold of hearing for very low frequency tones underlines the difficulties of producing the necessary stimuli. Even today, one is left with the uneasy impression that the apparent lower limit of the hearing mechanism may be a reflection of the shortcomings of the experimenters' equipment, rather than a true limit of the ear itself.

Imai (1907) made an exhaustive study of the threshold of hearing for frequencies below 30 Hz. His sound source was an electrically driven tuning fork 460 mm long with a prong cross-section of $10 \times 20$ mm. By systematically weighting the prongs, frequencies ranging from 30 Hz to 12 Hz were obtained. When the fork was placed as close to the ear canal as the vibrations allowed Imai was able to report that a vibration fundamental of 12 Hz could be detected.

Vance (1914) repeated Imai's experiments. The sound source was also a fork. However, Vance was well aware of the shortcomings of his source in that it produced overtones which were much more easily discerned than the fundamental. To minimise this defect Vance relied on thorough training of his observers. Apparently it took many hours of listening to the tones from the tuning forks before the individual felt any degree of certainty in detecting the fundamental immersed in its various overtones.

The thresholds reported by Vance and Imai indicated strongly the possibility that man could detect periodic acoustical stimulations below 20 Hz. Although, merely because of the high harmonic content of the signal, the data could be suspect. The severe problem of high signal purity delayed further work until 1932. Even then, the electrodynamic earphones of the day could not be relied upon to operate as required under the severe conditions imposed when attempting to produce intense low frequency signals. Brecher (1934) used a novel method to produce intense low frequency tones. His apparatus consisted of a closed box, one side of which was formed by a membrane. The centre of the membrane was mechanically driven by an eccentric cam, producing intense pressure variations within the closed cavity. This cavity was directly coupled to the observer's ear. Brecher reported the first true measurement of very low frequency thresholds. His observations are so consistent with present-day observations that they deserve to be recorded here. For frequencies around 25–30 Hz Brecher described the auditory sensation as one of hearing a relatively weak rumble, associated with an unpleasant tickling and feeling of vibration in the ear. Below 25 Hz the tonal character of the sensation gradually fell away until the observer could detect separate pressure peaks. The limit of tonality was 18 Hz. When the stimulus frequency was reduced below 18 Hz separate "puffs" were heard and slight pain was felt in the ear. Brecher called the critical region, around 18 Hz, the *fusion frequency*. He experimented down to around 7 Hz and concluded that the limit of detectability of low frequency tones had not been reached. When he examined a linear plot of his data he suggested that the sound levels would become impossibly high at about 5–6 Hz, where his plot of pressure versus frequency would approach the vertical asymptotically. His threshold data for one subject over the frequency region of around 7–15 Hz are shown in Fig. 1, and his subjective descriptions are summarized in Table I.

Once the advantage of Brecher's approach to high sound pressure levels at low frequencies was appreciated, the system was developed and refined by several workers. Wever and Bray (1936) used a pistonphone to provide the required pressure variations. This pistonphone worked into an enclosed volume formed by the pathway of two acoustic filters. One filter, a five-section low pass acoustic filter, had a roll-off frequency of 100 Hz, the second, a rubber tube, provided attenuation for frequencies above 3 kHz. Their combined response was sufficient to render the motor noise inaudible at the observation point. The observer was isolated from the equipment noise vibration by being seated in a quiet room. The stimulus was presented to the subject's earpiece by rubber tubing through the wall of the room. For safety reasons the investigators decided to limit the maximum sound pressure level to 30 dB re 1 bar (104 dB re 0.0002 $\mu$ bar), although much higher levels had been used prior to this work (Brecher, 1934). Nevertheless, they reported most interesting subjective descriptions of low frequency stimuli which have been included in Table I.

In the same year Békésy (1936) published the results of a most careful examination of low frequency phenomena. The problem of harmonic distortion was recognised and studied in detail. Two sound sources were used; a pistonphone and a thermophone. The thermophone was mounted directly in the subject's ear with an airtight seal. Included in the sealed system was a sensitive manometer incorporating a rubber membrane. By monitoring the amplitude displacement of a beam of light reflected from this membrane, pressure measurement was possible at threshold levels for frequencies below 50 Hz.

The pistonphone source could also be used with this sensing manometer. The source fluctuations in this case underwent severe filtration by various mechanical filters and were free of harmonics when presented to the subject.

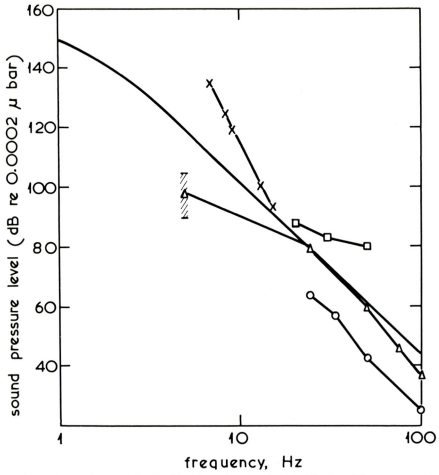

*Fig.* 1 Comparison of threshold data prior to 1961. □ Finck, 1961, monaural; ⩸ Wever and Bray, 1936, monaural; △ Corso, 1958, monaural; ○ Robinson and Dadson, 1956, binaural, free field; —— Békésy, 1936, monaural; × Brecher, 1934, monaural.

Békésy's combination of pure fundamental and direct threshold measurement technique was a major contribution to low frequency experiments. With this technique he examined thresholds of hearing

TABLE I: Subjective descriptions and effects of stimulus at near threshold levels

| Frequency region (Hz) | Observer | | | | | | |
|---|---|---|---|---|---|---|---|
| | Imai (1907) Vance (1914) (Pure tone) | Brecher (1934) (Pure tone) | Wever and Bray (1936) (Pure tone) | Békésy (1936) (Pure tone) | Gavreau (1966) (Pure tone) | Yeowart et al. (1967) (Pure tone) | Yeowart (1969) (Octave band noise) |
| Above 25 | | Weak rumble, unpleasant tickling in the ear | Tone character established | | | | 125 Hz—sounds like banded noise 63 Hz—fluctuating tone 32 Hz—traffic rumble |
| 25–20 | | Tonal character gradually falls away | Noisy flutter | Above 18 Hz tonal character | | Smooth, tonal | |
| 20–15 | | Separate "puffs" below 18 Hz—the fusion frequency | Thrusting effect | | | | 16 Hz—Traffic rumble, buffeting, fluctuating flutter |
| 15–10 | Weak fundamental detected at 12 Hz | | Pumping sound, pitch lower than at 5 Hz | Below 18 Hz, separate pulses discernible | | Rough, popping effect from 5 Hz to 15 Hz | |
| Below 10 | | | Pumping noise, "choo-choo", chug-chug | | 7 Hz sounds like a motor boat or tractor | Below 5 Hz, chugging, whooshing | 8 Hz—Rough, peaky tone 4 Hz—Separate random peaks |

down to 1 Hz, and masking and tactile phenomena associated with low frequency stimulation. Perhaps the only obvious criticism of this study that can be made concerns the small volume of air enclosed in the equipment. Physiological noise must be accentuated by this small volume, heartbeat being a significant source of interference below about 5 Hz. This physiological noise could have reduced the sensitivity of the ear in this frequency region.

Interest in the low frequency field declined after 1936 and until recently the Békésy data have stood, unverified. The initial interest in the field was stimulated by quests to understand and define the limits of the hearing mechanism. Brecher, for example, performed his experiments because the then existing information on the threshold of hearing and the threshold of pain, when extrapolated, intersected at 20 Hz. Brecher's inference from this information was that below 20 Hz no sound could be heard. His experiments discounted this position.

In recent years the advent of high-powered jet and rocket engines have provided intense low frequency sounds. Air-conditioning systems in large bays can in some circumstances generate significant noise output below 20 Hz. These modern and exotic sources have restimulated interest in low frequency noise phenomena.

Robinson and Dadson (1956) as part of an experiment to determine the equal loudness contours for pure tones down to 25 Hz reported thresholds of hearing in the low frequency region. The experimenters were attempting to measure free field thresholds, and to overcome the problems of presenting a progressive plane wave to the observers at 25 Hz, found it necessary to use a low frequency duct, which had been constructed for low frequency microphone calibration. This duct had a square cross-section of $60 \times 60$ cm and an overall length of 6.8 m. A double fibre glass wedge occupied 5.2 cm of its length. The driving unit was a single 46 cm cone loudspeaker. The subject's head and shoulders were enclosed in the duct. The threshold measurement technique adopted to determine the minimum audible field was to switch the tone on and off at irregular intervals of a few seconds while decreasing the sound level in 2 dB steps. The procedure was then repeated at levels staggered by 1 dB from the previous steps. The data for a group of 90 subjects are included in Fig. 1.

Corso (1958) performed threshold measurements down to 5 Hz with what has since become a typical approach to low frequency experiments. By this time electrodynamic loudspeaker technology had progressed to the point where the device could be used as a source instead of the fundamentally noisier mechanical piston. Corso used an electrodynamic driver connected to a rigid diaphragm in the wall of a plywood enclosure. The diaphragm which had a diameter of 10 cm was driven by a moving coil of 14 mm diameter, centred in a magnetic field of 1 T. The system was resonant at 200 Hz and to damp this resonance Corso drilled holes in the plywood enclosure. The subject's ear was coupled to the enclosed volume by a short brass tube which was sealed into the meatus by a mixture of modelling clay and vaseline.

Only total harmonic distortion measurements on the acoustic signal were reported. This distortion reached a maximum of 3% at 5 Hz. Unfortunately, total harmonic distortion is not a sufficiently sensitive indicator of the purity of a low frequency signal if one wishes to observe an unbiased threshold measurement. The distortion products must be below their respective thresholds. Therefore information on the apportionment of the total harmonic distortion across the harmonic frequencies is essential. This information would have been most valuable in the present case since the single threshold below 25 Hz which was reported showed poor agreement with Békésy's data. In fact the reported 5 Hz threshold fell in the region vaguely defined by Wever and Bray (1936).

Some data have been contributed to the threshold of hearing in the low frequency region by Finck (1961) as part of a low frequency masking experiment. His source was a loudspeaker driving a $5.6 \times 10^{-2}\,\text{m}^3$ triangular prismatic cabinet. The stimuli were presented to the subject via rubber tubes 6 mm in diameter. Figure 1 contains his three threshold measurements on a group of five observers.

Gavreau *et al.* (1966) reported a brief study of biological effects of very low frequency acoustic stimulation. Using a closed column 24 m long and 30 cm diameter driven by a loudspeaker he was able to report that a 7 Hz fundamental was audible (see Table I).

In 1964 Yeowart began a systematic study of the very low frequency region. At that time the threshold of hearing was not known with any precision. Figure 1 indicates the disparity of both absolute threshold values and the behaviour of the threshold with changing frequency. In view of the sparse data available it therefore seemed that a study of the low frequency threshold, particularly below 20 Hz would be valuable. Investigation of the commercially available earphones indicated that none was capable of handling the frequency range considered. It was therefore necessary to develop earphones for the purpose. The first requirement of the design was clearly a large power handling capacity. Also the volume of the earphone should be larger than usual to avoid the problem of physiological noise (heartbeat etc.) which would be set up in a small enclosed volume around the ear. To avoid significant signal distortion and loss of low frequency response the system had to be well sealed, including the area where the equipment contacted the subject's head. Figure 2 shows the final design chosen for the headset. The 30 cm diameter loudspeaker unit was mounted onto a 0.6 cm aluminium plate, thereby enclosing a volume of about 1 litre between the cone and the plate. A hole of 2.5 cm diameter led to a conventional ear defender

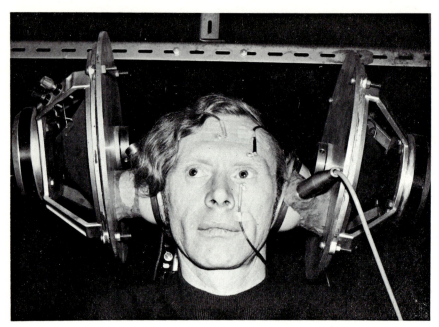

*Fig.* 2 Low frequency headset (Yeowart *et al.*, 1967).

cup. An airtight seal between the subject's head was obtained by moulding on to the edge of the ear defender a 3 cm thick surround of soft rubber. Two such units were mounted on a supporting structure so that both monaural and binaural experimentation could be undertaken.

As the acoustic system was large there was ample space to mount a monitoring microphone directly through the side of each ear defender cup. With suitable calibration direct measurement of the sound pressure level at threshold was possible for the lower frequencies examined. This simple method of direct pressure monitoring was possible since at the highest frequency used, the headset dimensions were $\lambda/14$, so it was reasonable to assume that pressure variations were uniform throughout the enclosed volume.

Figure 2 shows a liquid-filled surround which replaced the more massive rubber surround when sealing problems were not as critical.

A useful property of the stiffness loaded loudspeaker was the constant frequency response below about 100 Hz. Figure 3 shows this response which enabled noise as well as pure tone thresholds of hearing to be examined very easily.

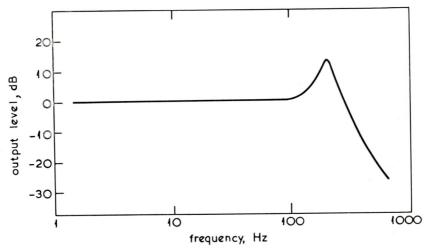

*Fig.* 3 Frequency response of headset.

General background noise from the equipment must be reduced below threshold. This background noise can be modulated by the low frequency stimulus and can give rise to incorrect and more sensitive thresholds due to the subject mistaking the modulated background noise for the fundamental. The noise level in the headset was reduced to that shown in Fig. 4 by inserting a low pass filter between the power amplifier and the loudspeaker coil. The frequency response in Fig. 3 includes the effect of this filter.

The importance of obtaining a good seal of the equipment on a subject's head is illustrated in Fig. 5.

The good seal conditions (solid line) were obtained initially. Then the application pressure of the headset to the subject's head was reduced until he reported poor contact with his head. A check, obtained by removing the subject from the headset and after a rest period putting him back in, demonstrates the repeatability of the good seal conditions (crosses) and the effect of a poor seal. The importance of the seal is most critical below 20 Hz. This problem could have been the cause of Corso's low threshold point at 5 Hz. His subject could have heard air leak hiss from the damping holes in his equipment, rather than the fundamental tone.

The threshold-determining technique used was the method of limits, in which the signal level was first raised from below threshold until the subject indicated that he could hear it, and then slowly lowered until he indicated that it was inaudible. The threshold was taken to be the mean of five upper and five lower limit determinations.

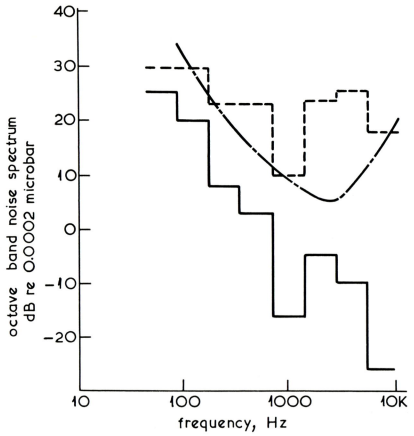

*Fig.* 4 Octave band noise level in the equipment with and without filter, compared with B.S. 2497: (1954) MAP threshold. – – – – without filter; —— with filter.

For these experiments the headset was located in a soundproofed and damped room, isolated from structural vibration by a floating floor.

Harmonic distortion measurements were taken for a variety of frequencies and sound levels. The rate of fall-off of the harmonic content of the signal is compared with the monaural threshold data obtained using this apparatus in Fig. 6. The nearest any particular harmonic approached its threshold was 20–30 dB below the threshold under consideration. For most of the frequency range considered the harmonics were considerably more than 30 dB below the threshold. More important, however, was the fact that throughout the entire range the harmonic content of the signal fell off with frequency at a

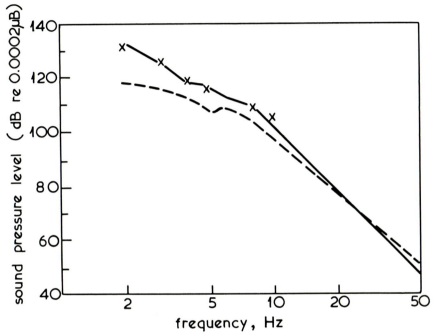

Fig. 5 Effect of earphone seal on measured threshold. —— good seal conditions; – – – – bad seal conditions; × good seal conditions (check).

greater rate than the threshold curve increased in sensitivity. The separation between the threshold of hearing and the harmonic distortion of the signal supported the position that no significant lowering of the measured threshold occurred because of signal impurity. The detailed results, including the number of ears involved in this monaural threshold determination, are to be found in Table II. A more detailed account of the experimental procedure can be found in Yeowart *et al.* (1967).

On release from the apparatus the subject was asked to describe the stimulus. The descriptions varied with frequency but could be split into three distinct regions (see Table I).

Once the monaural data were collected it was necessary to extend the threshold techniques to binaural application. Preliminary experiments were performed with a group of four subjects. The same sound pressure

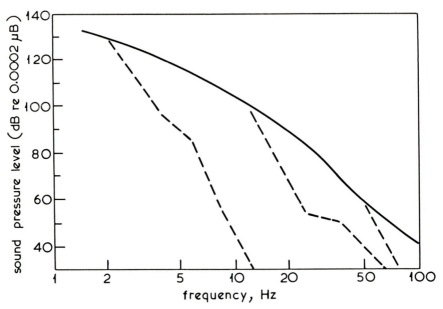

*Fig.* 6 Harmonic content of stimulus for various frequencies – – – –, compared with measured thresholds ——.

TABLE II: Monaural pure tone data (Yeowart *et al.*, 1967)

| Frequency (Hz) | Threshold (dB re 0·0002 μ bar) | Standard error of mean | Number of ears |
|---|---|---|---|
| 100 | 44.26 | 1.85 | 14 |
| 50 | 58.61 | 2.02 | 15 |
| 25 | 83.00 | 1.80 | 17 |
| 20 | 89.49 | 2.06 | 17 |
| 15 | 97.38 | 1.57 | 17 |
| 10 | 104.10 | 1.20 | 29 |
| 8 | 108.52 | 1.28 | 29 |
| 6 | 115.00 | 1.29 | 29 |
| 5 | 117.09 | 1.47 | 29 |
| 4 | 120.51 | 2.36 | 12 |
| 3 | 125.54 | 2.36 | 12 |
| 2 | 130.94 | 2.04 | 12 |
| 1.5 | 132.28 | 1.60 | 10 |

level was presented to both ears simultaneously for frequencies in the range 100 Hz to 5 Hz. The thresholds obtained showed a similar trend to the monaural pure tone data, but were several decibels more sensitive. Once the possibility of a binaural advantage over monaural listening at these low frequencies had been established a more detailed examination was executed. Because of the small difference sought (between binaural and monaural thresholds) it was necessary to examine both the monaural and the binaural thresholds at the same sitting.

A subject was placed in the apparatus and the monaural threshold for each ear determined. Equal sound pressure levels were then presented to both ears simultaneously and the binaural thresholds were measured. The experiment then continued with an attempt to fix the binaural threshold for equal sensation levels at each ear. The difference in sensitivity between the two ears, if any was found, was introduced between the two headsets by means of a calibrated attenuator. The final threshold of the series was taken.

Three types of threshold had been measured:

| Monaural thresholds— | obtained directly for each ear. |
| Binaural thresholds— | determined with the same sound pressure level applied to both ears. |
| Equalised binaural thresholds— | determined with the same sensation level applied to both ears. |

From these data the following two quantities were determined:

(a) Binaural advantage: This was the difference between the mean monaural threshold and the binaural threshold.

(b) Equalised binaural advantage: This was obtained from the difference between the monaural threshold for one ear and the equalised binaural threshold for the same ear.

The overall mean values for the two quantities were $3.1 \pm 0.19$ dB for the binaural advantage and $2.81 \pm 0.19$ dB for the equalised binaural advantage (Yeowart, 1972). Figure 7 shows the equalised binaural advantage plotted against frequency. The uncertainty in the advantage was found to be greatest between 20 Hz and 25 Hz, which is the frequency region where the tonality of the signal is breaking down. The binaural threshold data appear in Table III.

Because the headset had a constant frequency response below 100 Hz it was possible, with little difficulty, to extend the work on pure tone thresholds to include thresholds for octave bands of noise.

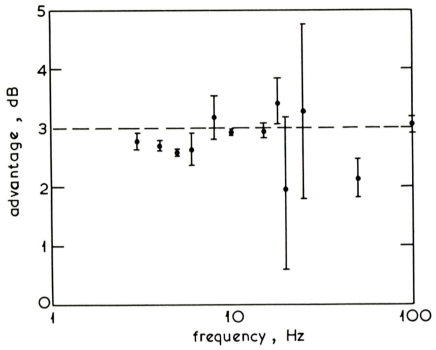

*Fig.* 7 Equalised binaural advantage.

TABLE III: Binaural headphone data (Yeowart and Evans, 1974) for five observers

| Frequency (Hz) | Threshold (dB re 0·0002 μ bar) | Standard error of mean |
|---|---|---|
| 100 | 31.4 | 0.8 |
| 50 | 44.9 | 1.2 |
| 25 | 76.4 | 1.1 |
| 20 | 84.2 | 1.8 |
| 18 | 87.7 | 2.6 |
| 15 | 91.9 | 1.6 |
| 10 | 97.7 | 2.0 |
| 8 | 104.7 | 1.2 |
| 6 | 106.6 | 2.8 |
| 5 | 110.3 | 2.5 |

The subjective descriptions of the noise bands followed the same pattern as the pure tone descriptions in that a frequency was reached where an impression of roughness became apparent (see Table I).

Several points of interest emerged from a comparison of the monaural tone data with the monaural noise data. The noise thresholds exhibited a similar trend with frequency to that established for the pure tone case. The change in slope of the auditory function around 18 Hz was still in evidence, although not quite so pronounced as in the pure tone

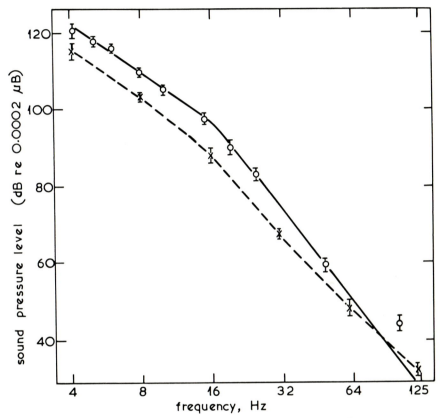

*Fig.* 8 Tone versus noise threshold data. ○ — ○ monaural tone data; ×−−−−× monaural octave band noise data.

case. When comparison was made on the absolute level of the thresholds it appeared that a frequency-dependent separation in sensitivity occurred, in such a way that for the lowest frequencies examined the noise thresholds were several decibels more sensitive than those for pure tone. In Fig. 8 one can see that this difference disappears above 63 Hz. Because these data were collected separately, a more detailed examination of the noise–tone difference was undertaken where both noise and tone data were collected during the same experimental session. The separation of the two thresholds was now much clearer, the significance levels shown in Fig. 9 vary smoothly with frequency

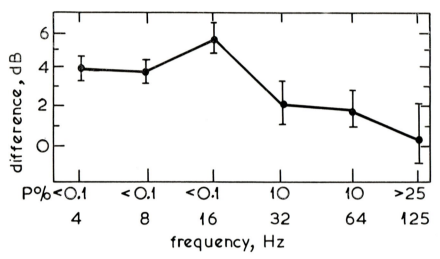

*Fig.* 9 Tone versus noise threshold difference.

from not significant at 125 Hz ($> 25\%$) to significant at 16 Hz and below ($< 0.1\%$).

Various possible explanations of the difference established between the tone and noise thresholds have been considered (Yeowart *et al.,* 1969). Variation of the skirt slopes of the low frequency octave filters (Tempest and Yeowart, 1966) did not effect the noise thresholds so that one could discount the possibility of inadequate frequency selectivity of the filters. It was also possible that detection of the higher frequency components within the pass band of the filters could have occurred. Since the threshold of hearing is more sensitive at the higher cut-off frequency of the filter than the lower, one could have obtained a more sensitive threshold if the threshold were expressed in terms of the centre frequency of the filter. A comparison of the noise band thresholds with the tone thresholds at the upper frequency limit of the filter did indeed effectively eliminate the difference for the lower frequency bands (below 16 Hz). However, this explanation led to the conclusion that the measured noise–tone difference should be greatest in the regions where the thresholds were changing most rapidly with decreasing frequency, i.e. around 125 Hz. Since, in fact, the difference was insignificant at that frequency, this explanation was discarded. The hypothesis which appeared to explain the difference in thresholds for tone and noise, and was also consistent with the subjective descriptions of the stimuli, was that the observers were able to detect separate pressure peaks in the noise signal, when these peaks were long enough for the ear to respond, i.e. below about 15 Hz. An analysis of the amplitude properties of banded noise suggested that if an observer accepted 0.5–1 pressure pulse per second as being characteristic of the 4 Hz octave band, then a noise to tone advantage of between 1.7 dB and 3.3 dB was possible. Simulation of the actual detection process with a detector with a time constant of 200 m, suggested differences of up to 4 dB were possible, dependent on the observers threshold criteria. These values agreed quite well with the experimental value of 4.1 ± 0.5 dB obtained for the lowest octave band, as shown in Fig. 10.

The programme of low frequency experimentation was then extended to a larger source which allowed whole-body immersion in the sound field. A low frequency chamber was developed with a capacity of 1250 litres, (Fig. 10). The chamber could accommodate a subject with a sufficient margin of comfort but because the system was sealed, an experimental session had to be limited to 20 minutes, by which time the atmosphere in the chamber needed some revitalisation. Six 0.46 m diameter loudspeakers were bolted over 0.27 m holes in three upright faces of the chamber using airtight seals. The fourth face formed the door, again constructed in such a way as to be airtight when closed. Two Perspex windows in the door provided for subject observation.

The frequency response of the amplifier and chamber is shown in Fig. 11. Below 25 Hz the response was constant to within ± 0.5 dB. The first peak in the curve at 40 Hz corresponded to the mechanical resonance of the stiffness loaded loudspeakers (with a free air resonance of 35 Hz); the succession of resonances are due to the chamber response. Below 25 Hz the wavelength is very much greater than the maximum internal room dimension and the pressure changes may be assumed constant throughout the volume. Under these conditions, direct measurement of the sound field was possible, and noise or tone experiments were feasible.

Threshold measurements for a group of twelve observers are reported in Table IV. A harmonic analysis of two typical stimuli at an spl of 130 dB are shown in Table V. The harmonics fell off at a greater rate than the threshold of hearing so one can assume that the reported data were uninfluenced by the signal distortion.

At the National Physical Laboratory Whittle et al. (1972) constructed the low frequency pressure chamber shown in Fig. 12. The enclosed

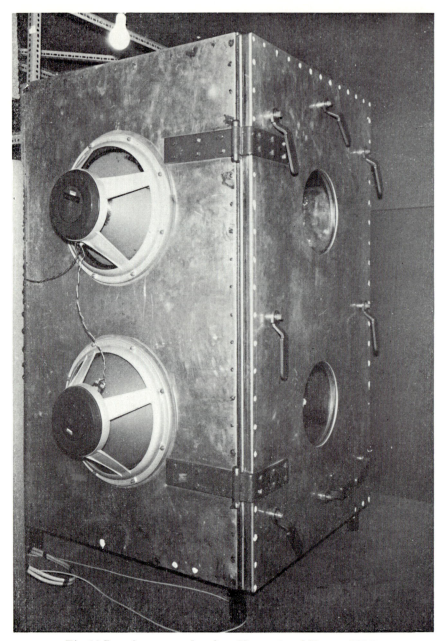

*Fig.* 10 Low frequency chamber (Yeowart and Evans, 1974).

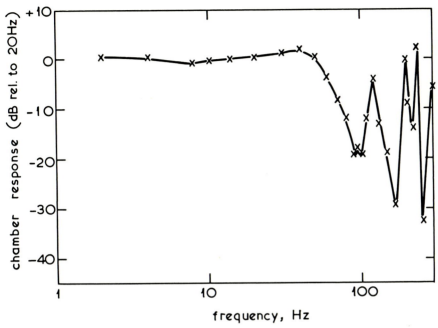

*Fig.* 11 Frequency response of low frequency chamber (Yeowart and Evans, 1972).

TABLE IV: Binaural thresholds for whole-body stimulation
(Yeowart and Evans, 1974) from twelve observers

| Frequency (Hz) | Threshold (dB re 0·0002 µ bar) | Standard error of mean |
|---|---|---|
| 20 | 85.2 | 0.6 |
| 15 | 92.1 | 0.4 |
| 12 | 97.0 | 0.6 |
| 10 | 99.5 | 0.6 |
| 8 | 102.4 | 0.7 |
| 5 | 111.1 | 0.6 |
| 4 | 112.4 | 0.8 |
| 2 | 121.4 | 0.5 |

volume was large enough for the subject to be comfortably seated
(about 0.8 m³). The internal chamber dimensions were 1.2 × 0.6 m base
with a height of 1.48 m. The enclosure was formed of rendered concrete
blocks and equipped with a steel-lined wooden inner door. A steel pipe

of internal diameter 65 mm and a length of 465 mm communicated with the enclosed volume of the chamber and various sound sources.

TABLE V: Harmonic content of Chamber stimuli (Yeowart and Evans, 1974), fundamental at 130 dB spl

| Fundamental (Hz) | Distortion products (dB below fundamental) | | | | |
|---|---|---|---|---|---|
| | f 1 | f 2 | f 3 | f 4 | f 5 |
| 16 | 34 | 45 | 63 | 69 | 77 |
| 7·5 | 38 | 46 | 58 | 61 | 70 |

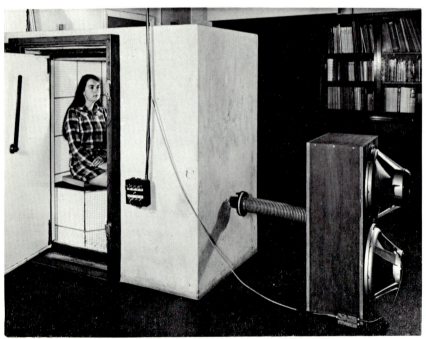

*Fig.* 12 Low frequency chamber, National Physical Laboratory, Teddington. (Crown copyright reserved.)

In their experiments on the threshold of hearing and equal loudness relationships careful attention was paid to the harmonic distortion present in the signal. The data reported in Table VI indicate that the

TABLE VI: Harmonic content of Chamber stimuli (Whittle *et al.*, 1972)

| Fundamental | spl dB re 0·0002 μ bar | Relative level of harmonic (dB) | | |
|---|---|---|---|---|
| | | f 1 | f 2 | f 3 |
| 3.15 | 139 | − 33 | − 32 | − 57 |
| 6.3 | 136 | − 41 | − 43 | − 66 |
| 12.5 | 125 | − 52 | − 61 | − 72 |
| 25 | 108 | − 52 | − 63 | − 66 |

harmonics present in the test tone fell off more rapidly than the threshold of hearing with increasing frequency. The measured thresholds are shown in Fig. 13.

## III. Comparison of Recent Binaural Threshold Data

The threshold data described earlier in this chapter and illustrated in Fig. 1 are not included in the following discussion. The reasons for this omission are various. Much of the earlier work below 50 Hz used low frequency sources which produced an unknown amount of harmonic distortion, or significant mechanical noise; these thresholds are therefore suspect. Békésy's data do not fall into this category but his reported low frequency data were acquired using one subject only.

Figure 13 contains the following data. The monaural headphone data of Yeowart *et al.* (1967) reduced by 3 dB to align the data with binaural reception (Yeowart, 1972), binaural headphone data (Yeowart, 1972), binaural chamber data (Yeowart and Evans, 1974) and binaural chamber data from the N.P.L. (Whittle *et al.*, 1972).

When one considers the four separate experiments with their differing subjects and technique the final agreement is remarkable. A spread of ± 3 dB encompasses all the data below 25 Hz.

Visual inspection of the data suggested that they split naturally into two distinct frequency regions on each side of 20 Hz. In these regions the variation of the threshold of hearing and the logarithm of the frequency could be adequately described by a linear relationship.

The least squares regression lines to the available data had slopes of 22.2 ± 3.5 dB/octave for frequencies above 20 Hz and 12.3 ± 0.9 dB/octave below 20 Hz. The cross-over point between the two regimes appears to be 92.0 dB spl at 15.5 Hz. A satisfactory engineering description to the threshold data below 100 Hz and above about 2 Hz may be obtained by constructing lines of the required slopes above and below the cross-over point.

Whittle *et al.* (1972) point out that the reported chamber data at 25 Hz and 50 Hz do not coincide with the M.A.F. data appearing in

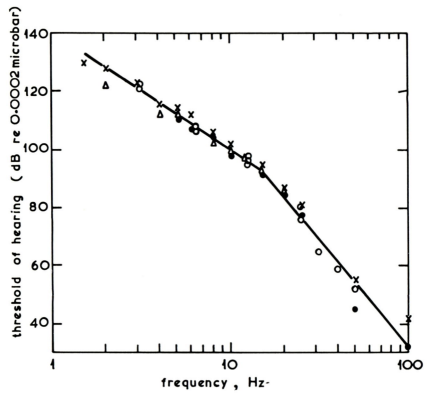

*Fig.* 13 Comparison of recent threshold data. × monaural headphone data −3 dB (Yeowart *et al.*, 1967); ● binaural headphone data (Yeowart, 1972); △ binaural chamber data (Yeowart and Evans, 1974); ○ binaural chamber data (Whittle *et al.*, 1972).

ISO R226 (1961). At 50 Hz the authors demonstrated that the difference could be encompassed by effects of subject training and threshold seeking technique. For the 25 Hz data, however, the major difference occurred when the subject was transferred from the pressure chamber to an anechoic chamber, technique and practice being relatively unimportant. The difference in hearing sensitivity, between low frequency stimuli presented by a chamber and stimuli presented in an anechoic room, is puzzling.

## IV. Low Frequency Equal Loudness Relationships

When the results of several investigations are compared, one can safely conclude that the behaviour with frequency of the threshold of hearing has been established down to several hertz. The equal loudness relationships in the same frequency region are somewhat less consistent. The problem probably has its source in the differing methodology of the two contributors to the field.

Stevens (1972) generated equal loudness relationships in more usual frequency regions by comparing some 25 sets of data. Below 25 Hz available data were sparse and the little that did exist appeared to corroborate Stevens' extrapolation of the loudness contours to an apparent convergence point of 1 Hz and 160 dB spl. Using this convergence point Stevens evolved a series of ground rules which allow one to construct equal sensation contours down to 1 Hz. Briefly the rules are as follows:

> Between 3150 Hz and 8000 Hz perceived magnitude is constant. Above 8000 Hz the contours rise at the rate of 12 dB/octave. Below 3150 Hz the contours rise at 6 dB/octave to 1250 Hz. Between 400 Hz and 1250 Hz perceived magnitude is constant.
>
> From 80 Hz to 400 Hz the contours behave as follows. Below 76 dB at 400 Hz the contours converge to a common point at 1 Hz, 115 dB. Between 76 dB and 121 dB at 500 Hz the contours have a slope of −4.5 dB/octave. Above 121 dB at 400 Hz the contours converge to a point at 1 Hz, 160 dB.
>
> All contours below 80 Hz converge toward 1 Hz and 160 dB, and thus do not affect the slope change with frequency at about 15.5 Hz established experimentally for the threshold of hearing.

Whittle *et al.* (1972) attempted to establish equal loudness contours in the low frequency region by experimentation. The physical equipment has been described previously in connection with their threshold determinations. Equal loudness tests were made by the method of constant stimuli. The stimuli were presented in sequence A0B0A0B, where A represents a fixed sound level, B a variable sound level and 0 a period of silence. A and B each had a duration of 2 s with rise and fall times of 100 ms. Because of experimental problems a step procedure for comparing loudness was chosen. The starting point was 50 Hz and was paired with 25 Hz. The mean sound pressure level at 25 Hz judged to be equally loud as the 50 Hz reference was used in a comparison with 12.5 Hz and so on.

When the threshold and equal loudness data from this experiment were compared to the relevant international standards (ISO R389, 1964, and ISO R226, 1961) several problems became obvious. Firstly, the shape of the present loudness contours differed in the range 50 Hz to 25 Hz from the ISO curves. The larger discrepancy appeared in the threshold data, the present data being far less sensitive at 50 Hz and 25 Hz.

Whittle *et al.* (1972) demonstrated that most of the threshold discrepancy was due to threshold measuring technique and subject practice at 50 Hz. Below this frequency the explanation was less obvious. Whittle *et al.* felt justified in adjusting their threshold contours for a conjunction with the ISO threshold at 50 Hz and for the lower frequencies, adjusting by an amount which was proportional to the separation of the loudness contours.

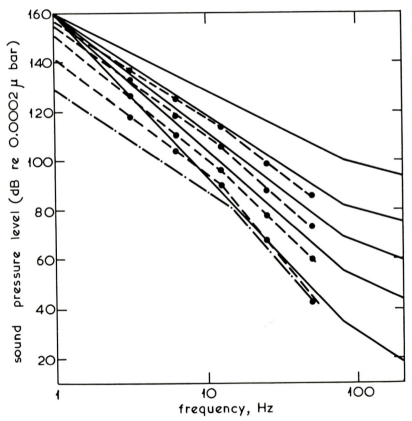

*Fig.* 14 Equal loudness contours at low frequencies. —— constructed from Stevens (1972); ● – – – – ● Whittle *et al.* (1972); —.—.— adjusted threshold (zero loudness) from Yeowart (1972).

Figure 14 compares equal loudness contours derived from the ground rules of Stevens (1972) with the threshold and equal loudness contours of Whittle *et al.* (1972) and Yeowart and Evans (1974). The two-segment linear representation of the threshold derived by Yeowart (1972) has been adjusted to coincide with Whittle's modified threshold at 50 Hz, the same adjustment occurring for all frequencies.

Stevens' linear extrapolation seems to be consistent with the experimental data both at threshold and for levels of up to about 70 phons for a significant portion of the low frequency range. There is, however, a small but consistent discrepancy between the experimental data and Stevens' extrapolation below about 15 Hz. The experimental results show a consistent change in slope below 15 Hz which is not reflected in Stevens' extrapolation. One is led to the conclusion therefore that the convergence point of Stevens' contours of 160 dB at 1 Hz, while being most convenient in drawing equal sensation contours, does not adequately describe the detailed frequency behaviour of the hearing mechanism below about 15 Hz. Stevens' zero loudness contour, for example, in Fig. 14 is seen to be some 20–30 dB too insensitive at 1 Hz. These differences will obviously be important only when the noise under consideration is dominated in loudness by frequency components lower than 15 Hz. While this situation is unlikely, it does seem that, for the sake of completeness, an additional segment, the seventh, would bring Stevens' loudness contours into line with existing information in the low frequency regime.

## V. Low Frequency Equal Annoyance Relationships

Stevens (1972) demonstrated that in the frequency range 50 Hz to 10 kHz there is no significant difference between an equal loudness contour and a contour of equal noisiness. Below 15 Hz, however, some recent work at the University of Salford has shown that a group of nine unpractised subjects would readily judge the annoyance of a low frequency signal, but objected when they were asked to judge the loudness of the same signal. The subjects insisted that the low frequency tones were detected as a combination of physical sensation and sound, and that the tone may not be very loud but it was most certainly annoying. Co-operation from this vociferous group of students could only be obtained when the experiment was conducted under the instruction of equal annoyance.

The results of a brief examination of low frequency equal annoyance contours are shown in Fig. 15. Signal distortion was at least 15 dB below the generalised threshold reported by Yeowart and Evans

4

(1974). Unfortunately, the threshold of hearing for this group was not measured. It does appear though that annoyance increases very quickly indeed at low frequencies, to the extent that at 3 Hz a just audible signal was judged to be as annoying as a signal with a frequency

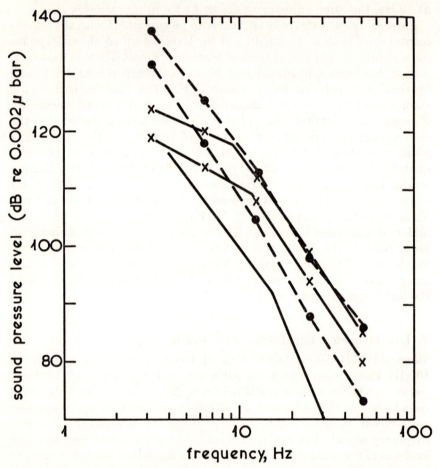

*Fig.* 15 A comparison of equal loudness and equal annoyance contours at low frequencies. ● – – – – ● loudness (Whittle *et al.*, 1972); ×——× annoyance; —— generalised threshold (Yeowart and Evans, 1974).

of 50 Hz at a level of 25 dB above threshold. Once the tactile sensations become obvious (below 10 Hz) there is a dramatic departure between the equal loudness contour of Whittle *et al.* (1972) and the equal annoyance contour described here. This departure is shown in Fig. 15.

## VI. Summary of Low Frequency Equal Loudness and Equal Annoyance Contours

Accurate description of low frequency loudness and annoyance is not yet possible. There still exist several unexplained and unquantified effects in the low frequency region. Stevens' linear extrapolation of the equal loudness contours is now known to be inconsistent with existing experimental data. The experimental data themselves present a dilemma in that at the higher frequencies (above 25 Hz) the zero loudness contour does not coincide with previously determined thresholds. Whittle *et al.* circumvented this problem by applying an arbitrary correction to the threshold data. Finally, the old problem of instructional sets appears to have been resurrected. At higher frequencies it has been adequately shown that there is no significant difference between an equal annoyance and an equal loudness judgment when sound levels are compared. However, when the stimulus frequency is below 10 Hz there does seem to be a measurable difference between judgments made under the two types of instruction. Before reliable conclusions can be drawn concerning the low frequency region, further research would be advantageous in clarifying the usefulness of low frequency chamber techniques for obtaining data on presumed free-field listening conditions and also in deciding whether a real difference exists between annoyance and loudness judgments.

## REFERENCES

Békésy, G. von (1936). Reported in "Experiments in Hearing", pp. 257–261 (McGraw-Hill, 1960).
Brecher, G. A. (1934). *Pflügers Arch. f. d. ges. Physiol.* **234**, 380–393.
B.S. 2497: (1954). British Standards Institution, London.
Corso, J. F. (1958). *Am. J. Psychol.* **71**, 367–374.
Finck, A. (1961). *J. Acoust. Soc. Am.* **33**, 1140–1141.
Gavreau, V., Condat, R. and Saul, H. (1966) *Acustica* **17**, 1–10.
Imai, M. (1907). Unpublished data, reported by Vance (1914).
ISO R226 (1961).
ISO R389 (1964).
Robinson, D. W. and Dason, R. S. (1956). *Brit. J. Appl. Phys.* **7**, 166–181.
Stevens, S. S. (1972). *J. Acoust. Soc. Am.* **51**, 575–601.
Tempest, W. and Yeowart, N. S. (1966). *Electr. Eng.* **38**, 397–399.
Vance, T. F. (1914). *Psychol. Monog.* **16**, 104–114.
Wever, E. G. and Bray, C. W. (1936). *J. Psychol.* **3**, 101–114.
Whittle, L. S., Collins, S. J. and Robinson, D. W. (1972). *J. Sound Vib.* **21**, 431–448.

Yeowart, N. S. (1968). *Electr. Eng.* **40**, 212–214.
Yeowart, N. S. (1972). *Proc. Brit. Acoust. Soc.* **1**(3), Paper 71, 103.
Yeowart, N. S. and Evans, M. J. (1974). *J. Acoust. Soc. Amer.* **55**, 814–818.
Yeowart, N. S. and Jones, K. L. (1972). "The comparative loudness of low frequency pure tones", Electrical Engineering Project Report, University of Salford.
Yeowart, N. S., Bryan, M. E. and Tempest, W. (1967). *J. Sound Vib.* **6**, 335–342.
Yeowart, N. S., Bryan, M. E. and Tempest, W. (1969). *J. Sound Vib.* **9**, 447–453.

# 4. Low Frequency Noise Annoyance

*M. E. Bryan*

## I. Annoyance, Loudness and Noisiness

It is well known that the annoyance or disturbance which any particular source of noise is going to cause is difficult to predict. As has been pointed out (Noise, Final Report, 1963) the practical way of doing this is the cumbersome method of the social survey. Therefore in trying to predict the response of the community to the noise from such things as aircraft, surface transport and industry, an assessment is made of the loudness or noisiness of the noise to which people are exposed. The implicit assumption seems to be that annoyance or disturbance grows with the loudness or noisiness of the noise and a measure of either of these latter quantities will give a reliable measure of the former quantities. Indeed figure seven (p. 202) of the report (*op. cit.*) presents data comparing the growth of "subjective intrusiveness" (a measure of annoyance) and "subjective noisiness" with the level of aircraft noise measured on the dB(A) scale and on the PNdB scale. It is seen that there is a fairly linear relationship between the subjective assessment of the noise (on either rating scales of intrusiveness or noisiness) and the objective measure of that noise in dB(A) or PNdB.

Stevens (1972) stated that "the evidence from experiments in several laboratories suggests that loudness and noisiness may be considered essentially synonymous". He went on to propose the unit of perceived level of loudness or noisiness (PLdB) for assessing and predicting the annoying effects of noises. Later in this paper Stevens reviewed the work on comparisons of the annoyance and of the loudness of noises and concluded "a single composite weighting function should prove adequate to the needs of noise evaluation". It appears then that a fair assessment of the annoyance which a noise has may be made from the evaluation of its loudness or noisiness on one of the numerous scales available. These may have been developed from laboratory studies such as PLdB or be one of the empirical scales, such as dB(A) or noise rating number (NR) aimed specifically at predicting community response (Schultz, 1972). If the noise exceeds a certain level on these various scales then it can be assumed that it is likely to cause annoyance.

However, there may be certain classes of noise for which these assessment procedures are unsatisfactory and where estimates of the loudness or noisiness of a noise are unsatisfactory predictors of the annoyance caused.

## II. Low Frequency Annoyance

Data are presented in this chapter from a variety of situations where the annoyance due to predominantly low frequency noise is considerably greater than that predicted from the commonly used noise assessment procedures. It is hoped to show that for this type of noise the existing procedures are, at best, inadequate and, at worst, inappropriate, and that the proposed relationship which exists between annoyance and loudness or noisiness for noises of predominantly mid and high frequency energy content is no longer valid. A common characteristic of these noises, which arise in transportation, in the work environment and in the home environment, is that there is a fairly rapid fall in sound pressure level with increasing frequency. The data to be presented in this chapter have been collected over the past 7 years and represents about 5% of the problems dealt with by the Salford University audiology group in their capacity as noise consultants to industry etc.

Generally speaking it has been found that existing noise assessment procedures, such as dB(A), NR etc. are satisfactory in estimating the reaction of the community to noise, although not of course in predicting individual reaction (Moreira and Bryan, 1972). It is because of certain similarities in the characteristics of the low frequency noises, and the consistent way in which they cause greater annoyance than the criteria predict, that the case is made out for giving such noises special consideration. Such noise spectra, usually associated with large mass high speed air flows, were undoubtedly much less common 10 or 20 years ago, when much of the work on noise assessment procedures appears to have been done, than they are today. It is hardly surprising that conventional criteria do not adequately deal with this type of noise—they were never intended to. However, in recent years surface transportation speeds have increased considerably, both in motor vehicles as a result of the introduction of motorways and on the railways due to the introduction of powerful electric and diesel locomotives. The use of large oil-fired boilers has become common in industry, as has the use of large air-conditioning plants. All these sources have energy predominantly below 100 Hz, have steeply falling frequency character-istics, and they have all given rise to considerably more annoyance than would be predicted by loudness and noisiness assessments.

### III. Low Frequency Noise Sources

The evidence that low frequency noise gives more annoyance than existing criteria predict comes from three different sources. Except for the case of noise inside vehicles the problems have given rise to strong adverse public reaction.

The three situations are: (1) Transportation; motor vehicle and train interiors, (2) The Work Environment; an electronics factory and a biology laboratory and (3) The Home Environment; due to neighbour-ing industrial plant. Each situation will be considered in turn and case histories described in detail. Their mutual characteristics will then be compared and conclusions about low frequency noise drawn.

### A. MEASUREMENT TECHNIQUE

In all three situations the same measurement technique was used. This has been described in detail elsewhere (Tempest and Bryan, 1972). Essentially the technique consists of determining the noise spectrum in octave bands from 2 Hz to 16,000 Hz. Two systems are used; (a) direct measurements of the noise levels in the octave bands from 32 Hz to 16,000 Hz using a Bruel and Kjaer sound level meter (type 2203) with octave filter set and (b) indirect measurements of the noise in the 2 Hz to 32 Hz bands obtained by use of a portable magnetic tape recorder (UHER 4000 L) fed via an FM converter from a Bruel and Kjaer sound level meter (type 2204) fitted with microphone cartridge (type 4145). The frequency response of this sytem is 1.5 Hz to 1200 Hz. The levels of the noise in the low frequency range are determined in the laboratory by feeding the tape recorder via a demodulator to a 2 Hz to 32 Hz octave filter set and Bruel and Kjaer valve voltmeter. Circuits of the modulator and demodulator have been published by Tempest and Bryan (1969).

Calibration of both systems is carried out by the use of a Bruel and Kjaer pistonphone (type 4220). A further check on the accuracy of the recording system is obtained by comparing the sound pressure level in the 32 Hz band by direct measurement with the sound pressure level as determined by the indirect measurement technique. Agreement of these two levels within two decibels is considered a satisfactory indication that the FM recording system is working correctly.

This system was developed for use in measuring noise levels in transportation environments when it was realised that conventional measurements down to 32 Hz gave a poor indication both of the annoyance of the noise and of its correct spectrum. In other words much of the energy of the noise lay below this frequency and it seemed likely that it would be necessary to measure noise to much lower frequencies if a true understanding of how annoyance arises in transportation were to be reached. Subsequently the low frequency measuring system was found to have applications to problems in the work and home environments where conventional measurement and annoyance assessment techniques were found to be inadequate in predicting actual annoyance.

## B. ASSESSMENT OF ANNOYANCE

The procedure followed is to assess the usefulness of some of the existing annoyance criteria in predicting the degree of annoyance found. In the case of the transportation noises the assessment of the reaction is based upon the observations of acoustic consultants with many years' experience in dealing with a wide variety of noise annoyance. In the case of the home and the work environments the reaction is a representative response of the exposed population and does not arise from isolated individuals who show high noise sensitivity. The reaction was that of at least 20% of the population and so it is fairly clear that the response was a result of the unusual nature of the noise. The significance of interindividual differences in sensitivity to noise is discussed in Moreira and Bryan (1972).

The following noise annoyance criteria were employed, dB(A), noise rating number (NR) (International Standards Organisation, 1971), British Standard 4142 procedure (1967) and Perceived Level (PLdB) (Stevens, 1972). The first three criteria were used because of their widespread currency (in the U.K. at least), whilst the last and more complex measure of subjective reaction, that of PLdB, was included because it had been especially modified with extended frequency weighted contours down to 1 Hz. Thus, one might anticipate, it should give a better prediction of subjective reaction to low frequency noises than the other criteria. The NR method does not have contours extending below 32 Hz whilst the dB(A) rating gives very little weight to frequencies below about 64 Hz.

## IV. Annoyance in Transportation

Noise levels were measured, annoyance was noted, and predicted annoyance was calculated according to the above criteria inside five different passenger cars and inside a multiple-unit diesel train. All vehicles were travelling at sustained speeds of between 48 km/h and 113 km/h.

## A. PASSENGER CARS

The adequacy of the dB(A), NR and PLdB measures in predicting subjective reaction to noise was tested under three conditions.

(a) The growth of annoyance was compared with the increase in predicted annoyance within the cars as the speed was increased. All the vehicle windows remained closed.

(b) The increase in annoyance was compared with the increase in predicted annoyance when a window or quarter light was opened. Measurements were made at different sustained speeds.

(c) The annoyance inside four vehicles travelling at three different sustained speeds was rated by the testers on a subjective scale ranging from "quiet" to "unbearable" (1–6) and compared with the ratings given by the three criteria.

At the time of testing the passenger cars were a fairly representative sample of the range of vehicles available from U.K. manufacturers and were all in good or excellent mechanical condition. In ascending order of engine size they were:

  (i) 1 litre (four-seater) saloon,
 (ii) 1.5 litre (five-seater) estate car,
(iii) 2.25 litre, four-wheel drive (diesel) utility vehicle (hard-top—no sound insulation),
(iv) 3 litre (six-seater) saloon,
 (v) 4 litre (eight-seater) limousine with passenger division.

### 1. *Growth of Annoyance with Speed*

Figures 1, 2 and 3 show the noise spectra at different sustained speeds for three of the vehicles; the 3 litre saloon, the 2.25 litre utility vehicle and the 1 litre saloon respectively. In all cases the windows of the vehicles were closed. The figures all show the same general pattern; most of the noise energy lies below 125 Hz, where it remains flat with falling frequency down to 2 Hz. Above 125 Hz there is a fall-off of noise level with frequency at the rate of about 6–10 dB/octave. It becomes clear why octave band pressure levels above 32 Hz are considerably lower than the sound pressure level as given on the linear scale of a sound level meter for such vehicles. There is relatively little energy in the higher octave bands and I hope to show these bands play a relatively minor part in determining annoyance above speeds of 64 km/h.

The other interesting feature shown by the figures is the change which occurs in noise spectra with increasing speed. Taking Fig. 1 as being

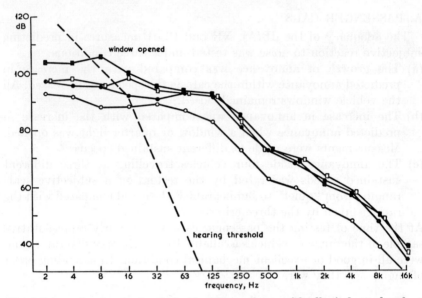

*Fig.* 1 Octave band noise levels inside 3 litre saloon, with all windows closed, at sustained speeds of 64 km/h (O—O); 97 km/h (●—●); 113 km/h (□—□); and with driver's window slightly open, at 113 km/h (■—■).

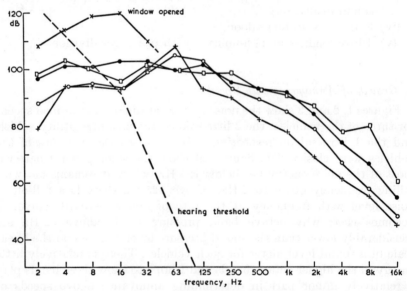

*Fig.* 2 Octave band noise levels inside 2.25 litre utility vehicle, with all windows closed, at sustained speeds of 48 km/h (+—+); 64 km/h (O—O); 80 km/h (●—●); 97 km/h (□—□); and with front passenger's window slightly open, at 97 km/h(×—×).

representative, it is seen that as the speed increases from 64 km/h to 97 km/h there is a 5–10 dB increase in noise level in all octave bands. However, when the speed increases from 97 km/h to 113 km/h the noise levels barely increase above 125 Hz whilst they increase by up to 10 dB below this frequency. As speeds increase above 80 km/h the outstanding effect on the noise spectra inside the vehicles is an increase in low rather

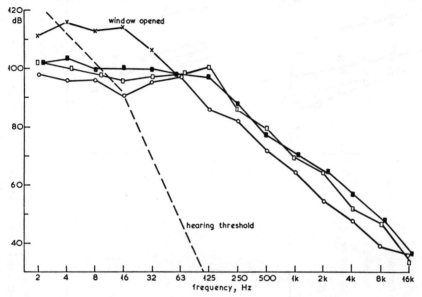

*Fig.* 3 Octave band noise levels inside 1 litre saloon, with all windows closed, at sustained speeds of 64 km/h (O—O); 97 km/h (□—□); 113 km/h (■—■) and with front passenger's window slightly open, at 113 km/h ( ×—× ).

than high frequency levels. Also at low speeds of around 48–64 km/h the figures show there is audible energy down to about 16 Hz; as the speeds increase to 97–113 km/h, noise down to the 8 Hz band is heard in all three vehicles.

On the question of the growth of annoyance with increasing speed it is not unreasonable to expect annoyance to grow with noise levels in much the same way as loudness or noisiness does. If this is the case, about a 10 dB increase in noise level on the appropriate scale should, for the average person, represent approximately a doubling of loudness or cause about a one unit increase in annoyance on a rating scale which passes from "quiet", (1); through "noticeable" (2); "intrusive" (3); "annoying" (4); "very annoying" (5); to "unbearable" (6). This is seen to be so in Fig. 4(a) for the rating of such noises as actual (i.e. not

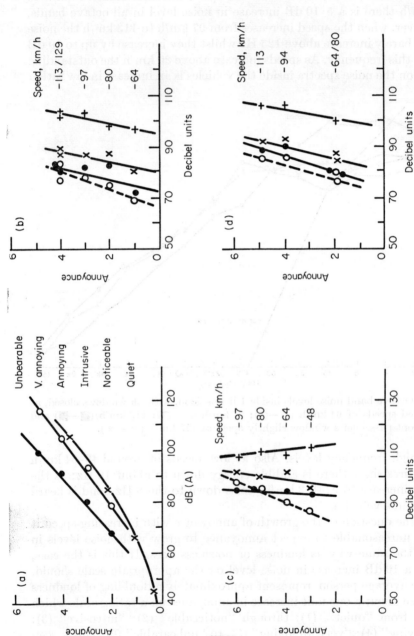

*Fig.* 4 Growth of actual annoyance compared with growth of sound pressure level, noise criteria and speed. (a) For aircraft noise etc. (O—O); 20s samples of traffic noise (●—●), and for 30m samples of traffic noise (×—×). (b) Inside 3 litre saloon; NR criterion (●—●); linear spl (+—+); dB(A) criterion (O– – –O); PLdB criterion (×—×). (c) Inside 1 litre saloon, symbols as in (b). (d) Inside 2.25 litre vehicle, symbols as in (b).

recorded) aircraft (Noise, Final Report, 1963) for recorded samples of aircraft, industrial and traffic noise, (Moreira and Bryan, 1972) and for 30 minute exposure to urban traffic noise (Johnson and Bryan—unpublished data). The three curves have much the same slope, varying from 11 to 14 dB/unit increase in annoyance, and have a mean slope value of 13 dB. The same is true for the growth of loudness or noisiness of other noises; there being, however, an exception in the external noisiness rating of individual motor vehicles (Noise, Final Report, 1963, p. 200), where the increase in level in dB(A) per unit increase in noisiness is only 8 dB.

However, the situation is apparently quite different for the growth of subjective response to the noise inside motor vehicles. As there seem to be no generally accepted criteria for acceptable levels inside transportation, assessments were made on the annoyance rating scale mentioned earlier by the same acoustics consultants who made the measurements. The growth of annoyance with noise level is so startlingly different from that of other noises that, even allowing for the idiosyncrasies of those making the judgments, it can only be attributable to the fact that we are dealing with an unusual type of noise. The growth of actual annoyance plotted against the noise criteria is given for the three vehicles in Figs. 4b, 4c and 4d. All three figures show the same pattern for the dB(A), NR and PLdB scales, i.e. there is a rapid rise for a moderate increase in noise level. For instance, for the 2.25 litre utility vehicle (Fig. 4(c)) at 48 km/h the annoyance rating is "intrusive" (or 3 on the rating scale) whilst by the time the speed has reached 97 km/h it has become "unbearable" (rating 6). The increases in dB(A), NR and PLdB values between these speeds are however only 10 dB, 1 dB and 6 dB respectively. This represents only about a 3 dB increase in noise level per unit increase in annoyance compared with a value of 13 dB found for other types of noise—see Fig. 4(a). The corresponding increases for the 3 litre saloon (Fig. 4(b)) and the 1 litre saloon (Fig. 4(d)) are 2.5 dB and 3 dB respectively.

Clearly the dB(A), NR and PLdB rating scales are of little value in predicting the growth of annoyance with increasing speed for motor car interiors. Recent work on the measurement of noise spectra inside a variety of heavy goods vehicle cabs shows that these are similar in shape to those inside motor cars (Tempest and Williams, 1975; Williams and Tempest, 1975). So it seems reasonable to assume that noise rating scales would also be inadequate in predicting annoyance in motor goods vehicles too. Although the Perceived Level (PLdB) has been especially modified to include spectra down to 1 Hz, and might therefore be expected to give a better prediction of annoyance to low frequency noises, it shows up no better than the dB(A) scale and the NR rating method which take little account of the low frequencies. It should be fairly self-evident that as all three criteria give only a 2–3 dB increase in noise level for unit increase in annoyance they are not likely to predict annoyance reliably. This magnitude of increase is about the size of the error likely in measuring the noise levels. Figures 4(b), 4(c) and 4(d) also show that a linear measure of the spl of the noise is no better in reflecting growth of annoyance.

## 2. *Effect upon Annoyance of Opening a Window*

The effect that opening a front window slightly at 97–113 km/h (by about 10–20 cm) or a quarter light has upon the noise spectra inside the vehicles is quite dramatic and is clearly shown in Figs. 1, 2 and 3. There is little or no increase in levels above 64 Hz but below this frequency there are increases of 10–20 dB. For instance, in the case of the 3 litre saloon (Fig. 1) there is now audible energy down to about 6 Hz at 113 km/h, whilst in the case of the 2.25 litre vehicle (Fig. 2) and the 1 litre saloon (Fig. 3) there is audible noise down to 4 Hz. However Table I shows that the average increases in the NR, dB(A) and PLdB noise ratings for the 3 litre, 2.25 litre and 1 litre vehicles respectively are less than 3, less than 1 and 3 whilst there are increases in overall spl of 2 dB, 18 dB and 8 dB respectively. However, the actual increase in annoyance upon opening a window or quarter light is generally one unit on the rating scale. In the case of the 2.25 litre vehicle (Fig. 2), at 97 km/h with both windows shut, the noise level is considered "unbearable", opening one window increases the noise level to the point where it becomes painful and distressing, yet this causes no more than a 1 dB increase in noise rating.

Most drivers will be well aware of the "buffeting" wind roar obtained upon opening their windows slightly at speeds in excess of 80 km/h, and concur that it leads to a significant increase in driver fatigue and annoyance. Table I clearly shows that the noise ratings do not predict anything like this increase in annoyance or noisiness. In some cases there is an actual decrease in decibel noise rating level—e.g. at 97 km/h for the 3 litre saloon the NR number decreases by 1 dB whilst the PLdB level decreases by 2 dB (the dB(A) level remains unchanged). The actual annoyance observed on the other hand increases from "intrusive" to "annoying".

Clearly, none of the three noise rating procedures seem able to predict, at all, the increase in annoyance caused by opening a window or quarter light in motor cars in which this causes a substantial increase in very low frequency noise level.

TABLE I: Actual and predicted annoyance inside three passenger vehicles

| Speed (km/h) | 3 Litre saloon | | | | | | | | | | 2.25 Litre vehicle | | | | | | | | | | 1 Litre saloon | | | | | | | | | |
|---|---|---|---|---|---|---|---|---|---|---|---|---|---|---|---|---|---|---|---|---|---|---|---|---|---|---|---|---|---|---|
| | NR | | dB(A) | | PLdB | | Lin | | Rating | | NR | | dB(A) | | PLdB | | Lin | | Rating | | NR | | dB(A) | | PLdB | | Lin | | Rating | |
| | WC | WO | WC | WO | WC | WO | WC | WO | WC | WO | WC | WO | WC | WO | WC | WO | WC | WO | WC | WO | WC | WO | WC | WO | WC | WO | WC | WO | WC | WO |
| 48 | 70 | — | 69 | — | 80 | — | 97 | — | 1 | — | 92 | 92 | 87 | 87$^a$ | 95 | 97 | 111 | 115$^a$ | 3 | 4 | | | | | | | | | | |
| 64 | 82 | — | 74 | — | 87 | — | 98 | — | 2 | — | 93 | 93 | 90 | 90 | 101 | 102 | 108 | 123$^a$ | 4 | 5 | 78 | — | 76 | — | 84 | — | 101 | — | 2 | — |
| 80 | 81 | 80 | 77 | 77 | 87 | 85 | 103 | 104 | 3 | 4 | 93 | 100$^a$ | 95 | 96$^a$ | 100 | 103 | 109 | 128$^a$ | 5 | 6 | 80 | — | 78 | — | 86 | — | 104 | — | 2 | — |
| 97 | 80 | 82 | 76 | 81 | 86 | 87 | 102 | 104 | 4 | 5 | 93 | 93 | 97 | 98 | 101 | 102 | 107 | 125$^a$ | 6 | 6$^b$ | 90 | 90 | 85 | 92 | 92 | 93 | 107 | 115 | 4 | 5 |
| 113 | 82 | — | 82 | — | 88 | — | 104 | — | 4 | — | | | | | 102 | | | | 6$^b$ | | 87 | 87 | 85 | 92 | 91 | 93 | 107 | 106 | 5 | 6 |

Actual rating of annoyance: 1 = Quiet; 2 = Noticeable; 3 = Intrusive; 4 = Annoying; 5 = Very annoying; 6 = Unbearable.
WC = Windows closed; WO = Windows open; Lin = Noise level on the linear scale of the sound level meter.
$^a$ Calculated; $^b$ Painful and distressing.

## 3. *Inter-vehicle Comparisons of Annoyance*

It is seen from an examination of Table II that the noise rating scales are much more successful in predicting differences in annoyance between vehicles than they are within vehicles. Four of the vehicles under test are placed in descending order of acceptability; the most acceptable vehicle at all speeds being the 4 litre limousine whilst the least acceptable was the 2.25 litre utility vehicle. Comparisons were made, for the windows-closed condition, at sustained speeds of 64 km/h, 80 km/h and 97 km/h. Table II shows that an increase in one unit on the annoyance rating scale corresponds to an increase in noise level of the dB(A), NR and PLdB scales of from 0 to 11 dB with a mean value of just under 5 dB. This compares with the 2 dB/unit rating increase found as speeds increase within any given vehicle, and suggests that these noise criteria scales may be of some value in predicting annoyance in inter-comparisons between different vehicles. Figure 5 shows a comparison of actual annoyance inside the four vehicles compared with the noise level as indicated by the dB(A), NR, PLdB and linear spl scales. The points are obtained by averaging the noise levels for the different vehicles for each value of annoyance rating. For instance on the dB(A) scale a noise rating of "annoying" (or 4) is obtained in the 1 litre car at 97 km/h, for a level of 85 dB, and in the 2.25 litre vehicle, at 64 km/h for a level of 90 dB. Thus the average dB(A) level corresponding to a rating of "4" is $(85 + 90)$ dB/2 = 87.5 dB. Figure 5 shows that the most linear relationship is obtained between actual annoyance and the dB(A) scale with the NR given the next most satisfactory relationship. The PLdB and linear noise measures give the least uniform increase with actual annoyance. In view of the simplicity of its measurement the dB(A) scale may therefore be the most suitable way available at the moment of predicting annoyance when comparisons are being made of noise inside different vehicles. From Fig. 5 it is seen that there is a mean value of 6 dB(A) increase per unit increase in annoyance rating for noise inside different vehicles. This value is of course just about half the increase, i.e. 13 dB/unit increase in annoyance, found for aircraft, traffic and industrial noise (see Fig. 4(a)). Interestingly enough, however, it is quite close to the value of 8 dB/unit increase in annoyance for the judgment of annoyance by curbside observers of single motor vehicles as reported in Noise, Final Report (1963), referred to earlier.

The data shown in Fig. 5 might serve as a basis for criteria of acceptable noise levels inside motor cars; as far as the author is aware there are no published recommendations for this. Thus the following criteria are proposed, though it must be remembered that Fig. 5 is based upon only four vehicles and upon a limited number of (albeit trained)

TABLE II: Noise ratings compared with four noise measures inside four passenger vehicles in descending order of acceptability for speeds of 64 km/h, 80 km/h and 97 km/h (windows closed)

| Vehicle | 64 km/h | | | | | 80 km/h | | | | | 97 km/h | | | | |
|---|---|---|---|---|---|---|---|---|---|---|---|---|---|---|---|
| | NR | dB(A) | PLdB | Lin | Rat | NR | dB(A) | PLdB | Lin | Rat | NR | dB(A) | PLdB | Lin | Rat |
| 4 litre saloon | 60 | 63 | 72 | 101 | 1 | 65 | 66 | 67 | 101 | 1 | 71 | 67 | 78 | 106 | 1/2 |
| 3 litre saloon | 70 | 69 | 80 | 97 | 1 | 82 | 74 | 87 | 98 | 2 | 81 | 77 | 87 | 103 | 3 |
| 1 litre saloon | 78 | 76 | 84 | 101 | 2 | 80 | 78 | 86 | 104 | 2 | 90 | 85 | 92 | 107 | 4 |
| 2.25 litre vehicle | 93 | 90 | 101 | 108 | 4 | 93 | 95 | 100 | 109 | 5 | 93 | 97 | 101 | 107 | 6 |

Rat = rating values—see Table I. Lin = spl on linear scale of sound level meter observers. The noise levels inside motor cars must be:

> below 91 dB(A)    if it is not to be "very annoying"
> below 85 dB(A)    if it is not to be "annoying"
> below 79 dB(A)    if it is not to be "intrusive"
> below 73 dB(A)    if it is not to be "noticeable"
> and   below 67 dB(A)    if it is to be considered quiet

In view of the rapid growth of annoyance with increasing noise levels an uncertainty of ± 3 dB might reasonably be put on the above figures.

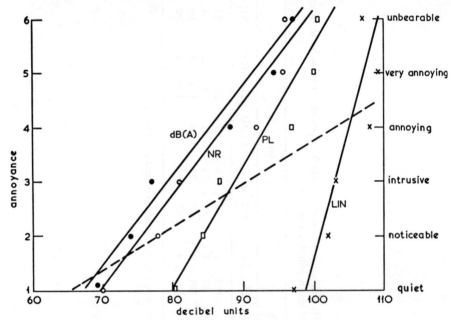

*Fig.* 5 Average growth of actual annoyance inside four passenger vehicles compared with growth of noise criteria and sound pressure level. NR criterion (O—O); dB(A) criterion (●—●); PLdB criterion (□—□); and linear spl (×—×) compared with growth of annoyance for traffic and aircraft noise (– – – – –) (data from Fig. 4).

Why do the rating scales work relatively well when inter-vehicle noise level annoyance comparisons are being made, but not when the growth of annoyance within a vehicle with increasing speed is being considered? An examination of Fig. 6 may go some way to providing an answer to this question. This figure compares the noise spectra for the four vehicles travelling at 97 km/h (with windows closed) and shows that there is a progressive increase in both noise spectra level and in annoyance from vehicle to vehicle. It is another matter whether the actual increase in noise rating adequately reflects the increase in annoyance.

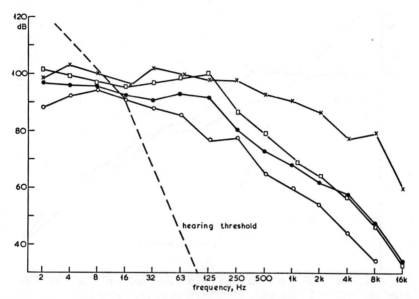

*Fig.* 6 Octave band noise levels inside four passenger vehicles, with all windows closed, at a sustained speed of 97 km/h. Four litre saloon (○—○), noise rated "quiet/noticeable"; 3 litre saloon (●—●), noise rated "intrusive"; 1 litre saloon (□—□), noise rated "annoying"; 2.25 litre vehicle (×—×), noise rated "unbearable".

## B. MULTIPLE UNIT DIESEL TRAIN

The other means of passenger transport in which noise spectra were obtained and an assessment made of the subjective acceptability of the noise was a British Rail multiple-unit diesel train. Measurements were made in both an (under-floor) motorised coach and an unmotorised coach (see Fig. 7).

The annoyance rating and noise levels in dB(A), NR, PLdB and linear dB for the two coaches are given in Table III. It is seen that the motorised coach was considered as being "very annoying" (rating 5) whilst the unmotorised coach was considered to be "slightly annoying" (rating 3/4). However, the differences in noise ratings of 4 dB(A), 1 NR and 2 PLdB are completely inadequate reflections of the difference in annoyance between the two coaches—see Table III. There are correspondingly small differences in noise spectra for the two coaches as is seen in Fig. 7. The largest differences occur in the 63 Hz octave band and below although they do not exceed 10 dB. Energy thus becomes audible in the 8 Hz band in the motorised coach compared with the

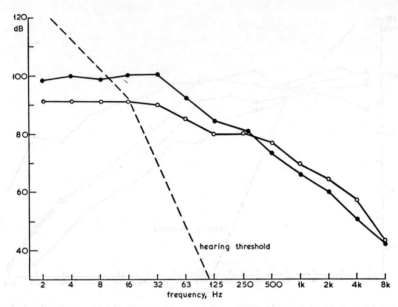

*Fig.* 7 Octave band noise levels inside British Rail multiple-unit diesel train at 64/80 km/h. Unmotorised coach (○—○), noise rated "slightly annoying"; motorised coach (●—●), noise rated "very annoying".

TABLE III: Noise criteria levels and annoyance rating inside motorised and unmotorised coach of B.R. DM-U train, 64/80 km/h

| Source | NR | dB(A) | PLdB | Lin | Rating |
|---|---|---|---|---|---|
| DMU (motorised) | 74 | 82 | 84 | 105 | 5 |
| DMU (unmotorised) | 73 | 78 | 82 | 94 | 3/4 |

For rating values see Table I.

16 Hz band in the unmotorised coach. Above this frequency the differences become progressively smaller with increasing frequency so it becomes unlikely that the difference in annoyance arises in this region. Another difference in spectra between the two coaches is the rate at which the noise falls with frequency; in the motorised coach this is 7.4 dB/octave compared with 5 dB/octave for the unmotorised coach.

Both the difference in low frequency noise level and in slope of spectra could be important in explaining the fairly considerable difference in annoyance. A similar result was obtained for speeds of 80–97 km/h.

As a final comment the acoustic consultants noted that in the various means of transport the unpleasantness rather than the loudness of the various noise environments seemed to determine the degree of acceptability. It will be shown in the following two sections on the work environment, and on the home environment, that low frequency noise sources seem to give rise to a different kind of disturbance or annoyance from that found due to normal noise sources which have little or no low frequency content.

## V. Annoyance due to Low Frequency Noises in the Work Environment

Two examples are given of noises occurring in the work environment which gave rise to considerable disturbance of employees, and whose spectra are similar to those in Section IV. In transportation they apparently arise due to the motion of the vehicle through the air, whilst in the work environment they arose due to the use of large extractor fans. There are a variety of circumstances in industry where high speed large mass airflows occur such as in blast furnaces, air-conditioning plants, large oil-fired boilers, air compressors etc. The two examples given here are particularly interesting and valuable since control conditions were available which made it possible to identify positively the low frequency noise source as the cause of disturbance.

The first example occurred in one of the buildings of an electronics factory. This building was single storey in construction and was divided into a number of bays by breeze block walls. The air-conditioning plant was installed on a concrete raft on the roof of one of the bays (bay 3); long air ducts carried the air to other bays. The remainder of the roofing was aluminium sheeting.

The building was new, well lit, spacious and looked a pleasant place in which to work. However, vigorous complaints had been received by the management from the workers in bay 3 that it was oppressive, and unpleasant to work in; some complained of headaches, others said that the place made them feel uneasy and that the noise of the air-conditioning was disturbing. There were no complaints from the adjacent and apparently identical bay 1. The management accepted that the workers complaints in bay 3 were genuine—indeed it was immediately apparent to the noise consultants when they inspected the two bays that bay 3 had a quite different atmosphere from that of bay 1. They too felt that the workers' complaints were valid and that the air-conditioning noise, although not loud, was exceedingly unpleasant. Noise spectra were obtained for both bays and are given in Fig. 8, the criteria noise levels are given in Table IV. The spectra have the classic low frequency noise shape with octave band levels reasonably flat up to 16–32 Hz, above this frequency the levels fall off with frequency at a rate of 6.3 dB/octave for bay 3 and 4.4 dB/octave for bay 1. There is very little difference in noise levels between the two bays, the levels being higher in the unacceptable bay 3 than those in the acceptable bay 1 in the 32 Hz, 63 Hz and 125 Hz octave bands by 13 dB, 8 dB and 6 dB respectively. At 1 kHz and above however the noise levels in bay 1 are higher than those in bay 3 by about 3–6 dB. The inadequacy of the noise criteria is brought out quite nicely in Table IV. This shows that the Noise Rating of bay 3 is only 2 dB higher than bay 1 (57 and 55 NR respectively); this is a completely inadequate reflection of the subjective difference between the two bays and both levels ought, according to the ISO criterion (45–75 NR) (1971), to be quite acceptable for this type of occupation. Neither the dB(A) nor the PLdB fares any better; in the case of the former, bay 3 is 1 dB *lower* than bay 1, and in the case of the latter, bay 3 is 2 dB higher than bay 1.

It is not clear which aspect of the noise spectrum is important in making bay 3 so much less acceptable than bay 1. The former has a steeper fall off in level than the latter at high frequencies (6.3 dB/octave as against 4.4 dB/octave) as well as having higher noise levels in the 32 Hz to 125 Hz octave bands. It is not yet clear which of these, if indeed either, is responsible for the greatly increased unpleasantness.

A very similar situation was found in a university radiochemistry building. Fume cupboards had been installed in several laboratories with unusually generous air flows. The staff in these laboratories complained when the extractor fans for these fume cupboards were in operation. They said such things as "the windows shook", "the noise makes you sleepy", "it is oppressive", "it makes you feel dizzy", or "the pressure is 2 atmospheres too high". Some refused to work in these laboratories when the fans were running. These complaints were made despite the fact that conventional noise reduction techniques had reduced the noise level in the laboratories with the fans running to 62 NR, 62 dB(A) and 70 PLdB. This is well within the ISO criterion (45–75 NR) and ought therefore to have been acceptable. Even more striking is the fact that the noise level fell very little with the fans turned off (by only 0 NR, 1 dB(A) and 3 PLdB), and yet no complaints were received for this condition. It was very clear to the noise consultants that the fans being on produced an unsatisfactory environment, although what aspect of the noise caused the disturbance was not very obvious. It was true that when the fans were on they produced a low

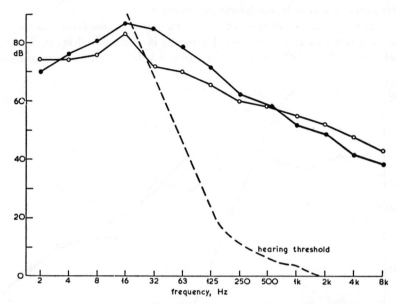

*Fig.* 8 Octave band noise levels inside electronics factory. Bay (1) (O—O), no complaints, 62 dB(A); Bay (3) (●—●), vigorous complaints, 61 dB(A).

TABLE IV: Noise criteria levels, observed and predicted reaction in electronics factory and radiochemistry laboratory due to fans

| Source | NR | dB(A) | PLdB | Lin | Observed reaction | Predicted reaction | Criteria [a] |
|---|---|---|---|---|---|---|---|
| Electronics factory | | | | | | | |
| Bay 1 | 55 | 62 | 68 | 82 | No complaints | No complaints | 45–75 NR |
| Bay 3 | 57 | 61 | 69 | 87 | Vigorous complaints | No complaints | 45–75 NR |
| Radiochemistry laboratory | | | | | | | |
| Fan off | 62 | 61 | 67 | 82 | No complaints | No complaints | 45–75 NR |
| Fan off | 62 | 62 | 70 | 91 | Vigorous complaints | No complaints | 45–75 NR |

[a] Suggested criteria ISO R1996 (1971).

level rumble which was not loud but was very intrusive and the laboratory became immediately oppressive.

A typical example of the noise spectra in one of the laboratories with and without the fume cupboard fans on is shown in Fig. 9. There is again very little difference in the noise levels for the two conditions.

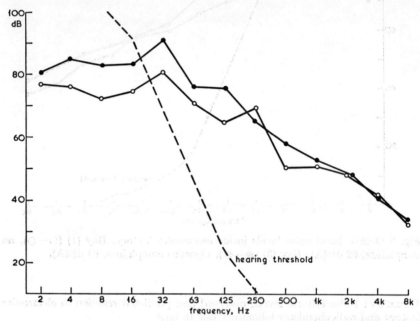

*Fig.* 9 Octave band noise levels inside radiochemistry laboratory. Extractor fans off (O—O), no complaints, 61 dB(A); extractor fans on (●—●), vigorous complaints, 62 dB(A).

These levels are greater with the fans on in the octave bands of 125 Hz and below; the difference reaching a maximum value of 10 dB in the 32 Hz band. One consequence of this would be to make energy audible down to about 16 Hz instead of only 32 Hz with the fans off. The slope of the noise spectrum with the fans on is greater than it is with the fans off (7.4 dB/octave as against 5.6 dB/octave). As in the case of the electronics factory, the unsatisfactory noise environment has a spectrum with a steeper slope than the satisfactory noise environment.

It might be worth pointing out that the noise spectra obtained in the work environment are similar to those found in transportation (see Section IV); however, the overall levels are lower, with sound pressure levels (on the linear scale) of 80–90 dB as compared with 90–120 dB in the latter case. This fact might be taken to suggest that the actual sound pressure level of the noises may not be a very important factor in determining annoyance compared with the actual shape of the spectrum.

## VI. Annoyance due to Low Frequency Noise in the Home Environment

Finally, three examples are given from the Salford Audiology Group's case book of neighbourhood noise nuisance which have caused considerably more disturbance than the criteria would predict, and where the noises were predominantly low frequency in nature. In the remaining cases the energy was predominantly above 100 Hz and there was usually good agreement between the criteria (dB(A) and NR) and the community response.

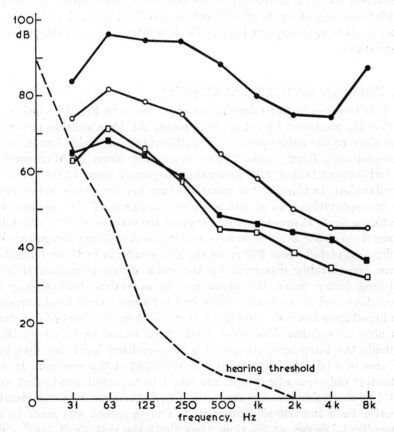

*Fig.* 10 Octave band noise levels due to Noise I, factory boiler; inside boiler house (●—●); on boiler house roof (○—○); 18 m outside boiler house (■—■); at 46 m outside complainants' houses (□—□).

## A. NOISE I: FACTORY BOILER

A large factory had recently converted its central heating boiler, of several million BThU/h, to oil firing. This is another example of a noise source consisting of a high speed flow of a large air mass. Two of the four residents who lived 45 m from the boiler house complained that the new noise disturbed them, particularly in the evenings. As Table V shows, outside the complainants' houses the noise level was 55 dB(A), which is also the maximum permitted level for evenings in that type of area. As the acoustic consultants' report said at the time, a serious nuisance would not have been expected but in this case the criteria were not an adequate reflection of actual annoyance.

Figure 10 shows how the spectrum of the noise changes from being relatively flat with frequency inside the boiler house, to one which falls with frequency at a rate of 5 dB/octave outside the aggrieved residents' houses. It is to be expected that this slope would be even steeper inside the houses.

## B. NOISE II. ASPHALT PLANT (ONE)

This increase in slope does occur as is shown in Fig. 11 which is for Noise II, produced by an asphalt plant. At 15 m outside this plant the slope of the noise spectrum is 6 dB/octave but inside houses where complainants lived, some 370 m away, the slope has increased to 9.2 dB/octave falling with increasing frequency from 32 Hz. This is a similar slope to those of the unsatisfactory low frequency noises found in transportation and in the work environment of the previous two sections. Noise II arose from a new plant for making asphalt which had opened up at the same time as a development of thirty bungalows was being completed some 370 m away. The residents in these bungalows were considerably disturbed by the noise of an 18 million BThU/h oil-fired boiler, when the plant was in operation, both during the weekdays and at weekends. They had petitioned their local authority to investigate the noise and the latter called in members of our group to give an opinion. The noise levels were found to be 51–54 dB(A) outside the bungalows compared with permitted levels for that type of area of 55 dB(A) (weekdays) and 50 dB(A) at the weekend. In this situation only sporadic complaints might be expected, but in fact some 50% of the residents were annoyed. The disturbance was considerably greater than the criteria anticipated. The comment was made in the consultants' report, at the time, that "both the ISO (draft 314E, 1963) and BS 4142 procedures in our opinion underestimate the problem in this case because of the low frequency nature of the noise". The residents stated that they felt that their houses were being shaken, which obviously worried them. It was in fact possible to feel the windows vibrating, but there was no detectable ground vibration.

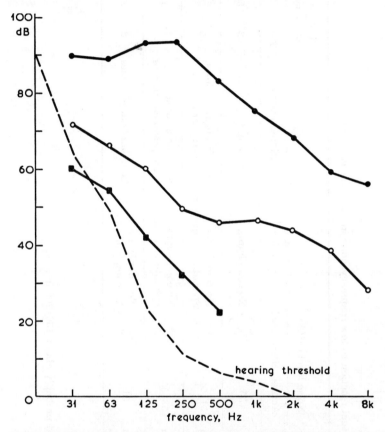

*Fig.* 11 Octave band noise levels due to Noise II, asphalt plant (one): 15 m from plant (●—●); 370 m from plant, outside complainants' houses (○—○); 370 m from plant, inside complainants' houses (■—■).

## C. NOISE III: ASPHALT PLANT (TWO)

A similar plant for making asphalt which produced Noise III opened up in a different part of the North-West, this time in an area of established houses. This again caused considerable annoyance in two areas; (a) of about 150–200 terraced houses some 230 m from the plant, and (b) in an area of about 10 detached bungalows and houses some 460 m from the plant. It can be seen from Table V that only in area (a) would sporadic complaints be expected at the weekends and during residents stated that they felt that their homes were being shaken, which obviously worried them. It was impossible to feel the window vibrations, but there was no detectable ground vibration.

TABLE V: Expected and actual reaction to low frequency noise in the home environment

| Noise source | Area | Noise level dB(A) | | Expected reaction | Actual reaction | Residents annoyed | |
|---|---|---|---|---|---|---|---|
| | | Actual | Permitted | | | No. | % |
| Noise I: Factory boiler | ? | 55 | 60[a] 55[b] } No complaints | | Complaints | 2 | 50 |
| Noise II: Asphalt plant | Suburban | 51–54 | 55[a] 50[c] | No complaints Sporadic complaints | Complaints at all times, vigorous action | 15 | 50 |
| Noise III(a): Asphalt plant | Suburban | 53–55 | 55[a] 50[bc] | No complaints Sporadic complaints | Sporadic complaints Widespread complaints | 15[d] | 47 |
| Noise III(b): Asphalt plant | Suburban | 51 | 55[a] 50[bc] | No complaints No complaints | Complaints at all times | 2 | 20 |

[a] Day time 8 a.m.–6 p.m.
[b] Evenings up to 10 p.m.
[c] Weekends.
[d] Only 32 households visited probably about 150–200 in area.

evening working when actual levels exceed the criterion by 3–4 dB. In fact there were sporadic complaints due to daytime working, and widespread complaints due to evening and weekend working. At area (b), where no complaints are predicted by the criteria at any time, there were complaints due to working at all times. These complaints were of

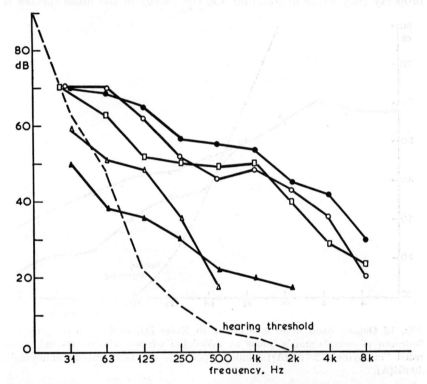

*Fig.* 12 Octave band noise levels, due to Noise III, asphalt plant (two): 69 m from plant (●—●); 230 m from plant, outside complainants' houses (a) (○—○); 230 m from plant, inside complainants' houses (a) (△—△); 460 m from plant, outside complainants' houses (b) (□—□); 460 m from plant, inside complainants' houses (b) (▲—▲).

unease caused by the noise which appeared as a low-pitched rumble inside the houses, and which it was not possible to "blanket out" with other sound. It was worse late at night or early in the morning when people were either prevented from sleeping or woken up by the noise.

Figure 12 shows that the shape and slope of the noise spectrum are similar to those of Noises I and II. Inside the houses in area (a) the slope is 10.5 dB/octave and in area (b) it is 5 dB/octave.

It was apparent from Noises I, II and III that the nuisance they caused was greater than either the British Standard 4142 (1967) in dB(A) or the ISO standard (NR) (1963) would predict. Both criteria underestimate annoyance by an amount corresponding to some 10–15 dB. Any explanation of this effect must be made in terms of the property they share in common, i.e. the energy in the noise spectra is

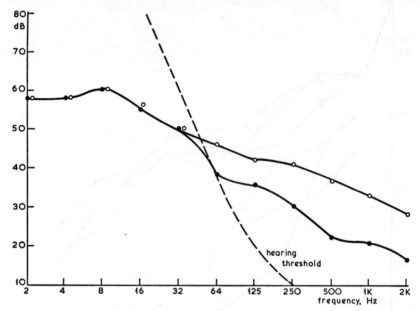

*Fig.* 13 Octave band noise levels, due to Noise III, asphalt plant (two): in bedroom of complainant's house at midnight; window closed (●—●), noise rated "annoying", 28 dB(A); window open (○—○), noise rated "annoying", 40 dB(A).

largely occurring at frequencies of 125 Hz and below by the time the noises have reached the inside of the complainants' houses. This fact is seen from an examination of Figs. 10, 11 and 12. Figure 13 shows the spectra for Noise II measured in one of the bedrooms of an aggrieved resident in area (b) for both the windows open and the windows closed. This shows that although no noise is audible below 64 Hz there is energy present down to 2 Hz and the energy levels below 64 Hz are the same for both windows open and closed. In this case opening the windows increased the dB(A) level from 28 to 40; however, subjectively, there was neither increase in annoyance nor loudness compared with when the windows were closed. This suggests very strongly that annoyance is being determined by the lowest audible frequencies of the noises.

## VII. Discussion

The aim of this chapter has been to bring together examples of noise from three different situations, transportation interiors, the work environment and the home environment, where current noise criteria at best give only a fair prediction, and at worst a completely inadequate prediction, of actual annoyance found. Sufficiently widespread annoyance has arisen in all three environments to conclude that it arose not from any peculiar sensitivity of individuals exposed but due to the type of noise producing the annoyance. The common characteristic of the different noise sources was that their energy was predominantly in frequencies of 125 Hz and below. A fairly adequate approximation to their noise spectra can be made by means of two straight lines. These are a horizontal line representing the energy below about 125 Hz (the turnover point) and a line with a slope of between 5 and 10 dB/octave representing the fall off in energy with increasing frequency about the turnover point. We feel intuitively that this rapid fall in energy with frequency may well provide a clue to explain the excessive annoyance caused by this rather unusual type of noise. Pink noise for instance has a fall-off of only 3 dB/octave (equal spl in each one-third octave band) and its annoyance can be adequately predicted by use of the PLdB scale (Stevens, 1972).

It is suggested that the slope of the noise spectra of these low frequency noises rather than their absolute levels may be important in determining annoyance because there is such a wide range in the latter (from 120 dB inside motor vehicles down to 60 dB inside the houses in the neighbourhood nuisance problems), yet the same type of extreme disturbance was produced at all levels. For this reason too, it seems unlikely that low frequency annoyance is due to the physiological effects (such as balance disturbance, etc.) reported elsewhere in this book, as these effects would seem to require levels in excess of 100 dB in the normal hearing subject.

Low frequency noises of the type of interest to us here can therefore be represented by two parameters; the turnover point (in Hz) and the slope (in decibels/octave). This has been done in Table VI for five of the noises which had been rated as subjectively acceptable and nine of the noises which had been rated as subjectively unacceptable. The main point of interest is that the mean turnover point and slope of the acceptable noises were 29 Hz and 5.7 dB/octave respectively, the corresponding values for the unacceptable noises were 68 Hz and 7.9 dB/octave respectively. The mean values of the turnover points and slopes differ at the 5% and $(5-1)\%$ levels of significance respectively. This suggests that differences in either or both parameters (which are

TABLE VI: Slope and turnover point values of spectrum for acceptable and unacceptable low frequency noises

| | Acceptable | | | | Unacceptable | | |
|---|---|---|---|---|---|---|---|
| Source | Slope (dB/octave) | Turning point (Hz) | Rating | Source | Slope (dB/octave) | Turning point (Hz) | Rating |
| 4 litre saloon, 64–97 km/h | 7.5 | 32 | Quiet/Noticeable | 1 litre saloon, 113 km/h | 9.1 | 125 | Annoying |
| 3 litre saloon, 64 km/h | 6.1 | 32 | Quiet | 2.25 litre vehicle, 64 km/h | 7.7 | 125 | Annoying |
| DMU unmotorised | 5.0 | 32 | Slightly/Annoying | 3 litre saloon, 113 km/h | 8.0 | 125 | Annoying |
| Electronics factory, bay 1 | 4.4 | 16 | No complaints | DMU motorised | 7.4 | 32 | Very annoying |
| Radiochemical laboratory, fan off | 5.6 | 32 | No complaints | Electronics factory, bay 3 | 6.3 | 32 | Vigorous complaints |
| | | | | Radiochemical laboratory, fan on | 7.4 | 32 | Vigorous complaints |
| | | | | Noise II inside home | 9.2 | ? | Very annoying |
| | | | | Noise III(a) inside home | 10.5 | ? | Very annoying |
| | | | | Noise III(b) inside home | 5.0 | 8 | Very annoying |
| Mean □ | 5.7 | 29 | | | 7.9 | 68 | |

quite small) are important in determining whether or not low frequency noise is going to be acceptable. The difference in the turnover point possibly just reflects the fact that the unacceptable noises tend to be about 10 dB greater in level than the acceptable noises (for an identical situation). The difference in slope between what is considered acceptable and what is considered unacceptable may be of more importance. The two idealised spectra are shown in Fig. 14. A difference in level of 10 dB at low frequencies has been assumed.

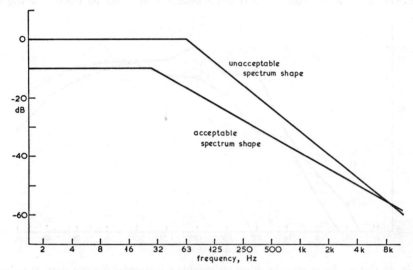

*Fig.* 14 Idealised shapes of noise spectra of the mean of five acceptable and of nine unacceptable low frequency noises.

The difference in mean slope values of only 2.2 dB/octave between those spectra which were considered acceptable and those which were considered unacceptable is quite small. This could be taken to suggest that subjects are very sensitive to slight changes of slope for low frequency noises. A possible explanation of why this might be so is found by examining the slope of the NR curves, the dB(A) weighting function and the PLdB curves in the region of interest (60–120 dB spl). Their respective loss of sensitivity with falling frequency in the range 1 kHz to 32 Hz is 7.6 dB/octave, 8.0 dB/octave and 6.4 dB/octave—the mean value being 7.3 dB/octave. Thus it is seen that the acceptable low frequency noises all, with one exception, have slopes less than the slopes of the noise-rating curves whilst the unacceptable ones all, with the exception of two noises, have slopes which are greater than those of the noise-rating curves (see Table VI).

5

The implications of these results are not altogether clear but one possible explanation of why high slope low frequency noises are particularly annoying might be as follows. The various criteria such as NR, PLdB etc. assume that noisiness, loudness or annoyance of a noise is predominantly determined by the octave or one-third octave band which has the greatest sound pressure level after weighting. The remaining octave bands are less important in determining the subjective response. If the noise has a spectrum with a slope of less than 7.3 dB/octave the most prominent octave bands will tend to occur at high

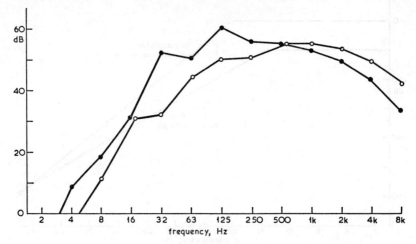

*Fig.* 15 Octave band spectra of an acceptable (electronics factory, bay 1) noise (○—○) and an unacceptable (radiochemistry laboratory, fan on) noise (●—●) after passing through an "A" weighting network. The loudness of the acceptable noise will be determined mainly by the 500 Hz and 1 kHz octave bands, whilst the loudness of the unacceptable noise will be determined by the 125 Hz octave band.

frequencies, i.e. above 125–250 Hz, and loudness etc. will be determined by these bands in the normal way. However, for spectra having slopes of greater than 7.3 dB/octave the most prominent octave bands will occur at or below 250 Hz and the subjective response will be determined by this unusual low frequency noise. We also know that loudness grows more rapidly in the frequency region below 250 Hz and for spl's above 60 dB (see Stevens, 1972); hence if these bands predominate their subjective effect will become even more enhanced than if the same (weighted) pressure levels occurred at higher frequencies.

The plausibility of this effect is illustrated in Fig. 15, which shows the spectra for bay 1 of the electronics factory and the fan-on condition in the radio chemistry laboratory (see Section V). The former noise has a slope of 4.4 dB/octave and is satisfactory and the latter's noise has a slope of 7.4 dB/octave and is unsatisfactory. The figure shows their respective spectra as they would be if they had passed through an "A" weighting network. The spectra of bay 1 now has a fairly flat spectrum with the predominant bands being 500 Hz, 1 kHz and 2 kHz. These bands will determine the annoyance and give the noise a fairly high-pitched sound. Whilst the spectra for the radiochemistry laboratory has the greatest spl in the 125 Hz band and annoyance will be determined by this band and give the noise a low-pitched sound. The same effect can be demonstrated with the other spectra of Table VI.

This, very tentative, explanation "ties up" with the subjective effects of the unacceptable noise spectra. It is apparent that people reacted badly to the type of noise which is audible as a low-pitched rumble. In the home environment, for instance, the cause of the noise may be not at all obvious to aggrieved residents, and indeed the source may be some distance away. Also in some cases, because of room resonances, these types of noises can be plainly audible inside a house (or only in certain rooms) and not audible outside. The complainants say the noise makes them uneasy and that it is disturbing to them. This may be partially due to the fact that it sometimes makes their house windows or some objects in their rooms vibrate, and they fear damage to their houses. All this suggests that the reaction is somewhat different from, and more extreme than, that due to more normal noise spectra.

There is very little in the literature about low frequency noise annoyance. Sharland (1968) has commented that "boiler rumble can be detected and has caused complaints when its octave band level is below the relevant NR level". His explanation of this effect is in terms of amplitude modulation below 100 Hz in the spectrum of the boiler rumble. Only further research can show which if either of the above two explanations is correct.

Clearly a great deal of this discussion is speculative with respect to the cause of excessive annoyance due to low frequency noise. There is little doubt that the effect is genuine and one where our existing criteria are of little value. However, it is not possible to say at this time with what measure of the spectra they should be replaced to obtain a more accurate prediction of low frequency annoyance. The next stage is a laboratory study of low frequency annoyance using noises of different spectrum shape and slopes etc. From such work it ought to be possible to deduce suitable criteria for the adequate prediction of low frequency annoyance.

## REFERENCES

British Standards Institution (1967). BS 4142. London.

International Standards Organisation (1963). Draft Proposal 314 E, Technical Committee 43, Acoustics, Switzerland.

International Standards Organisation (1971). Recommendation R 1996, 1st edn., Switzerland.

Johnson, M. and Bryan, M. E. (unpublished data).

Moreira, N. M. and Bryan, M. E. (1972). *J. Sound. Vib.* **21**, 449–462.

Noise, Final Report (1963). Cmnd 2056, Her Majesty's Stationery Office, London.

Schultz, T. J. (1972). "Community Noise Ratings", Applied Science, Barking, U.K.

Sharland, I. J. (1968). *Phil. Trans. R. Soc. Lond., Series A* **263**, 291–297.

Stevens, S. S. (1972). *J. Acoust. Soc. Am.* **51**, 575–601.

Tempest, W. and Bryan, M. E. (1969). *Electron. Engng* **39**, 87–89.

Tempest, W. and Bryan, M. E. (1972). *Applied Acoustics* **5**, 133–139.

Tempest, W. and Williams, D. (1975). "Noise and the Lorry Driver", paper read at the Institute of Acoustics Conference, Salford University 23/24 January.

Williams, D. and Tempest, W. (1975). *J. Sound Vib.* **43**, 97–107.

# 5. Physiological and Psychological Effects of Infrasound at Moderate Intensities

*Margaret J. Evans*

## I. Introduction

Although the first scientific studies of infrasound and its effects were made as long ago as World War I, the subsequent years have yielded very little information on the subject. Until recently the examination of human reaction to infrasound was confined to determining the threshold of hearing at these low frequencies, indeed, it was widely held that sounds below 20 Hz could not even be heard.

In the past decade interest in the various phenomena associated with infrasonic acoustic stimulation has rapidly increased as high energy, low frequency pressure oscillations have become common in the development of aircraft and space-craft propulsion units. The thrust at lift-off of space-rockets is in the multi-million pound range, so the turbulent mixing of exhaust gases with the surrounding atmosphere, and the aerodynamic noise, have peak acoustic outputs in the frequency range below 20 Hz. Consequently problems concerning the physical and psychological well-being of astronauts arose, and N.A.S.A. sponsored work in the early 1960's concentrated on the effects of very high intensity infrasound on trained forces personnel (Mohr *et al.*, 1965; Alford *et al.*, 1966). Research workers became aware that the problem was not confined only to high intensities when draughtsmen refused to work in offices close to the test-bed of the Concorde engines. They complained of nausea, dizziness, lethargy and a general inability to concentrate. It was concluded that these unpleasant and unusual symptoms were due to the presence of infrasound in the engine's noise spectra.

## II. Physiological Effects

It seemed to be theoretically possible that the infrasonic stimulus might produce disturbances of the static and dynamic organs of balance—the otoliths and semi-circular canals, as acoustic signals below 20 Hz are within the normal frequency range of these organs.

This hypothesis has been investigated by Evans and Tempest at the University of Salford (Evans *et al.*, 1971; Evans and Tempest, 1972), using infrasonic stimulation down to 2 Hz at levels of up to 145 dB spl for both aural and whole-body exposure.

## A. AURAL EXPOSURE

Because of the power required, and the very low frequencies involved, conventional headphones were completely inadequate for producing intensities up to 145 dB spl and a special headset was designed (Yeowart *et al.*, 1967) consisting of 2–15 watt 30 cm loudspeakers. Each loudspeaker was mounted on an aluminium plate coupled directly to ear-defender cups (Fig. 1). The headphones, driven by a specially designed low frequency amplifier and filter system, had a working frequency range of 1–200 Hz, and could deliver sound pressure levels up to 146 dB. The acoustic system was large enough to permit the mounting of a monitoring microphone in the side of each ear-defender cup, which could be used to measure the actual sound pressure level at the subject's ear.

### 1. *Detection of Effects*

The basic premise of this work was that infrasonic stimulation could possibly disturb the organs of equilibrium in normal human subjects.

When an animal or human experiences motion, real or apparent, each eyeball rotates in the opposite direction to the perceived motion. This action is clearly directed towards maintaining a steady image on the retina and produces a change in the corneo-retinal potential. If the motion persists, the eyes upon nearing the limit of their travel will rapidly flick in the direction of motion and then resume their compensatory motion. This periodic movement is termed "nystagmus" and is a sensitive and reliable indication of balance disturbance. If the changes in corneo-retinal potential are monitored using skin electrodes a characteristically shaped trace is observed (Fig. 2). This technique of electronystagmography was used by Evans *et al.* (1971) and Evans and Tempest (1972) to detect signs of balance disturbance in their subjects.

### 2. *Nystagmographic Results*

Each subject sat in the test apparatus for periods of 15 minutes. No measurements were made during these periods, this was in order to condition the subject to the test environment so that nervous responses

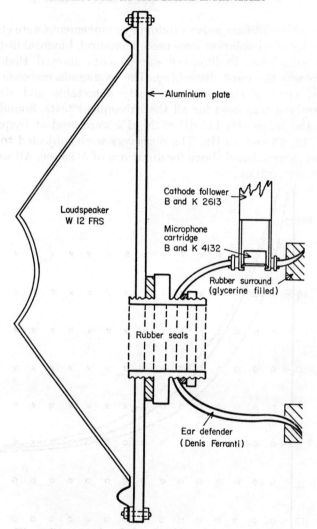

← Aluminium plate

Cathode follower
B and K 2613

Microphone
cartridge
B and K 4132

Loudspeaker
W 12 FRS

Rubber surround
(glycerine filled)

Rubber seals

Ear defender
(Denis Ferranti)

*Fig.* 1 Cross-sectional sketch of low frequency headset.

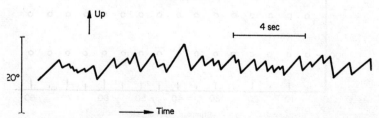

↑ Up

4 sec

20°

→ Time

*Fig.* 2 Typical vertical nystagmic response to binaural "antiphasic" infrasonic stimulation.

such as blinking and excessive random eye movements were eliminated. Three modes of stimulation were used, monaural, binaural in-phase and binaural antiphase. Preliminary experiments showed that binaural antiphase was the most disturbing. The nystagmic response obtained from this type of stimulus was easily detectable and stable, and consequently it was used for all the subsequent tests. Sound pressure levels in the range 100–145 dB re 20 μPa were used at frequencies of 2, 4, 5, 7, 12, 15 and 20 Hz. The observers were subjected to stimulus intensities as mentioned above for durations of 5–85 sec. All were tested in the sitting position.

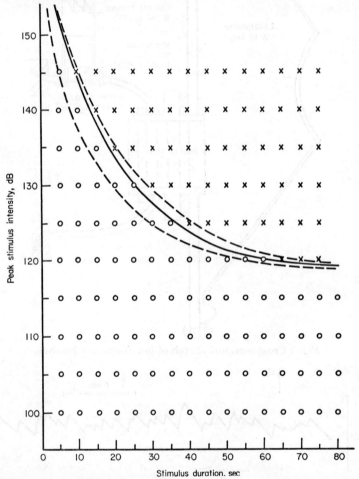

*Fig.* 3 Threshold curve for vertical nystagmus induced by a 7 Hz binaural stimulus: × response; ○ no response; ––––– region of uncertainty.

(a) *Nystagmus threshold*: As well as sound pressure level, the effects of stimulus duration and frequency on the threshold of the onset of nystagmus were examined. After the initial conditioning period each subject was exposed to a series of infrasonic pure tones at a fixed frequency from 100 dB spl to 145 dB spl in 5 dB steps for durations of 5–85 sec. For this full investigation 7 Hz was chosen as Gavreau *et al.* (1966) had suggested that this was possibly the most disturbing frequency, being close to the natural resonance frequency of many of the internal body organs and being the same frequency as the alpha brainwaves. Only one stimulus was used at each sitting to avoid any possibility of overlap effects. Figure 3 shows the combined results for all the subjects. If the combination of a particular stimulus duration and intensity did not produce a nystagmic response in the subject this pair of co-ordinates was marked with an open circle, if the nystagmic response was positive, with a cross. Hence the graph does not represent an absolutely determined threshold curve but the interface between co-ordinates giving positive and negative nystagmic responses. The series of tests was repeated at frequencies of 2, 4, 5, 12, 15 and 20 Hz. Figure 4 shows the threshold curves obtained, these were plotted in the same manner as the curve for 7 Hz.

The variation of the nystagmic threshold with frequency is shown in Fig. 5. The mean threshold level at each frequency for a 60 sec duration was obtained from the above curves and hence the sound pressure levels are subject to a 5 dB uncertainty.

(b) *Response duration*: The duration of the nystagmic response was taken as the time from when the nystagmus was clearly present until it was not easily recognised. Figure 6 shows the relationship between the duration of the stimulus and the duration of the recorded nystagmic response. No relationship was found between the duration of the nystagmus and the intensity or frequency of the stimulus.

(c) *Type of nystagmus*: In all the cases the nystagmus induced by infrasonic stimulation was of the slow phase first type, with the slow component representing the upward movement of the eyes and the fast phase the rapid downward return to the normal position. The frequency of the nystagmus was independent of the frequency of the stimulus, and of the order of 1 beat/sec. This was not entirely stable, a typical trace contained nystagmic beats varying from 1.5 beats/sec to 0.7 beat/sec.

(d) *Latency*: Unlike some forms of vestibular stimulation, the nystagmic response and the stimulus were not synchronised, although they were closely correlated in duration. There was a variable latency period between the onset of the nystagmic response and the onset of the stimulus. This latency period varied from stimulus to stimulus and, slightly, from subject to subject, although it was constant for each subject for each particular stimulus of a given frequency and intensity. Generally the higher the intensity the greater was the amplitude of the nystagmus and the shorter the latency period.

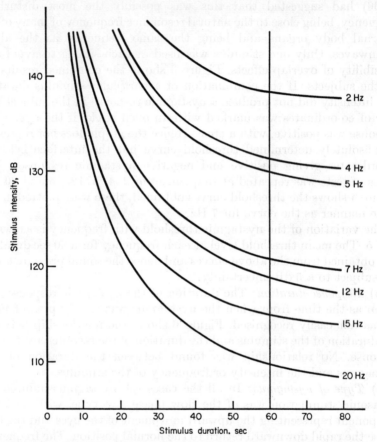

*Fig.* 4 Threshold of vertical nystagmus induced by pure infrasonic tones.

## 3. *Subjective Responses*

After each exposure the observers were asked to record any subjective effects they had experienced and their descriptions of the stimuli. The subjective descriptions of the stimulus varied with frequency, as one would expect, and generally fell into three categories:

(i) Frequencies above 20 Hz were described as smooth and tonal.

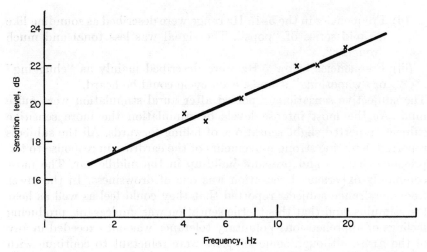

*Fig.* 5 Variation of nystagmus threshold with frequency for a 60 sec stimulus duration.

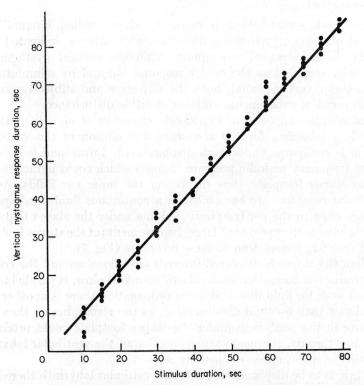

*Fig.* 6 Vertical nystagmus response duration *vs* stimulus duration.

(ii) Frequencies in the 5–15 Hz range were described as sounding like a rapid series of "pops". The signal was less tonal and much "rougher".

(iii) Frequencies below 5 Hz were described mainly as "chugging" or "whooshing" sounds, each cycle could be heard.

The subjective sensations reported after aural stimulation were quite mild. At the most intense levels of stimulation the more sensitive subjects reported slight sensations of falling forwards. All the subjects reported detecting strong movements of the eardrum in response to the pressure changes and pressure build-up in the middle ear. The most commonly experienced sensation was one of drowsiness. In the lower frequency range subjects reported that they could feel as well as hear the stimulus, and that this tactile sensation was unpleasant, producing feelings of apprehension. Voluntary tolerance was not exceeded in any of the cases, although some subjects were reluctant to continue with longer duration exposures.

## 4. *Interpretation of Results*

This work showed that infrasound, when applied binaurally to normal observers, produces a disturbance of balance, indicated by a clearly defined vertical nystagmus. Although vertical nystagmus is classically regarded as the ocular response induced by stimulation of the anterior vertical canal, both the objective and subjective results of this series of experiments indicate otolithic disturbance.

The results support the hypothesis (Reschke *et al.*, 1970) that a possible mechanism for the acoustical stimulation of the vestibular system is perilymph/endolymph displacement. Infrasound is regarded as low frequency periodic pressure changes which could induce motion in the stapes footplate thus displacing the inner ear fluids. As the vestibular receptors are suspended in a continuous fluid-filled system, and are close to the perilymphatic volume under the stapes footplate, it is reasonable to expect that large displacements of the stapes footplate could result in stimulation of these receptors (Fig. 7).

When the stapes is displaced inwards fluid flows around the cochlea and produces deformation of the elastic round window. If parallel to this normal path for fluid flow and wave propagation there is another high impedance path for fluid displacement, as the results imply, then high pressure in the perilymph under the stapes footplate could produce a fluid flow through the membranous portion of the vestibular labyrinth resulting in deformation of the hair cells.

If fluid is to be displaced through the vestibular labyrinth there must be some elastic structure allowing volume displacement or an outlet through which fluid could flow. Such a pathway exists via the endo-lymphatic duct to the endolymphatic sac.

To recapitulate; the speculation is that there are two pathways for fluid flow through the labyrinth when pressure is applied to the oval window, one through the cochlea and the other via the perilymph through the endolymphatic duct to the endolymphatic sac, this second pathway would have a much higher mechanical impedance and probably

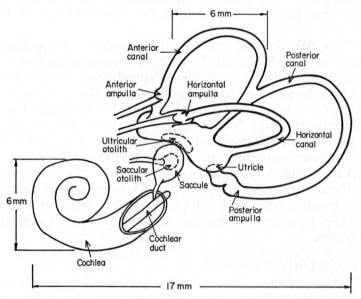

*Fig.* 7 Ventro-lateral view of the left human labyrinth.

such a high resistive component as to limit any appreciable fluid displacement and potential vestibular displacement to low frequency or static pressure changes. Therefore the audio-frequency stimulation would result in no appreciable fluid displacement through the vestibular apparatus due to this low-pass characteristic of the second pathway.

Support for this speculation is as follows:

(a) The long response time latencies which were observed suggest that there is a high resistance to fluid flow.

(b) Differences in latency as a function of stimulus intensity suggest that fluid flow through the endolymphatic duct occurs more readily following intense stimulation than following moderate stimulation.

(c) The observation that stimulus integration occurs for low intensity/duration stimulation suggests a complex highly resistive pathway.

The more intense physical stimulation produces a higher rate of fluid flow causing more intense physiological stimulation as well as a shorter latency.

(d) The change in the shape of the auditory threshold at low frequencies suggests that some change in the detection process occurs at around 16 Hz. It is possible that in this region the fluid flow ceases to be through the cochlea only.

This theory assumes that the nystagmus arises from the otolith system but the possibility that it arises from the semi-circular canals cannot be overlooked.

The distinction drawn between the function of the static and dynamic vestibular organs is inadequate for the explanation of many observations concerning the response to vestibular stimulation. For example, if a person is subjected to sufficient angular acceleration he becomes dizzy and falls, these sensations indicate both canal and otolith stimulation and disturbance, hence indicating that the otolith organs may have some influence on the occurrence of nystagmus. It is suggested that the otolithic organs exercise some control over the semi-circular canals and act in an inhibitory fashion on the occurrence of nystagmus under normal conditions. When a normal subject is exposed to infrasound, the otoliths are stimulated as described above, this inhibition is removed and vertical nystagmus arising from the anterior vertical semi-circular canal occurs.

## B. WHOLE-BODY EXPOSURE

The subjective effects of whole-body exposure to infrasound were also investigated by Evans and Tempest (1972). A low frequency pressure chamber was constructed of 6 mm aluminium plate mounted on a frame of 2.5 cm² section steel, and with a capacity of 1.23 m³ it could accommodate a subject with a sufficient margin of comfort. Six 46 cm diameter loudspeakers with sealed cones were mounted, using airtight seals over 27 cm diameter holes in three upright faces of the chamber. The fourth upright formed the door, again constructed in such a way that it was airtight when closed. Two heavy duty Perspex windows were let into the door for subject observation or illumination as required. The maximum undistorted sound pressure level obtainable was 137.5 dB.

The group of subjects who had taken part in the previously described series of experiments underwent a series of discrete exposures at frequencies from 0 to 20 Hz and intensities from 100 to 137.5 dB spl. After each exposure they were asked to record their subjective impressions, which are presented below:

### (1) *Frequency range 2–5 Hz: spl range 100–125 dB*

(a) Movement of the eardrum in response to the pressure changes.
(b) Pressure build-up in the middle ear.
(c) Difficulty in swallowing, all subjects were persistently trying to swallow as a mechanism for pressure release.
(d) Slight post-exposure headaches which were not persistent.

### (2) *Frequency range 2–5 Hz: spl range 125–137.5 dB*

(a) Movement of the eardrum.
(b) Difficulty in speaking and voice modulation.
(c) Chest wall vibration.
(d) Swaying sensations as if falling.
(e) Lethargy and drowsiness.
(f) Slight tinnitus at frequencies above 10 Hz.
(g) Post-exposure headaches and fatigue.

### (3) *Frequency range 5–15 Hz: spl range 125–137.5 dB*

(a) Movement of the eardrum.
(b) Middle-ear pain.
(c) Difficulty in speaking and voice modulation.
(d) Severe chest wall vibration.
(e) Severe abdomen vibration and associated feelings of nausea.
(f) Falling sensations.
(g) Lack of concentration and drowsiness.
(h) Tinnitus.
(i) Severe post-exposure fatigue and headaches.

### (4) *Frequency range 15–20 Hz: spl range 125–137.5 dB*

(a) Severe middle-ear pain.
(b) Respiratory difficulties—gagging sensations. In one case spasms of uncontrollable coughing developed.
(c) Nasal cavity vibration.
(d) Persistent eye watering.
(e) Tinnitus.
(f) All subjects experienced sensations of fear including excessive perspiration and shivering, these symptoms decreased with successive exposures.
(g) Severe post-exposure fatigue and headaches.
(h) In two cases (both female) cutaneous flushing.

Voluntary tolerance was not exceeded in any of the cases although at higher frequencies and intensities, i.e. at the higher sensation levels, the subjects were approaching this point, and were reluctant to continue with the longer duration exposures.

The problems of whole-body exposure to infrasound have been investigated more fully by Hood *et al*. (1972), who also used a low frequency pressure chamber (Leventhall and Hood, 1972) of a different design and utilised both random noise and pure tone stimulation, but concentrated mainly on the psychological effects. The stimulus was produced by four 38 cm speakers mounted in the walls of the chamber and driven by a 300 W amplifier. The maximum spl obtained was 126 dB for random noise and 145 dB for pure tones. In the latter case a tunable neck mounted on the side of the chamber was used to form a Helmholtz resonator which could be tuned over a range of 3 Hz to 18 Hz.

Field measurements made by Hood and Leventhall (1971) indicated that it would be useful to perform experiments in a random noise field at levels of 110 dB and 120 dB with a control level of 80 dB. The high frequency cut-off of the spectrum used was 15 Hz, low frequency fall-off was compensated by tuning the system to 3 Hz. This gave a flat response from 2 Hz to 15 Hz. The neck also provided a method of ventilation using a small fan which circulated air into and around the chamber. This gave a background noise level of 80 dB which made the chamber interior independent of variation of low frequency noise levels in the laboratory. A 70 dB(A) random noise field was used to mask intruding audio noise.

Two sets of physiological tests (Hood *et al*., 1972) were performed on a group of 11 normal subjects aged between 21 and 43. The first was a simple balance task adapted from the Sommer and Harris Rail Task (Sommer and Harris, 1970). The subjects were required to balance on a 2.5 cm wide rail with their eyes open, their feet positioned in a heel-to-toe fashion and arms folded across their chests. The time was measured from the moment that the subject assumed the correct position until it was violated by unfolding the arms, lifting a foot, and/or stepping off the rail. The task was terminated after 60 sec if the subject was still balanced on the rail. The subject's score was the total time in seconds that he balanced during 10 trials giving a maximum of 600. The times were measured using an electronic counter. Only a small decrement of about 9% was observed. This does not conflict with the results of Evans and Tempest (1972) as the rail test is a very insensitive measure of balance disturbance and the disturbances recorded by Evans and Tempest were small, especially at levels of less than 120 dB.

Attempts were also made to assess the auditory effects of infrasound by auditory screening of the subjects before and after exposure to infrasound. The audiograms showed that at 110 dB there was no temporary threshold shift after 90 min. At 120 dB 28.5% of the sample showed a temporary threshold shift (TTS) of 10 dB in the mid-frequency range.

## III. Psychological Effects

The psychological effects of infrasound are more intense under whole-body stimulation. Evans and Tempest (1972) recorded sensations of drowsiness, lethargy and lack of concentration in their subjects after exposure to moderate levels of infrasound, and feelings more akin to fear and panic at the higher levels when the physiological effects became more subjectively apparent. Hood *et al.* (1972) studied these sensations quantitatively using standard psychological tests of reaction time etc.

### 1. *Manual Dexterity Test*

This test was designed to measure the decrement in performance in the subject's manual dexterity. The test consisted of transferring nuts from one bolt to another. The results obtained were inconclusive and Hood *et al.* (1972) concluded that the experiment as designed was not sensitive enough to detect any decrement in performance. It is also possible that the subjects had not reached maximum proficiency in the the test under normal conditions before starting the experiment with the result that their performance was continuously improving due to learning during the test.

### 2. *Pointer Following Test*

To measure co-ordination, visual acuity and reaction time, a pointer following test was designed. The image of a suitably adapted centre reading moving coil meter was projected on to a window in the chamber. The output from a low frequency random noise generator was used to drive the pointer. The subject was provided with a steering wheel which was connected by a pulley system to a pointer which could move along the same path as the line image of the meter pointer. The subject was instructed to follow the lime image with the pointer. The wheel was also connected to a potential divider giving a voltage output proportional to the displacement of the pointer from the centre of the screen. The signals from the potential divider and the meter were scaled and subtracted by feeding into a differential amplifier; the output from the amplifier was proportional to the distance between the line and the pointer. This output was full-wave rectified and fed into an integrating voltmeter; the digital output was proportional to the subject's error in following the pointer. The test was performed for periods of 10 min and the integrator score noted every 60 sec. Of the subject sample 86% showed a significant performance decrement at 110 dB but at 120 dB only 28% showed a decrement. Hood *et al.* (1972) suggested that this was due to the masking of the 110 dB of infrasound by the 70 dB background white noise, but at 120 dB the infrasound was above the threshold of hearing and this extra stimulus increased the arousal of the subject and hence improved his task performance.

### 3. *Reaction Time Test*

A simple single-button reaction time test was performed 50 times. This was chosen in preference to a multiple-choice test because of the large spread of values given by such a test. The results indicated a general increase in reaction time at 110 dB, but at 120 dB only three of the subjects showed a decrement in performance. Hood *et al.* (1972) again attributed this to the increase in the subject's arousal level.

### 4. *Number Recognition*

This test was primarily designed to detect any changes in visual acuity due to exposure to infrasound. A series of numbers were flashed onto a screen which formed part of the chamber window, for a duration of 0.006 sec a number. The subject was told to record the number. The light intensity, exposure time and speed of the number flash were adjusted until the subject just started to make mistakes under normal conditions. The test was repeated in the infrasonic field using digits 1–9 in a random sequence repeated 100 times. The frequency at which the numbers were flashed was kept constant, and the subjects were warned before each flash by a short buzz.

Only one subject showed a performance decrement at 120 dB and he also complained of watering eyes during the test. Hood *et al.* (1972) assumed that this was totally unconnected with the exposure to infrasound and so dismissed the result as anomalous, but Evans and Tempest (1972) indicated that this is one of the possible subjective effects of infrasound and this result could possibly be regarded as relevant.

### 5. *Measurement of Channel Capacity*

The purpose of this test was to measure the amount of information capable of transmission by the subject, who is regarded as an information channel, and the effect of noise on the channel when overloaded. A matrix containing a single dot was flashed onto the screen for $\frac{1}{30}$ sec. The subject was told to indicate the position of the spot; the greater the order of the matrix, the more the information which the subject had to transmit to give the correct answer. The matrices used were $3 \times 3$, $4 \times 4$, $6 \times 6$ and $8 \times 8$, all had the same external dimensions. There were 125 observations made at a constant flashing rate.

No performance decrement in the noise field was noted, but it is possible that the warning buzz caused an atypical response due to an instantaneous raising of the arousal level.

## 6. *Complex Subsidiary Task Test*

The previously described sets of tests all indicated that the main response to the infrasonic field above 120 dB was one of subject arousal. To measure performance decrement where subject arousal occurs requires a more complex task. Hood *et al.* (1972) developed a subsidiary task technique for this purpose. This consisted of two tasks, a primary and a secondary task. Priority attention was ascribed to the primary task and the subject was required to perform the secondary task when possible.

The primary task used was the pointer following test, the subject was required to perform this task with one hand and the secondary task was a simple single-button reaction time test, the subject's reaction time was measured at random intervals averaging to one every 30 sec. Again the results obtained were rather confusing. Theoretically there should have been a decrement in performance for the secondary task and an improvement in the performance of the primary task. Of the six subjects used two performed in this manner; one appeared to regard the secondary task as the primary task and showed a decrement in performance of the primary task and an improvement in the secondary task, and the other three showed a performance decrement in both tasks, which for one subject was greater in the primary task and for the other two greater in the secondary task. Generalising, the presence of infrasound caused a performance decrement of 6% in the primary task after 60 min and of 4% in the secondary task after 30 min at an spl of 120 dB. No explanation of these results was offered.

## 7. *Complex Balance Task*

Hood suspected that the results of the simple balance task could also be interpreted in terms of subject arousal and developed a more complex task to investigate this hypothesis. Two beams of width 2.5 cm and 1.9 cm were used and the test was performed on them alternately followed by a subsidiary task. There was an appreciable decrement in performance of around 20% in the infrasound field.

## 8. *Comparison with the Effect of Alcohol*

The performance decrements noticed in the above tests were similar to the effects to be expected when the subjects have a sufficiency of alcohol and Hood *et al.* (1972) suspected that infrasound may be of a similar character, and that the two effects might interact. Three tests were performed simultaneously; the primary test was the pointer following task, the excursion amplitude of the pointer was reduced so

TABLE I: Comparison of the effects of alcohol and infrasonic noise on task performance

| Condition | Primary task | | Central reaction time | | Peripheral reaction time | |
|---|---|---|---|---|---|---|
| | Mean score | Change in mean (%) | Mean score | Change in mean (%) | Mean score | Change in mean (%) |
| Quiet, no alcohol | 226 | — | 0.439 | — | 0.495 | — |
| Quiet, alcohol | 250 | 10.5 | 0.441 | 7.1 | 0.555 | 12.2 |
| Noise, no alcohol | 249 | 9.9 | 0.470 | 0.6 | 0.505 | 2.2 |
| Noise, alcohol | 270 | 19.5 | 0.478 | 7.7 | 0.588 | 15.7 |

as to present a smaller field of view to the subject. The subsidiary tasks were central and peripheral reaction time tests in which the subjects were required to observe and monitor flashing lights at the centre and periphery of the field of view. Four test conditions were used in random order: (a) Quiet, no alcohol, (b) Quiet, alcohol, (c) Infrasound, no alcohol and (d) Infrasound, alcohol. The infrasound condition was a sound field of a random noise at 115 dB in the frequency range 3–15 Hz. The alcohol condition was two double measures of 70° proof spirit consumed 30 min before the start of the test. The results are presented in Table I.

It can be seen from these results that the subjects generally show a deterioration in performance with noise and alcohol exposure. For the primary task, the pointer following test, the single stimulus condition produced a performance decrement of around 10% and the joint stimulus condition about 20%, showing that there is no interaction between the effects and that the influences are additive. The central and peripheral reaction time tests showed the same results.

## REFERENCES

Alford, B. R., Jerger, J. F., Coats, A. C., Billingham, J., French, B. O. and McBrayer, R. O. (1966). *Trans. Acad. Ophth. Otol.* **70**, 40–47.

Evans, M. J., Bryan, M. E. and Tempest, W. (1971). *Sound* **5**, 47–51.

Evans, M. J. and Tempest, W. (1972). *J. Sound Vib.* **22**, 19–24.

Gavreau, V., Condot, R. and Saul, H. (1966). *Acustica* **17**, 1–10.

Hood, R. A. and Leventhall, H. G. (1971). *Acustica* **25**, 10–13.

Hood, R. A., Leventhall, H. G. and Kyriakides, K. (1972). *Proc. Brit. Acoust. Soc.* **1**, No. 3, Paper 71–107.

Leventhall, H. G. and Hood, R. A. (1972). *Proc. Brit. Acoust. Soc.* **1**, No. 3, Paper 71–101.

Mohr, G. C., Cole, J. N., Guild, E. and von Gierke, H. E. (1965). *Aerospace Medicine* **36**, 817–824.

Reschke, M. F., Parker, D. E. and von Gierke, H. E. (1970). *J. Acoust. Soc. Am.* **48**, 913.

Sommer, H. C. and Harris, C. S. (1970). Aerospace Medical Research Laboratory, Report No. AMRL–TR–70 26.

Yeowart, N. S., Bryan, M. E. and Tempest, W. (1967). *J. Sound Vib.* **6**, 335–342.

# 6. Effects of Intense Infrasound on Man

*H. E. von Gierke* and *C. W. Nixon*

## I. Introduction

Major noise problems are typically associated with exposure to acoustic energy which is actually heard. Infrasound may pose additional problems for man even though it is not perceived as auditory sensation in the usual sense. Although customarily defined as acoustic energy at subaudible frequencies, auditory perception of infrasound does occur at high sound pressure levels (Yeowart *et al.*, 1967, 1969).

A wide variety of effects of infrasound exposures on humans has been observed in experimental situations and reported as subjective symptoms in day-to-day living (Green and Dunn, 1968; Stevens, 1971; Bryan and Tempest, 1972; Evans and Tempest, 1972; Hood *et al.*, 1972). Changes in hearing sensitivity of a temporary nature have been measured after exposure to noise containing intense infrasound. Mechanical effects on the middle ear system may include drum membrane responses and aural pain as well as aural distortion of speech reception (von Gierke *et al.*, 1953). Infrasound stimulates and is absorbed by systems and organs of the body other than the ear which may be adversely influenced by excessive exposure (Mohr *et al.*, 1965). Vestibular disturbances, respiratory effects, performance decrements and even modification of the alpha rhythm have also been attributed to infrasound exposure. If, and to what extent, the low levels of infrasound experienced during routine living and occupational activities might influence human performance, health and well-being, is still an open question. However, experience with very intense infrasound clearly suggests potentially adverse effects on man and the need to define exposure limits in line with generally applied preventive medicine principles.

Infrasonic energy acts upon, and enters the body from, airborne and structure-borne sources. Although in most noise environments the airborne sound pressure levels are too low to result in any appreciable energy levels in the body, except the ear, intense infrasound can result in clearly noticeable vibration of body parts and resulting biological effects. The mismatch between the characteristic acoustic impedance of air and the body surfaces prevents large amounts of energy from entering the body (von Gierke, 1972). However, the lower the frequency the more energy from an airborne sound wave is absorbed by the body surface. If body parts are in contact with liquids containing sound energy or with structures such as machinery or buildings, the situation is quite different, and most of the energy is transmitted to the body. Once the energy is inside the body the nature of the source makes little difference with respect to its biological effects. In this respect bioacoustic and vibration research share a common concern for the energy in the body tissues, its subsequent effects and means for its control within safe and acceptable limits (von Gierke, 1972).

## II.  Sources of Infrasound

Infrasound is generated by various events in nature, by numerous man-made systems, by routine living activities and is experienced by everyone in varying degrees. Infrasound typically occurs in natural environments at relatively low levels as a result of events such as thunder, air turbulence, volcanic activity, winds, large waterfalls, ocean waves and the impact of waves on beaches (Stevens, 1972). Natural activities such as walking, jogging and swimming as well as travelling in an automobile at high speeds can produce the same low frequency pressure fluctuations as infrasound, although they are technically better identified as "pseudosound" if they are not propagating as sound waves through the air. (For example, a 15 cm up-and-down motion of a human head during jogging produces in the ear a pressure fluctuation of 90 dB re 0.00002 N/m² at the running frequency of, for example, 1 Hz although there is no sound wave in the air.) However, infrasound from man-made sources occurs at relatively greater magnitudes, appears to be growing both in terms of levels of intensity and in incidence of exposure, and is propagated over great distances with relatively little energy loss. The high-powered propulsion systems of aircraft and space vehicles, ships, air heating and cooling units, compressors and transformers in closed spaces and the like, all produce infrasound. Figure 1 provides an example of the relative levels of low frequency and infrasonic rocket engine noise as a function of distance from the launch site. Infrasound rarely occurs in the absence of other acoustic energy or of mechanical forces such as vibration and acceleration. The extent to which effects attributed to infrasound may in fact be caused by some other component of the total mechanical force environment is a question which has not been approached. The systematic analysis of the influence of infrasound and the definition of acceptable exposures must consider the combined and interactive effects of the total stimuli in the environment.

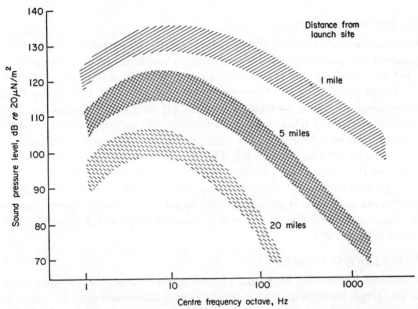

*Fig.* 1 Rocket launch noise: infrasound levels vs distance from launch site. Adapted from Cole and Powell (1962).

Infrasound energy is also contained in the power spectrum of impulsive noise such as some explosive noises, blast waves and sonic booms from supersonic aircraft. Many original estimates of the potential biological effects of large amplitude infrasound waves were based on data available from biological blast research (White, 1968).

Infrasound is considered to be intense, irrespective of the source, when levels approach the pain threshold of the human ear, when the threat of other potential adverse effects exists, and when subjective reports include symptoms such as general unpleasantness, nausea and disorientation. The percentage of the population affected by intense infrasound is much smaller than the part generally affected by acoustic energy. As a consequence, much less research has been conducted on the effects of intense infrasound on man than on the more obvious and direct effects of acoustic energy on the auditory system. There are not many comfort and safety criteria on man's exposure to infrasound.

Well-supported exposure limits are needed to ensure reliable task performance, comfort, safety and protection from interference and personal injury during exposure to intense infrasound. Systematic laboratory and field research to establish these limits has only been started within the past decade.

### III. Investigative Methods

Various methods may be employed in efforts to establish relationships between infrasound exposure and human response. Such relationships must be based on accurate descriptions of human responses as well as of the physical stimuli. Experimental, observational and theoretical approaches to these questions include (1) empirical studies in field environments, (2) laboratory experiments, (3) subjective reports and observations of adverse effects and (4) biodynamic models to explain responses to intense infrasound. The problem of providing appropriate infrasound environments in which physiological responses and behaviour may be measured and observed has been approached in two general ways. One approach is to utilise infrasound as it exists in present noise environments and the other is to generate infrasound using special laboratory devices.

### A. FIELD ENVIRONMENTS

Intense infrasound as found at specific locations in jet engine noise fields, large transformer and compressor rooms etc. may be used as experimental environments in which volunteers experience the infrasound exposure, and their responses, as recorded, are related to the measured exposure characteristics. The use of infrasound as found in field environments is a practical consideration, particularly when the data and results are to be applied to the personnel working in that particular environment. It is also economical from the signal generation cost standpoint, but perhaps most important is that it may be the only infrasound source available to many experimenters. On the other hand, field environments require the experimenter to move the investigation to the location of the infrasound and usually only a specific exposure condition, or set of conditions, are available and consequently a systematic study of a range of conditions is not possible. The infrasound, which is of primary interest, is typically only one component of the total noise and vibration environment and it is almost impossible to reduce or eliminate the other noises present, which, in effect, contaminate the infrasound. Consequently, observed effects are not clearly related to the infrasound as much as to the overall noise environment, unless the stimulus is very well controlled. Comprehensive research can be conducted using field environments by selecting a number of different locations which collectively provide the range of exposure conditions to be investigated, as was done by Mohr *et al.* (1965).

## B. LABORATORY EXPERIMENTS

In the laboratory, a variety of facilities and devices has been designed and constructed with the capability and/or purpose of producing infrasound for animal and human research. Table I contains a summary

TABLE I: Descriptions of representative facilities and devices used for infrasound research

| Investigator | Facility | Generator | Operation | Performance |
|---|---|---|---|---|
| Békésy (1960) | Thermophone | Loudspeaker coupled via manometer | Beating of two A.C. signals inside thermophone capsule; frequency response down to 1 Hz | $10^4$–$10^5$ dyne/cm² sound pressure |
| Benox (von Gierke *et al.*, 1953b) | Pistonphone and mercury manometer | Motor-driven pistonphone; manual control manometer | Alternating pressures up to 50 Hz | 165 dB alternating pressure; 180 dB static pressure |
| Mohr *et al.* (1965) | Whole-body enclosures; free field; jet engine; high pressure air source; low frequency test chamber | Hydraulic loudspeakers; high velocity air flow; low frequency siren | Normal operating modes for various devices and facilities | Discrete tones and bands of noise at levels of 150–154 dB |
| Nixon (1973) | Pistonphones | Coupled to ear via closed tube | Motor-driven alternating pressures | 165 dB + alternating pressure |
| Leventhall and Hood (1972) | Whole-body pressure chamber, 91 × 122 × 183 cm | Four 15 m diameter loudspeakers: 300 W amplifier | Operates as a Helmholtz resonator tunable over range of 3 Hz to 18 Hz | 145 dB for single frequency; 126 dB for noise band |

TABLE I—*continued*

| Investigator | Facility | Generator | Operation | Performance |
|---|---|---|---|---|
| Yeowart *et al.* (1967, 1969) | Monaural/ binaural head- phones from 0.3 m diameter loudspeakers | Earmuff drivers worked into volume of 1 litre | Response is flat up to 200 Hz | Maximum spl is 150 dB at 1 Hz |
| | Whole-body 1200 litre cabinet | Six 0.46 m diameter loudspeakers on sides of chamber | Electro- dynamic | Maximum spl is 140 dB |
| Johnson (1973a, b) | Whole-body chamber 1.5 m³ | Hydraulic- driven 1.8 m piston and 46 cm piston | Alternating pressures, 0.5–30 Hz | 1.8 m piston: 172 dB (0.5– 10 Hz) falling to 158 dB at 30 Hz 46 cm piston: 144 dB (1– 10 Hz) falling to 135 dB at 20 Hz |

of descriptions of several such facilities which have been used for infrasound and hearing research. Pistonphones and manometers may be used to produce aural exposures of alternating pressures as well as very high static pressures (von Gierke *et al.*, 1953; Hansen, 1955). Very intense levels of infrasound are possible with these devices coupled directly to the ear. Whole-body pressure chambers, which totally enclose the subject, usually employ several large loudspeakers as the signal generators. One unique system, a 1.5 m³ whole-body chamber (Dynamic Pressure Chamber), employs hydraulically driven pistons of 1.83 m and of 46 cm diameter as the signal generators (Fig. 2) (Johnson, 1973b). Infrasound signals of 172 dB at 0.5 Hz to 8 Hz decreasing in level to 158 dB at 30 Hz are produced by the primary system, as shown in the performance profile in Fig. 3. (It must be kept in mind that these pistonphone-type chambers usually produce only the pressure effects of an infrasound wave. The velocity effects are not simulated in such facilities and have so far not been studied. There is good theoretical reason for the assumption that they are less important than the pressure effects.) The method of using infrasound generators in the laboratory avoids many of the problems and limitations of field studies and allows

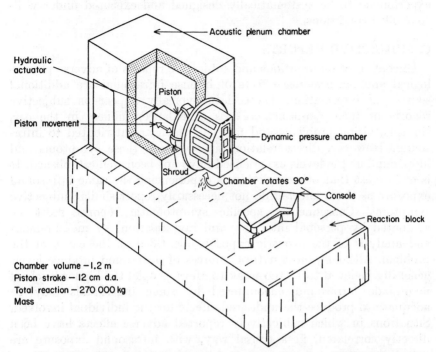

*Fig.* 2 Pictorial view of the Dynamic Pressure Chamber (DPC) system.

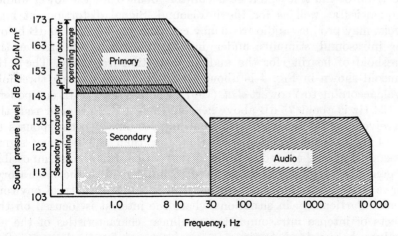

*Fig.* 3 Performance profile of the Dynamic Pressure Chamber showing the operational envelopes of the primary infrasound, the secondary infrasound and the audiofrequency systems.

experiments to be systematically designed and executed under well-controlled conditions.

## C. SUBJECTIVE REPORTS

Uncontrolled observations and subjective reports of adverse physiological and performance effects of intense infrasound are additional sources of information. These data typically appear as subjective reports of such symptoms as loss of balance, fullness in the ear, tinnitus, vision problems and fatigue, which are attributed to infrasound. However, direct relationships between these symptoms and infrasound at the levels experienced have not been well established. It is of interest that other individuals experiencing the same infrasound exposure as those affected do not necessarily report similar subjective symptoms. Consequently specific symptomatic reports must be evaluated by personal interview and investigation, by measurement and analysis of the acoustic exposure identified as the cause of the problem. Although most natural sources of infrasound produce levels generally believed to be too weak to affect people, the higher levels of man-made infrasound encountered by some individuals may be adequate to produce the undesired effects for the individual involved. Situations in which subjectively reported adverse effects have been directly correlated, in a causal way, with infrasound exposure are extremely rare.

It is extremely important for field and laboratory studies that the spectrum of the test signal be accurately defined for the lower audio-frequencies as well as for the infrasound. Signal distortion, at high levels, may produce audio-frequency components only 15–20 dB below the infrasound stimulus under investigation and well above the threshold of hearing for the audible distortion frequency. The 4 Hz sinusoid shown in Fig. 4 is about 15–20 dB above hearing threshold level, according to Yeowart et al. (1967), whereas the 107 dB component at 124 Hz is about 75 dB above hearing threshold. It is clear that the perceived 124 Hz signal may have an impact on subject responses to the 4 Hz exposure, perhaps even greater than the primary signal depending upon the response under investigation. It is almost impossible to generate very intense distortion-free infrasound in the laboratory, nor is such infrasound likely to be of importance in natural environments. Particularly in situations where the interest is focused on the effects of intense infrasound, the nonlinear characteristics of the air produce harmonic distortions in an intense infrasound wave after several wavelengths of propagation. Consequently it is essential that infrasound stimuli be accurately measured and analysed so that

interpretation of human responses can be made with full knowledge
of the total spectrum to which the observers were exposed. Without

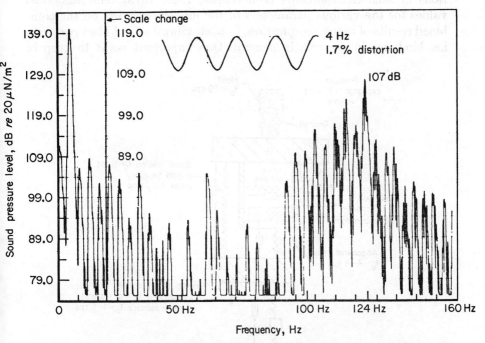

*Fig.* 4 Frequency distortion of a 4 Hz signal at 140 dB sound pressure level.

this information, human responses to the higher frequency energy may
be erroneously attributed to infrasound.

## D. BIODYNAMIC MODELS

Biodynamic models can be used to understand the response of the
human body to infrasound based on knowledge of how energy is
received, transmitted and absorbed by the various body tissues.
Considerable work has been done in this area over the past 20 years,
which allows the characterisation of the physical response of the body
to vibrating energy for the whole frequency range from semi-static
loading to ultrasonic frequencies. The dynamic response of composite
body structures to shock vibration and blast inputs can so be understood and predicted. Biodynamic models for the whole-body and
various subsystems have been developed and are in practical use.

A lumped parameter model of the human body of the type illustrated
in Fig. 5 can, for example, be used to predict and understand the

response of the respiratory system to infrasound and blast waves, and to analyse the coupling between chest wall and abdominal wall vibrations in such environments (von Gierke, 1968, 1973). The numerical values for the various parameters of the model are based on the combined results of human respiration, impact, vibration and blast research, i.e. biodynamic research in general. One important point to keep in

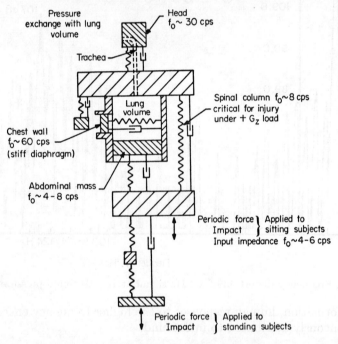

*Fig.* 5 Lumped parameter model of the human body describing its response to longitudinal impact, vibration, blast or infrasound exposure.

mind in applying these results to infrasound considerations is the fact that at these low frequencies the acoustic energy is propagated through the body system in the form of transverse shear waves and not in the form of longitudinal compression waves. In general, throughout the frequency range of interest the vibratory response of body parts can be described in terms of lumped parameter systems as in the example presented in Fig. 6.

Other biodynamic models of interest include the various models of the middle and inner ear (Zwislocki, 1962; Mundie, 1963). They are not only of interest to an understanding of the auditory response at these low frequencies and to an estimate of tympanic membrane rupture at extremely high intensities, but also to a prediction of the harmonic distortion produced in the middle and inner ear, i.e. for an estimate

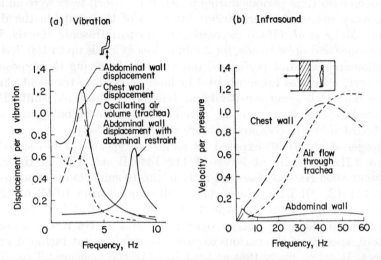

*Fig.* 6 The theoretical response of the thorax–abdomen system of the lumped parameter model is illustrated in (a) for longitudinal whole-body vibration and in (b) for infrasound excitation.

of the audible distortion components one must expect even for an ideal distortionless sinusoidal infrasound input at the tympanic membrane.

## IV. Physiological and Performance Effects

Over the past decade experience with human exposure to infrasound has demonstrated that man is quite resistant to adverse effects from this very low frequency energy. On the other hand, very intense levels of infrasound have been accompanied by behavioural responses. In many instances, investigations of responses have included auditory, whole-body or general physiological, vestibular, performance and respiratory effects. Generally, the studies deal with short-term exposures, which may or may not have been repeated, and not with chronic exposure.

## A. EFFECTS ON HEARING ACUITY

### 1. *Audition*

Some early observations of possible infrasound effects on hearing were not described in terms of hearing sensitivity for audiometric test frequencies. Tonndorf (personal communication) reported on the effects of infrasound in the diesel rooms of submarines on the hearing of crew members. Depression of the upper limits of hearing was demonstrated by decreased time periods during which tuning-fork tests were audible. Recovery occurred after various intervals of time outside the diesel room. Mohr *et al.* (1965) exposed subjects to infrasonic signals, both pure tones and noise bands, for 2 min or less at levels up to 150–154 dB. Audiometry was not performed immediately following the exposures; however, measures taken about 1 hr later showed no transient change from normal hearing sensitivity or temporary threshold shift (TTS). In the latter work an exposure signal was experienced only once, while on-board submarine exposures were experienced daily.

Jerger *et al.* (1966) exposed 19 males to repeated 3 min signals of from 2 Hz to 12 Hz at levels of 119–144 dB spl. TTS in the range of 3000–8000 Hz was observed in 11 of the 19 subjects for exposures of 137–141 dB. All TTS values were small ranging from 10 dB to 22 dB. The author indicates that the 7–12 Hz exposures at high levels did produce considerable energy over the 100–4000 Hz range. Unfortunately, spectra of the various exposure signals are not included in the report. It seems likely that at least some of the measured TTS, if not most of it, may have been caused by the upward spread of energy in the exposure signals.

A number of studies of TTS and infrasound have been conducted in our laboratory using pistonphones and a large pressure chamber as signal generators. Using a pistonphone coupled tightly to the ear via an ear-muff, Nixon and Johnson (1973) investigated effects on hearing threshold levels of 14 Hz at 140 dB and 18 Hz at 135 dB for 30 min exposures. Some subjects experienced no changes in hearing for standard audiometric test frequencies due to the exposures, while others showed various amounts of TTS, with one subject showing a maximum 20 dB change at one test frequency in one ear.

In another series of investigations, Johnson (1973b) measured the effects of short duration auditory exposures of 135–171 dB at 0.5–12 Hz and whole-body exposures of 135–144 dB at 1–20 Hz. The pressure chamber shown in Fig. 2 which provides whole-body exposures to infrasound at levels as high as 172 dB was used to generate the stimuli. Exposure durations varied from 26 sec of 7 Hz at 171 dB to 30 min of 4 Hz, 7 Hz and 12 Hz at 140 dB. The various exposure parameters, effects on hearing, if any, and recovery are itemised in Table II.

It is clear from the data contained in Table II that TTS has been measured following infrasound exposures at moderately intense levels. The observed changes in hearing threshold levels at standard audiometric

TABLE II: Summary of representative human exposures to infrasound and reported hearing response

| Investigator | Exposure | Hearing response | Recovery |
|---|---|---|---|
| Tonndorf | Submarine diesel room 10–20 Hz, no level given | Depression of upper limits of hearing as measured by number of seconds a tuning fork was heard—no conversion to MAP | Recovery in few hours outside of diesel room |
| Mohr et al. (1965) | Discrete tones; narrow band noise in 10–20 Hz region; 150–154 dB exposures of about 2 min | No change in hearing sensitivity reported by subjects; no TTS measured about 1 hr post exposure | |
| Jerger et al. (1966) | Successive 3 min whole-body exposures, 7–12 Hz; 119–144 dB | TTS in 3000–6000 Hz range for 11 of 19 subjects (TTS of 10–22 dB) | Recovery within hours |
| Nixon (1973) | Pistonphone coupled to ear via earmuff; 18 Hz at 135 dB. Series of six 5 min exposures in rapid succession | Average TTS of 0–15 dB after 30 min exposures | Recovery within 30 min |
| Nixon (1973a) | Pistonphone coupled to ear via earmuff. 14 Hz at 140 dB. Six individual exposures of 5, 10, 15, 20, 25 and 30 min | Three experienced subjects: no TTS in one; slight TTS in one; 20–25 dB TTS in one | Recovery within 30 min |
| Johnson (1973b) | Ear only: pressure chamber coupled to ear via tuned hose and muff | | |
| | 171 dB (1–10 Hz), 26 sec, 1 sub[a] | No TTS | |
| | 168 dB (7 Hz), 1 min, 1 sub | No TTS | |
| | 155 dB (7 Hz), 5 min, 2 sub | No TTS | |
| | 140 dB (4, 7, 12 Hz), 30 min, 1 sub | 14–17 dB TTS | Recovery within 30 min |
| | 140 dB (4, 7, 12 Hz), 5 min, 8 sub | 8 dB TTS for 1 subject | Recovery within 30 min |
| | 135 dB (0.6, 1.6, 2.9 Hz), 5 min, 12 sub | No TTS | |
| | 126 dB (0.6, 1.6, 2.9 Hz), 16 min, 11 sub | No TTS | |

[a] sub = subject(s)

TABLE II—*continued*

| Investigator | Exposure | Hearing response | Recovery |
|---|---|---|---|
| | Whole body: all exposures, 2 sub: | | |
| | 8 min at 8 Hz at spl's of 120, 126, 132, 138 | No TTS | |
| | 8 min at 1, 2, 4, 6, 8, 10 Hz at 144 dB | No TTS | |
| | 8 min at 12, 16, 20 Hz at 135–142 dB | No TTS | |

test frequencies have been small and recovery to pre-exposure hearing levels has been rapid for the few situations in which TTS did occur.

In the experimental investigations just described, some harmonic distortion and/or masking were introduced above threshold levels in the low audio-frequency region. These signals must be expected to produce greater effects on the ear at audio-frequencies than the infrasound. However, it can be assumed that any effects of the composite signals would be no greater than those of the infrasound alone. In fact, the infrasound would be expected to have relatively less effect on the ear than the higher frequencies at which overtones occurred. This assumption becomes more tenable in view of the low incidence and small amounts of TTS observed. Further support is found in the absence of any patterns of TTS behaviour, that is, no consistent auditory responses were observed for frequency, intensity, ears affected and the like. Temporary changes in human hearing due to distortion-free infrasound have not been demonstrated. The conditions under which aural distortion, occurring in the ear due to intense infrasound, may produce TTS in the audio-frequency range have yet to be defined.

## 2. *Effects of Impulsive Noise on Hearing*

Sonic bangs, generated by aircraft in supersonic flight, have been alleged to affect human hearing adversely. The sonic bang is an impulsive sound with peak acoustical energy in the infrasound region. The energy density spectra of idealised sonic bangs of different duration are shown in Fig. 7 (Nixon *et al.*, 1968). The maximum energy, with a roll-off of 6 dB/octave, is found at about 20 Hz for a fighter-type aircraft ($T = 0.04$ sec) and goes down to below 2 Hz for supersonic transport-type aircraft ($T = 0.4$ sec). Such bangs must be considered as infrasound signals on the basis of the energy density spectra.

Sonic bangs experienced in the community range from about 25 N/m²
to 96 N/m² on average. Field investigations and experience with
exposure of humans to sonic booms as intense as $6.91 \times 10^3$ N/m² have
revealed no adverse effects on hearing. During a study at White Sands,
New Mexico, on "Structural Response to Sonic Boom", personnel

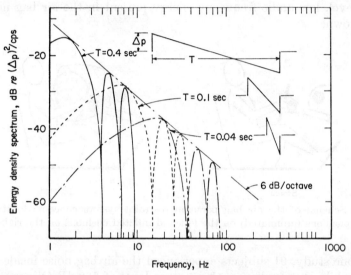

*Fig.* 7 Calculated energy density spectra of idealised sonic bangs of different
duration.

experienced about 30 sonic bangs daily over two 30 day periods
separated by 1 month (Sonic Boom Structural Response Test Programme, 1965). Sonic bangs were increased in intensity from about
$2.4 \times 10^2$ N/m² early in the programme to $1.34 \times 10^3$ N/m² late in the
study. Audiometric data collected at frequent intervals showed no
changes in hearing due to the intense exposures. At Tonopah, Nevada,
individuals experienced sonic booms on the ground at levels of
$2.40 \times 10^3$ N/m² to $6.9 \times 10^3$ N/m² with no adverse effects on the hearing
(Nixon *et al.*, 1968). On the basis of these as well as other data on sonic
boom exposure of humans, it may be concluded that the intense
infrasound present in high level sonic booms does not constitute a
problem for the human auditory system.

A relatively new car passenger safety device involves the use of
large hollow cushions which are concealed collapsed in the dashboards
of automobiles and which, when the car encounters a forward crash,
rapidly fill with gas and occupy the space between the front of the car

and its occupants to cushion their forward impact (Fig. 8). The extremely
rapid deployment of these prototype systems was accompanied by an
intense impulsive noise which was heard by the occupants. For purposes
of our discussion, the frequency content of the air bag inflation noise
can also be generally described by the idealized spectra of Fig. 7,
showing maximum energy at the lowest infrasound frequencies. Some
high level, low audio-frequency energy present in the air bag noise is
not shown.

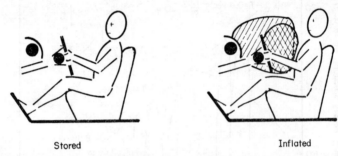

Stored                                                    Inflated

*Fig.* 8 Schema of the air bag personal restraint system concept: locations of
stored cushions (uninflated) on the left and inflated cushions on the right.

In one study, 91 subjects experienced the air bag noise inside a test
automobile at a median peak pressure level of 168 dB (Nixon, 1969).
Analysis of the air bag noise indicated the presence of acoustical
energy in the low audio-frequency regions. About 50% of the subjects
experienced some TTS with about 95% of these recovering pre-
exposure threshold on the same day. About 5% required a little longer
to recover with one subject showing a slight shift at one frequency for
several months.

In another study, the air bag impulse noise was separated into its
component parts—a low frequency pressure pulse, associated with
displacement of the internal volume of the automobile by the inflating
bag, and a high frequency noise burst, associated with activation of the
system, gas flow turbulence and the bag unfolding (Sommer and
Nixon, 1974). Volunteers were exposed to each of three noises, the low
frequency pressure pulse, the high frequency noise burst and the
composite air bag noise (both components simultaneously). The results
shown in Fig. 9 indicate that maximum TTS was caused by the noise
burst, no TTS was caused by the pressure pulse and for the total signal
the noise burst effects were reduced by the pressure pulse resulting in
less TTS than for the noise burst alone.

Although the sonic bang and the air bag inflation noise may not satisfy a strict definition of infrasound, the very intense infrasound components certainly qualify them for consideration. There is no clear-cut evidence that the infrasound in either of these signals in any way adversely affects the ear. On the other hand, it is suggested that the infrasound components may act to ameliorate undesirable effects of

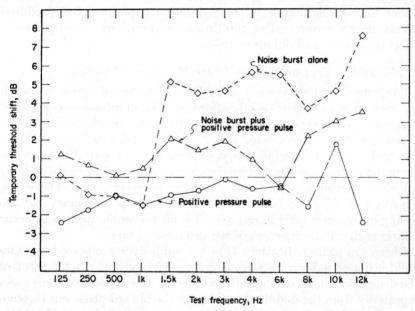

*Fig.* 9 Temporary auditory threshold shift produced by various components of simulated air bag noise.

higher frequency energy. Certainly, there is clear evidence that loading the middle ear system with static pressure or very slow pressure changes (von Gierke and Warren, 1953; von Gierke *et al.*, 1953; Hansen, 1955) does reduce transmission of acoustic energy to the inner ear and may be considered protective. Whether or not intense infrasound might serve to reduce the adverse effects of intense audio-frequency energy on the ear is a subject worthy of further investigation.

## B. OTHER EFFECTS ON THE AUDITORY SYSTEM

Infrasound may stimulate the auditory system at levels of sufficient magnitude to cause, first, tactile sensation and, finally, aural pain (von Gierke *et al.*, 1953; Békésy, 1960). During the whole-body and aural exposures to infrasound, particularly below about 5 Hz, subjects may report the unmistakable sensation that the eardrum membrane is being mechanically massaged at levels of 120 dB and above. At lower intensity levels, perception of the sensation, which is not unpleasant, becomes less noticeable within a little time. At higher intensity levels, subjects occasionally report the sensation as being initially unpleasant; however, this too appears to dissipate during continuation of the exposure. Massage of the drum membrane system by infrasound, at rather high levels and/or for long duration exposures, has produced effects clearly recognised at the drum membrane by investigators as injection (Nixon and Johnson, 1973).

### 1. *Middle Ear Pressure Change/Drum Membrane Retraction*

Subjects almost universally describe a sensation of "pressure build-up" or change in the ear shortly after initiation of infrasound exposure. This sensation is reported by many subjects at around 126 dB and by virtually all persons evaluated at 132 dB. This "fullness" is experienced for both aural and whole-body exposures. The sensation remains throughout the exposure and persists for some time afterwards in many subjects. Ventilation of the ear during exposure may relieve the sensation of fullness; however, the relief is only temporary for the feeling of pressure quickly returns. This phenomenon appears to occur a little earlier than injection of the drum membrane.

There are some indications that the subjectively reported pressure build-up is actually a pressure decrease. The cyclical displacement of the drum membrane during infrasound exposure appears to force gases repeatedly from the middle ear cavity on the inward phase out through the collapsed Eustachian tube. The negative pressure created by this action is not automatically equalised on the alternate phase of the cycle and drum membrane retraction will likely occur. The specific exposure conditions under which drum membrane retraction occurs have not been defined. There is some evidence that drum membrane retraction acquired during infrasound exposures may not be due entirely to a negative pressure in the middle ear. During exposures to 14 Hz at 140 dB, all subjects exhibited mild retraction. After the exposure each individual ventilated the middle ear system via the Valsalva manœuvre, under the active observation and guidance of an otologist. Following confirmed ventilation or pressure equalisation, the retracted drum condition remained and persisted for some time afterwards. A temporary change in the activity of the middle ear muscle system is believed to account for the persistent retraction; however, this assumption remains to be investigated. One consequence of this retraction phenomenon is that even with positive ventilation following exposure, prior to audiometric testing, some retraction may remain and indicate a slightly elevated threshold.

The efficiency of middle ear sound transmission to the inner ear is reduced when this system is retracted. As an investigator, one must consider the advisability of having experimental subjects periodically ventilate the middle ear system during studies of infrasound since different effects would be expected from exposure of a retracted as opposed to a non-retracted drum membrane system. Regardless of the exposure, it is critical that the middle ear system be adequately ventilated prior to measurement of post-exposure hearing threshold levels. A retracted middle ear system will show reduced sensitivity which may be attributed to sensorineural effects.

A vascular injection of the eardrum membrane may be observed during and following exposure. This injection is similar to that produced by therapeutic massage of the drum membrane. The degree of injection may be slight or severe in which case it is highly visible all along the handle of the malleus and in the folds. Although slight injection may be caused by many different factors, it is not considered "abnormal". Severe injection, however, must be recognised as a positive indication of over-exposure.

## 2. *Aural Pain*

Pain in the ear is related to displacement of an otherwise normal middle ear system beyond its mechanical limits of normal operation. Aural pain is not directly related to sensitivity, as evidenced by the fact that normal and hard-of-hearing persons have the same average aural pain thresholds. Likewise, it is not associated with, and not a warning for, sensorineural hearing loss which can become very severe without any experience of pain. At infrasonic signals, pain may be experienced at levels which pose no risk to hearing.

Thresholds for aural pain are summarised in Fig. 10. The data of von Gierke *et al.* (1953) and of Békésy (1960) are highly consistent. One data point on the figure represents a condition where one subject reported pain from a pistonphone exposure of around 140 dB at 14 Hz, which disappeared after a few minutes and did not return during the 30 min exposure at that level. It appears that the pain threshold might be elevated a few decibels, 2–3 dB, with high level exposure experience of the subject. The pain threshold appears to be about 140 dB around 20 Hz rapidly increasing to about 162 dB at 2 Hz. Pain produced by static pressure on the ear, either positive or negative, appears between 175 dB and 180 dB. Any form of aural pain during infrasound exposure must be considered an indicator that the tolerance limits of the mechanical elements of the auditory system have been reached and the exposure should be terminated and avoided in the future.

Tympanic membrane injury may occur as a result of intense acoustic exposures which drive the middle ear system beyond the mechanical limits of its normal modes of operation and which may exceed the

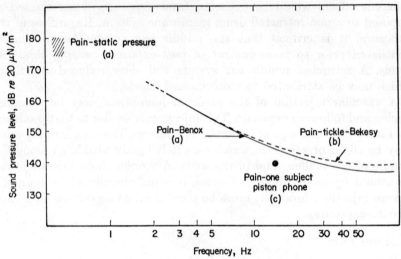

*Fig.* 10 Thresholds of aural pain for infrasound and for static pressure.

rupture strength of the membrane itself. Severe middle ear damage is usually accompanied by some inner ear damage as well. Drum membrane ruptures usually heal with little residual effect on hearing; however, ossicular chain and inner ear effects may be much more persistent. On the basis of various damage risk data, the threshold for human tympanic membrane rupture occurs at average pressure changes of around $4.15 \times 10^4$ N/m² to $5.53 \times 10^4$ N/m².

## 3. *Speech*

Effects of infrasound exposure on voice communication primarily affect the talker but may also influence speech reception. High intensity infrasound may influence various functions involved in speech production. Amplitude modulation of the voice during speech production is obvious at very low frequencies as a result of the chest being driven by the infrasound, and is reported by almost everyone exposed to infrasound. Choking, coughing, gagging sensations, chest wall vibration and modulation of respiratory rhythm, all of which may influence speech production, have been reported for whole-body exposures below 50 Hz and at levels up to 150 dB. On the basis of subjective judgments of face-to-face speech reception during studies involving intense whole-body infrasound exposures and of measurements from an objective study, some general conclusions are warranted. Intense infrasound modulates speech in such a way that the talker appears to be experiencing whole-body vibration. Speech intelligibility under such vibration has been studied extensively (Nixon, 1962; Nixon and Sommer, 1963). However, major decrements in speech communication efficiency are not observed in spite of the changes perceived by the listener. Whether or not the infrasound-modulated speech is more susceptible to masking by audiofrequency signals, as is the case with some vibrated speech, has not been investigated.

On the listener's ear the infrasound exposure must lead to a slight modulation of the hearing acuity by the infrasound frequency; the pressure changes modulate the transmission characteristics of the middle ear for static pressure changes. However, these effects should only become noticeable at infrasound levels above 140 dB.

As a consequence of the generally satisfactory intelligibility or efficiency observed, refined studies of face-to-face speech communication in infrasound have not been pursued. On the other hand, some subjects report minor difficulty in understanding speech listening through headphones during whole-body infrasound exposure (Nixon, 1973). This observation has not been examined to determine if the reduced efficiency is due to the headphone system, the auditory mechanism or a combination of the two factors.

### 4. Hearing Protection

Exposure to intense infrasound may occur at hearing tolerance limits where potential hazards exist or at lower levels which pose no hearing risk but are subjectively disagreeable. Effective hearing protection is highly desirable in either case. Classically, earplugs have provided good performance across the audio-frequency range, whereas ear-muff protector performance decreases with decreasing frequency.

Subjective reports of ear protector effectiveness in intense infrasound indicate that good insert-type earplugs provide appreciable attenuation of the acoustic energy. Earmuff-type protectors appear to provide negligible protection and on occasion are reported to amplify the noise under the muff. Earmuffs, which are suspended from lightweight spring tension headbands, were noticed to vibrate visibly against the sides of the subject's head during infrasound exposure. When worn over insert earplugs, earmuffs appeared to experienced listeners to add attenuation obtained by the wearer to that provided by the earplugs.

An experimental investigation of earmuff effectiveness in infrasound, using both a subjective and a physical method, confirms the subjective observations reported above (Nixon *et al.*, 1967). Good earmuff protectors provide about 18 dB of sound protection between 20 Hz and 100 Hz and very little protection in the infrasound region as shown in Fig. 11. Theoretically airtight insert-type earplugs will give constant

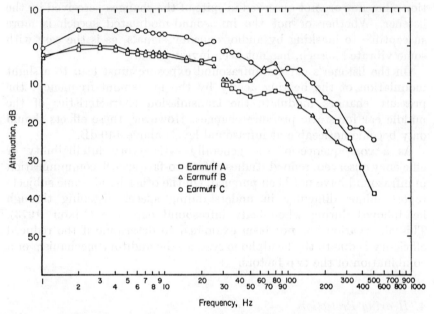

*Fig.* 11 Earmuff hearing protection against infrasound and low frequency energy.

attenuation over the whole infrasound region of over 20 dB (von Gierke and Warren, 1953). For optimum protection in sound fields below 20 Hz, good insert earplugs are recommended for short duration exposures; good insert earplugs in combination with good earmuffs are recommended for intense exposures of long duration.

## V. Whole-body Effects

### A. SUBJECTIVE SYMPTOMS

Clear-cut whole-body responses to infrasound, other than the auditory system, appear only at very intense exposure levels. Mohr *et al.* (1965) conducted what is believed to be the first systematic, controlled study of whole-body exposures of human subjects to high intensity infrasound and very low audio-frequency energy. This study remains somewhat of a classic, providing the only available technical information on human responses to the various exposure stimuli. A variety of different noise sources was acoustically analysed and several were shown to contain intense infrasound components. The facilities at the Wright–Patterson Air Force Base,* Dayton, Ohio, and at the National Aeronautics and Space Administration, Langley Research Center, Langley, Virginia, which were used as infrasound and very low frequency experimental sound fields, are described in Table III. Broad

TABLE III: Facilities and field environments used in the study reported by Mohr *et al.* (1965)

| Facility | Energy source | Environment |
|---|---|---|
| Aerospace Medical Research Laboratory High Intensity Sound System | 14 kW electrodynamic loudspeaker system housed in 142 m³ room | [a]110 dB at 20 Hz; the low end of the spectrum peaked at 80 Hz |
| Turbojet engine, J57 with afterburner | Jet engine exhaust noise | [a]120 dB at 2 Hz; the low end of the spectrum peaked at 80 Hz |
| National Aeronautics and Space Administration 1.8 m × 2.8 m Thermal Structures Tunnel, Langley, Va. | Blowdown operation; broad-spectrum noise | [a]Energy levels up to 138 dB at 20 Hz |
| National Aeronautics and Space Administration Low Frequency Noise Facility, Langley, Va. | Hydraulic piston system; 4.3 m diameter diaphragm enclosed in a 6.1 m diameter cylinder steel chamber | Discrete tone exposures; 152 dB at 1 Hz to 140 dB at 18 Hz |
| United States Air Force Sonic Fatigue Facility | Low frequency siren | Discrete tone exposures; 148–154 dB at 40–80 Hz |

[a] Although infrasound (energy below about 20 Hz) is very intense, energy in the frequency range of 20–120 Hz was from 8 dB to 15 dB higher than the infrasound levels.

* The Dynamic Pressure Chamber described earlier was not available at the time of these experiments but was developed as a result of the Mohr *et al.* pilot study.

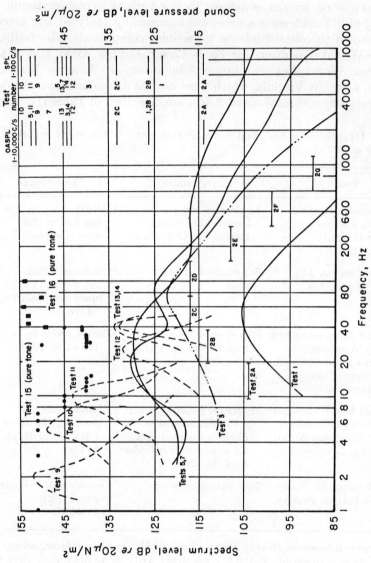

*Fig.* 12 Acoustic spectra and levels of the test exposures in the Mohr *et al.* study.

band noise, narrow band noise and discrete tones were employed as stimuli at levels above 150 dB. The actual spectra of sixteen test environments are shown in Fig. 12. (The environments investigated are not ones to which personnel must be exposed in industrial and aerospace operations.)

In the series of studies of the frequency range below about 50 Hz the maximum exposure levels (152 dB) did not reach the subjective, short term tolerance limits for the subjects wearing ear protection (subjects possessed intense noise exposure experience). Unusual subjective sensations were experienced which might prove alarming to a novice noise exposure observer; symptoms such as chest wall vibration, gag sensations and respiratory rhythm changes. Although the resonant frequency ordinarily cited for the human chest is around 60 Hz, energy below 30 Hz produced clear-cut modulation effects on respiration and speech. It was noted that subjective sensations rose in intensity rather rapidly as sound pressure levels were increased above 145 dB.

Above the infrasonic region, in the 50–100 Hz range, more acute symptoms were reported and the exposures were judged to be intolerable. Symptoms such as mild nausea, headaches, visual blurring, choking and coughing caused subjects to hesitate to consider submitting themselves to higher level and/or longer duration exposures. All subjects complained of marked post-exposure fatigue which was resolved by a night's sleep.

The general conclusion from this study asserted that noise-experienced personnel, wearing hearing protectors, can tolerate infrasound energy at sound pressure levels up to 150 dB for short durations (approximately 2 min) without threat to safety or well-being. The exposures from 50 Hz to 100 Hz were very likely approaching the subjective voluntary tolerance limit which could probably also interfere with reliable performance.

## B. PERFORMANCE

Adverse effects of brief infrasound exposure on performance have not been demonstrated. Discrete tones of 1, 3, 5, 6 and 7 Hz at a level of about 152 dB had no effect on visual acuity, finger dexterity and speech production. However, approximately equivalent levels of exposure at discrete frequencies of 43 Hz, 50 Hz and 73 Hz produced significant visual decrements described by both subjective and objective measures. Speech production was clearly modulated during all exposures between about 30 Hz and 100 Hz. However, no decrement in intelligibility could be attributed to the modulation effect. Effects of infrasound interference with performance reported at lower intensity levels may be comparable to audio-frequency effects which are, at best, unclear. The acoustic exposure is but one element in the conglomerate which actually determines individual performance and includes motivational factors, task difficulty, distraction, task loading, pacing, arousal and numerous other factors which may or may not be related to the acoustic stimulus. The present data do not support the suggestion that infrasound even at very intense exposure levels is detrimental to human performance.

## C. RESPIRATORY EFFECTS

The influence of infrasound on respiration varies with the frequency and intensity of the acoustical energy. The experience of respiratory symptoms in the human pilot studies led to detailed laboratory animal experiments which are still in progress.

Due to changes in body dimensions all mechanical resonances, such as the chest resonances, occur at different frequencies for small animals compared to humans. Therefore, animal data must be interpreted by applying appropriate scaling laws to the biodynamic model being used (von Gierke, 1968). Respiratory phenomena, for example, observed at a certain sound frequency in small animals must therefore be expected to occur at a corresponding lower frequency in man.

Anaesthetised animals (dogs) experienced a dramatic decrease and even cessation of respiration · at intense exposure levels (Johnson, 1973a). The results of a typical experiment in which whole-body exposure to infrasound was increased immediately to 172 dB (Fig. 13) show that normal respiration ceased until the stimulus was removed, and then it returned. No adverse effects or after-effects of the arrested active respiration, or of the infrasound-produced passive respiration, were observed in any of the animals. The growth of this effect can be seen in Fig. 14 where the decline of respiration accompanies stepwise increases in level of from 165 dB to 175.5 dB. The threshold of this effect occurred usually at 164–166 dB. Occasionally, on about one out of every five attempts, the respiration rate declines but does not cease. The use of infrasound for artificial respiration is suggested for consideration by these early observations.

Respiratory symptoms in humans were observed as respiratory rhythm changes during whole-body infrasound exposures below 50 Hz at levels up to 150 dB. The limits of voluntary tolerance were not reached by these exposures. Respiratory phenomena experienced in the range of 50–100 Hz at levels of 150–154 dB contributed to alarming symptoms which precluded further exposures of longer duration or

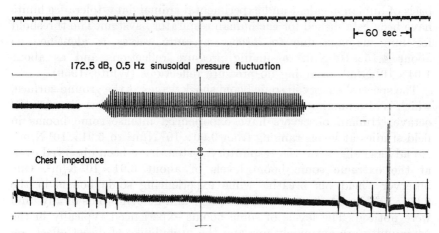

*Fig.* 13 Cessation of measurable canine respiration during exposure to intense infrasound.

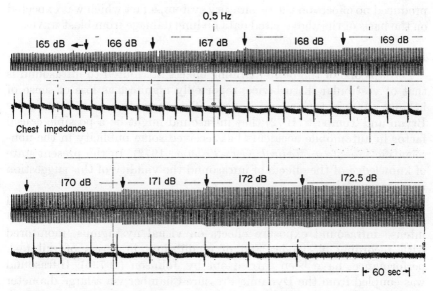

*Fig.* 14 Variations in canine respiratory responses corresponding to stepwise changes in levels of infrasound exposure.

higher levels. Preliminary voluntary tolerance was reached within the controllable exposure conditions utilised by the investigators.

Shock waves generated by blast and by sonic booms contain predominant energy at infrasonic and low audiofrequency regions. On the basis of human accident and experimental animal data, tolerance limits have been established for the human respiratory system. The threshold for lung damage due to intense pressure waves is identified as about $4.15 \times 10^4$ N/m² assuming pressure reflections and as about $1.04 \times 10^5$ N/m² assuming no pressure reflections (White, 1959).

The spectral energy in sonic boom shock waves at the ground surface, which is also maximum in the infrasonic range, rolls off at about 6 dB/octave. Human observers have experienced intense sonic booms in field studies at levels ranging from $9.60 \times 10^2$ N/m² to $6.91 \times 10^3$ N/m². No adverse effects on the respiratory system have been observed even at the extreme sonic boom levels of about $6.91 \times 10^3$ N/m². One observer "held his breath" while experiencing sonic booms in the $9.60 \times 10^2$ N/m² to $4.80 \times 10^3$ N/m² range and no symptoms of any kind were noticed. The levels of sonic booms experienced typically in the community are extremely low and the probability of direct effects on the respiratory system is essentially non-existent. Sonic booms, at the most intense exposure level experienced by humans up to now, have produced no effects on the respiratory system, a fact which was expected on the basis of the above-cited data on lung damage from blast waves.

## D. VESTIBULAR EFFECTS

Perhaps one of the more alarming effects attributed to infrasound is that of vestibular disturbance, reportedly manifest as loss of sense of balance, disorientation and nausea. The suggestion put forward by Bryan and Tempest (1972) that infrasound might be a possible causal factor in automobile accidents has received some publicity in the non-scientific press (e.g. *Medical News-Tribune*, 1972). In the present state of knowledge of the effects of infrasound the validity of this suggestion is controversial.

Visual nystagmus and postural equilibrium are commonly employed as measures of activation of the vestibular system. Investigations of intense infrasound exposure effects on visual nystagmus, monitored with recording electrodes and of equilibrium in terms of rail task performance, have been carried out by Johnson (1973b). Infrasound was coupled from the Dynamic Pressure Chamber via a large diameter flexible hose to short secondary hoses at the earmuff devices which enclosed the ears. Adjustment of the length of the coupling hose and of the secondary hoses allowed presentation to one or both ears and of phase differences in the signals to the two ears.

Visual nystagmus was studied on volunteers who experienced infrasound monaurally, bilaterally in-phase and bilaterally 180° out-of-phase at levels of 142–155 dB. Results are presented in Table IV, and may be summarised by the statement that visual nystagmus was not observed for any of the intense conditions investigated.

TABLE IV: Visual nystagmus during aural exposure to intense infrasound

| N | Frequency (Hz) | Intensity (dB) | Stimulus duration (min) | Ear | Finding |
|---|---|---|---|---|---|
| 2 | 7 | 142 | 2 | Monaural | No nystagmus |
| 2 | 0.6 | 142 | 2 | Monaural | No nystagmus |
|   | 1.6 | 142 | 2 | Monaural | No nystagmus |
| 2 | 2.9 | 142 | 2 | Monaural | No nystagmus |
|   | 7 | 142 | 2 | Monaural | No nystagmus |
| 2 | 0.6 | 142 | 2 | Bilateral | No nystagmus |
|   | 1.6 | 142 | 2 | Bilateral | No nystagmus |
| 3 | 7 | 145 | 5 | Bilateral (180° phase difference) | No nystagmus |
| 3 | 7 | 155 | 5 | Bilateral (180° phase difference) | No nystagmus |

Postural equilibrium, as indicated by ability to stand on narrow rails,* was evaluated for infrasound exposures at sound pressure levels ranging from 110 dB to 140 dB. Results are summarised in Table V (Postural Equilibrium). The numbers heading the four columns on the far right correspond to the conditions shown in the Frequency column. For example, in the 110 dB exposure series, number 1 refers to Control, number 2 to 0.6 Hz, number 3 to 1.6 Hz and number 4 to 2.9 Hz. The entries in the four columns are mean time in seconds that the subjects remained on the rails. Initial inspection and subsequent statistical treatment of these data reveal no effects of infrasound on postural equilibrium for the conditions evaluated. In spite of the appearance of a suggested trend in the 140 dB exposures, no significant differences were observed.

These investigations examined two sensitive indicators of vestibular system response, visual nystagmus and postural equilibrium. Acoustic energy from 0.6 Hz to 12 Hz was experienced at levels ranging from 110 dB to 155 dB. Clearly, no effects of these exposures on either

* Rail test has been used extensively in the study of human vestibular performance and may be interpreted as a "standard" measurement tool. It is described by Graybiel and Fregley (1963).

response were found for any condition tested. (Higher frequency sounds studied by the same methodologies resulted in clear vestibular effects starting at exposure levels of 105 dB (Harris and Sommer, 1968).) In view of this evidence one would not expect infrasound at the levels

TABLE V: Postural equilibrium during aural exposure to intense infrasound

| | | | | | Findings | | | |
|---|---|---|---|---|---|---|---|---|
| N | Fre-quency | In-tensity | Duration | Rails used | Control | 0.16 Hz | 1.6 Hz | 2.9 Hz |
| 4 | Control, 0.6, 1.6, 2.9 Hz | 110 dB | 10 min per con-dition, 30 min total | 4.45, 3.18, 1.91 cm | 33.7[a] | 32.4 | 35.2 | 37.0 |
| 12 | Control, 0.6, 1.6, 2.9 Hz | 125 dB | 10 min per con-dition, 30 min total | 4.45, 3.18, 1.91 cm | 39.3 | 41.5 | 39.2 | 39.7 |
| 12 | Control, 0.6, 1.6, 2.9 Hz | 135 dB | 6 min per condition, 18 min total | 3.18 cm | 43.7 | 44.4 | 40.8 | 45.2 |
| | | | | | Control | 4 Hz | 7 Hz | 12 Hz |
| 8 | Control, 4, 7, 12 Hz | 140 dB | 6 min per condition, 18 min total | 3.18 cm | 45.9 | 40.6 | 39.9 | 39.6 |

[a] Entries are mean time in seconds.

investigated and below to have any significant effect on human vestibular function. For further discussion of vestibular effects on animals, which cannot yet be quantitatively related to the human findings, see Chapter 7.

## VI. Preliminary Tolerance Levels

Limit levels for infrasound exposure may be prescribed on the basis of our experiments with auditory and whole-body responses. Our dis-cussion has revealed that human performance and vestibular function were not influenced by exposures as intense as 140–155 dB. Under some stimuli conditions auditory and respiratory effects were observed. The auditory system appears to be more sensitive to possible adverse effects of infrasound than the other systems evaluated, except for possible whole-body responses at intense exposure levels. Consequently, to define limit levels primarily in terms of the auditory system responses should also provide protection for the other, less susceptible, systems and functions. The tentative exposure limits were derived with respect to safety and interference with, and preservation of, general bodily functions. Subjective annoyance and/or comfort were not part of the considerations.

Tentative limit noise levels which may be considered as acceptable for 8 min exposures are 150 dB at 1–7 Hz, 145 dB at 8–11 Hz and 140 dB at 12–20 Hz (Fig. 15). These levels apply to discrete frequencies

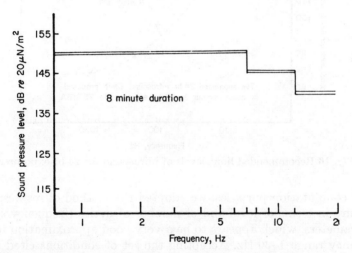

*Fig.* 15 Recommended limit levels of infrasound for 8 min exposures.

or octave bands centred about the stated frequencies. Maximum exposure duration is 8 min with 16 hr rest between exposures. The use of good insert earplugs may increase the permissible levels by 5 dB for the same exposure times by reducing the aural contribution to the overall response. Earplugs are strongly recommended for all intense infrasound exposures to minimise subjective sensations. Levels above 150 dB should be avoided even with maximum hearing protection until additional technical data are accumulated.

If one were required to specify safety criteria for long exposures to infrasound, some extrapolation would be called for in the absence of complete data. The proposed 24 hr exposure limits presented in Fig. 16 represent such an estimate. The data described earlier indicate essentially no effects at 20 Hz for exposures of 8 min at levels up to 141 dB. Using the equal energy rule of 3 dB per doubling or halving of time, and some rounding, and extrapolating from 8 min out to 24 hr reduces the limit level to about 118–120 dB at 20 Hz.

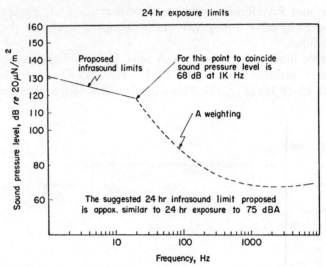

*Fig.* 16 Recommended limit levels of infrasound for 24 hr exposures.

For computation purposes, we adopted the method of respresenting exposure in terms of level and of number of cycles (frequency × time) as parameters, which appears to be a very good approximation for the frequency range 1–20 Hz. Accepting the set of conditions cited above as a base acceptable exposure, the formulation becomes:

$$\text{Limit spl} = 10\log\frac{t}{8\,\text{min}} + 10\log\frac{f}{20} + 141$$

Limit levels for selected frequencies of 1–20 Hz and exposure durations of 1–24 hr are contained in Table VI. The 24 hr duration levels are represented as the Proposed Infrasound Limits curve between 1 Hz and 20 Hz in Fig. 16 (24 hr exposure limits). As shown in that figure, the suggested 24 hr infrasound limit is approximately similar to a 24 hr exposure to 75 dB(A). One is reminded that limit values were derived by extrapolation and should be used with care. (Details of this method are described by Nixon and Johnson (1973).)

TABLE VI: Table of recommended maximum permissible exposures

| Duration (hr) | Frequency (Hz) | | | |
|---|---|---|---|---|
| | 1 | 5 | 10 | 20 |
| 1 | 145 | 138 | 135 | 132 |
| 8 | 136 | 129 | 126 | 123 |
| 24 | 131 | 124 | 121 | 118 |

## VII. Summary

This chapter has discussed methods for investigating infrasound effects on man, physiological and performance effects, subjective reports and preliminary limit levels of infrasound exposure. Major observations and findings are summarised in Table VII in terms of system or function and corresponding effects of the various infrasound exposures. It is clear that relatively little experimental data on infrasound are available, that man appears to be reasonably resistant to infrasound compared to audible sound and that the suggested limit levels for safe exposures may possibly be over-conservative. Limits with respect to comfort and

TABLE VII: Summary of auditory, whole-body and subjective effects of intense infrasound exposure

| System/Function | Tolerance and maximum effects |
|---|---|
| Auditory | |
| Audition | Small amounts of TTS observed at various audio-frequency signals for exposure durations of 20–30 min; adverse effects not expected for exposures up to 30 min at levels below 150 dB |
| Drum membrane/ middle ear | Threshold for middle ear pressure (fullness) around 130 dB; retraction occurs at levels above 120 dB and may be accompanied by vascular injection |
| Pain | Pain threshold is about 145 dB at 20 Hz, increasing to about 155 dB at 4–5 Hz and 165 dB at 2 Hz. Static pressure induces pain at 175–180 dB |
| Speech | Modulation of speech production begins around 130 dB and grows with increasing level; at maximum levels investigated (150–154 dB) modulation was significant with no degradation of speech efficiency (discrimination) in face-to-face situations |

TABLE VII—*continued*

| System/Function | Tolerance and maximum effects |
| --- | --- |
| Whole body | |
| Performance | No evidence of motor performance effects in field and laboratory studies at levels up to 154 dB |
| Vestibular | No effects demonstrated with human subjects at levels as high as 155 dB. Some animal effects at very high sound pressure levels; however, results not consistent |
| Respiratory Infrasound | Respiratory rhythm changes or modulation in humans begin around 130 dB. Normal respiration in dogs declines starting at 164–166 dB and ceases at levels around 172 dB while stimulus is on; no adverse after-effects |
| Sonic boom | No effects on respiration at sonic boom intensity levels as great as $6.9 \times 10^3$ N/m². |
| Blast | Threshold for lung damage identified as $4.15 \times 10^4$ N/m² pressure reflections, $1.04 \times 10^5$ N/m² assuming no reflections |
| Subjective | |
| Tolerance | Subjective voluntary tolerance not reached for brief exposures; unpleasant subjective symptoms experienced at levels above 150 dB |

annoyance cannot be established at the present time. However, all well-documented data support the tentative conclusion that infrasound, which is not subjectively perceived in some way, has no effect on performance, comfort and general well-being.

## REFERENCES

Békésy, G. von (1960). "Experiments in Hearing", McGraw-Hill, New York.
Bryan, M. E. and Tempest, W. (1972). *New Scientist* 16 March, pp. 584–586.
Cole, J. N. and Powell, R. G. (1962). "Estimated Noise produced by Large Space Vehicles as related to establishing Tentative Safe Distances to Adjacent Launch Pads and the Community", Aerospace Medical Research Laboratory, Wright–Patterson Air Force Base, Ohio, Report M–2, April.
Evans, M. J. and Tempest, W. (1972). *J. Sound Vib.* **22**, 19–24.
Graybiel, A. and Fregley, A. R. (1963). "A New Quantitative Ataxia Test Battery", BuMed Project MR005, 13–6001, Subtask 1, Report No. 107, and NASA Order No. R–37, Naval School of Aviation Medicine, Pensacola, Florida.

Green, J. E. and Dunn, F. (1968). *J. Acoust. Soc. Am.*, **44**, 1456–1457.

Hansen, R. G. (1955). "The Effect of Static Air Pressure in the External Auditory Meatus on Hearing Acuity", WADC TR–55–95, April.

Harris, C. S. and Sommer, H. C. (1968). "Human Equilibrium during Acoustic Stimulation by Discrete Frequencies", AMRL TR–68–7, Aerospace Medical Research Laboratory, Wright–Patterson Air Force Base, Ohio, May.

Hood, R. A., Leventhall, A. G. and Kyriakides, K. (1972). Some subjective effects of infrasound. *Proc. Brit. Acoust. Soc.* **1** (3), Paper 71–107.

Jerger, J., Alford, B., Coats, A. and French, B. (1966). *J. Speech Hearing Res.* **9**, 150–160.

Johnson, D. L. (1973a). "Effects of Infrasound on Respiration", presented at the 44th Meeting of the Aerospace Medical Association, Las Vegas, Nevada, May.

Johnson, D. L. (1973b). "Various Aspects of Infrasound", Proceedings of Colloquium on Infrasound, The National Centre for Scientific Research, 38–40 rue de General Leclerc, Paris, France.

Leventhall, H. G. and Hood, R. A. (1972). Instrumentation for infrasound. *Proc. Brit. Acoust. Soc.* **1** (3), Paper 71–101.

*Medical News—Tribune*, "Does Infrasound make Drivers Drunk?" 10 April, 1972.

Mohr, G. C., Cole, J. N., Guild, E. and von Gierke, H. E. (1965). *Aerospace Med.* **36**, 817–824.

Mundie, J. R. (1963). "The Impedance of the Ear—A Variable Quantity", U.S. Army Medical Research Laboratory, Ft. Knox, Kentucky, Report No. 576.

Nixon, C. W. (1962). *J. Auditory Res.* **2**, 247–266.

Nixon, C. W. (1969). "Human Auditory Response to an Air Bag Inflation Noise", Department of Transportation, FHA, Washington, D.C., March, PB–184–837, Clearinghouse for Federal Scientific and Technical Information, 5285 Port Royal Road, Springfield, Virginia 22151.

Nixon, C. W. (1973). "Human Auditory Response to Intense Infrasound", Proceedings of Colloquium on Infrasound, The National Centre for Scientific Research, 38–40 rue de General Leclerc, Paris, France.

Nixon, C. W. and Johnson, D. L. (1973). "Infrasound and Hearing", Proceedings of International Congress on Noise as a Public Health Problem, U.S. Environmental Protection Agency.

Nixon, C. W. and Sommer, H. C. (1963). "Influence of Selected Vibration on Speech (Range of 2 Hz–20 Hz and Random)", Aerospace Medical Research Laboratory, Wright-Patterson Air Force Base, TDR–63–49, June.

Nixon, C. W., Hille, H. K. and Kettler, L. K. (1967). "Attenuation Characteristics of Earmuffs at Low Audio and Infrasonic Frequencies", Aerospace Medical Research Laboratory, TR No. 67–27, May.

Nixon, C. W., Hille, H. K., Sommer, H. L. and Guild, E. (1968). "Sonic Booms resulting from Extremely Low Altitude Supersonic Flight: Measurements and Observations on Houses, Livestock and People", Aerospace Medical Research Laboratory, TR No. 68–52, October.

Sommer, H. C. and Nixon, C. W. (1974). "Primary Components of Simulated Air Bag Noise and their Relative Effects on Human Hearing", Aerospace Medical Research Laboratory, Wright–Patterson Air Force Base, Ohio, TR 73–52, November.

Sonic Boom Structural Response Test Programme, White Sands Missile Range, SST–65–4, Federal Aviation Agency, Office of Supersonic Transport, Washington, D.C., March 1965.

Stephens, R. W. B. (1971). "Very Low Frequency Vibrations and their Mechanical and Biological Effects", Seventh International Congress on Acoustics, 26G1, Budapest.

Stephens, R. W. B. (1972). Natural sources of low frequency sound. *Proc. Brit. Acoust. Soc.* 1 (3), Paper 71–105.

von Gierke, H. E. (1968). Response of the body to mechanical forces—an overview. *Ann. N.Y. Acad. Sci.* 152, 172–186.

von Gierke, H. E. (1972). "Non-auditory Effects of Ultrasonic, Infrasonic, and Vibratory Energy on Man", Conference on Acoustics and Societal Problems, Arden House, Harriman, New York, 18–21 June.

von Gierke, H. E. (1973). Dynamic characteristics of the human body. *In*: "Perspectives in Biomedical Engineering" (R. M. Kenedi ed.), Macmillan, London.

von Gierke, H. E. and Warren, D. R. (1953). "Protection of the Ear from Noise", Benox Report, Contract N6 ori–020, Task Order 44, ONR Project Nr. 144079, University of Chicago, December.

von Gierke, H. E., Davis, H., Eldredge, D. H. and Hardy, J. D. (1953). "Aural Pain Produced by Sound", Benox Report, Contract N6 ori–020, Task Order 44, ONR Project Nr 144079, University of Chicago, December.

White, C. S. (1959). "Biological Blast Effects", Lovelace Foundation for Medical Education and Research, U.S. Atomic Energy Commission, TID–5564, September.

White, C. S. (1968). The scope of blast and shock biology and problem areas in relating physical and biological parameters. *Ann. N.Y. Acad. Sci.*, 152, 89–102.

Yeowart, N. S., Bryan, M. E. and Tempest, W. (1967). *J. Sound Vib.* 6, 335–342.

Yeowart, N. S., Bryan, M. E. and Tempest, W. (1969). *J. Sound Vib.* 9, 447–453.

Zwislocki, J. (1962). *J. Acoust. Soc. Am.* 34, 1514–1523.

# 7. Effects of Sound on the Vestibular System*

*D. E. Parker*

## I. Introduction

Sound exposure may evoke several types of response from a person in addition to those directly related to hearing. Among these *non-auditory* effects of sound are responses which result from activation of vestibular system receptors.

## A. PURPOSE

My co-workers† and I are interested in describing the biomechanical and physiological mechanisms whereby sound affects the receptors of the vestibular system. The primary purpose of this chapter is presentation of our experiments with laboratory animals. Animal experimentation has been pursued to further our understanding of the effects of sound on the human vestibular system.

A general introduction to the vestibular system is presented in Section 1.B. Subsequent divisions of this initial section briefly review previous research concerning the effects of sound on vestibular receptors (Section 1.C) and present the basic anatomy and physiology necessary to understand our procedures and results (Section 1.D).

Section II summarises our research concerning the mechanisms of acoustical stimulation of the vestibular system. The section is divided according to the three classes of acoustical stimulation that we have

---

* Although this book is mainly concerned with infrasound, the effects of pressure transients and audio-frequency sound are considered in this chapter for two reasons. First, response mechanisms for infrasound should be deducible if we completely understand the mechanisms for vestibular reception of pressure transients and audio-frequency sound. Second, we have relatively little information regarding biomechanical and physiological vestibular responses to infrasound *per se*.

† M. F. Reschke and H. E. von Gierke have made major contributions to the research described in this chapter. S. Lopater, G. Bushweiler, R. Tubbs and G. G. Parker have helped collect and analyse data.

used: Section II.A describes responses to transient pressure changes at the ear drum (tympanic membrane), Section II.B presents our observations using infrasound stimulation, and Section II.C reviews our results with audio-frequency sound stimuli. The observations described in Section II were obtained from guinea pigs and monkeys. Unfortunately, the results observed with these two animal species frequently differ, at both the biomechanical and physiological levels.

Section III attempts to assess the significance of our animal studies. Established or possible differences in the anatomy of guinea pigs and monkeys that might illuminate the observed response differences are considered in Section III.A, and the implications of the observations for hypothetical mechanisms of acoustical vestibular stimulation are noted in Section III.B. Finally, the relationships between our animal data and observations with humans are noted (Section III.C).

## B. THE VESTIBULAR SYSTEM

The vestibular system has two distinct, yet interrelated functions. First, the vestibular system co-ordinates with other sensory systems in maintaining the spatial orientation of the body, including the head and eyes. Vestibular influences can be observed in several orientation reflexes (e.g. the counter-rolling of the eyeball when the head is tilted). The vestibular system is often presented as a postural control system because it makes important contributions to motor control of the body. This classification is not completely correct because the vestibular system also has a significant influence upon our spatial orientation perceptual system. This second function is associated with subjective awareness of (1) body orientation with respect to gravity and (2) body movement (within limits). Vestibular receptors contribute to perception of orientation and motion because they respond to linear and angular acceleration (gravity can be described as linear acceleration). Obviously many senses, including sight, hearing and touch, contribute to perception of spatial orientation. The contribution of the vestibular system to spatial orientation perception is clearly illustrated when signals from vestibular receptors are modified by disease or unusual stimulation.

One of the difficulties that we encounter in dealing with the vestibular system relates to the unusual nature of the sensations evoked by stimulation of vestibular receptors. I can think of no sensation that is uniquely correlated with vestibular stimulation in the way that visual sensations are associated with stimulation of the eye. For example, strong motion sensations may result from strictly visual inputs, as most of us have noticed while watching a "chase scene" in a cinema. Similarly, we encounter difficulties when we attempt to relate particular sensations uniquely to vestibular disturbances. For example, the symptoms of motion sickness can be evoked by unusual or intense vestibular stimulation; however, similar sensations can be evoked under many other conditions (e.g. alcoholic intoxication). Unless we have reason to believe that vestibular receptors are somehow stimulated, we are unable to attribute particular unpleasant sensations to the vestibular system.

Further information on the general nature of the vestibular system is available in Howard and Templeton (1966).

## C. BACKGROUND

Acoustical stimulation of vestibular receptors has been a topic of much confusion and controversy. Early research and theory concerning acoustical vestibular stimulation were obscured by failure to differentiate between the functions of the cochlear and vestibular portions of the labyrinth. Through the haze of conflicting observation and opinion, two main lines of development can be detected. One group of investigators proposed that the ability to localise sounds in space was associated with stimulation of the semi-circular canals. This sound localisation view of semi-circular canal function was supported during the present century by the work of Tullio. Another group of investigators advocated Flourens' position that the vestibular receptors were concerned with movement rather than with detection of acoustical signals. This second group of investigators recognised that sound can stimulate the vestibular receptors but noted that the responses elicited by sound stimuli were analogous to those produced by motion stimuli. In other words, the investigators who followed Flourens believed that sound can be considered an *inadequate* stimulus for the vestibular receptors. A summary of early work concerning acoustical vestibular stimulation can be found in Camis (1930).

During the period from 1930 to the present time, several investigators have reported responses indicative of vestibular stimulation following exposure of humans to high intensity acoustical stimulation. Nystagmus (involuntary oscillation of the eyeball clearly related to vestibular stimulation) has been observed following exposure to pure tones ranging from 200 Hz to 2500 Hz at intensities from 120 dB to 160 dB spl. Observers report sudden shifts or displacements of the visual field following stimulation at intensities of 115–130 dB spl with pure tones that have rapid onset rates. These visual field displacements are also thought to result directly from vestibular stimulation.

Dizziness, nausea and disturbances of postural equilibrium have been correlated with sound stimulation at intensities and frequencies lower than those which are required to evoke nystagmus or reports of visual field displacement. These responses are believed to reflect activation of vestibular receptors; however, the possibility that dizziness, nausea and equilibrium disturbance result from acoustical stimulation of physiological systems in addition to the one associated with vestibular receptors cannot be discounted. This matter is pursued further when the relationships between observations on animals and those with human beings are discussed in Section III.C. References for recent acoustical vestibular stimulation research can be found in Parker *et al.* (1968a) and Harris (1972).

## D. ANATOMY AND PHYSIOLOGY

It is convenient to think about the mechanisms between acoustical stimulation and physiological or behavioural vestibular responses in terms of three basic blocks, as illustrated in Fig. 1. Environmental

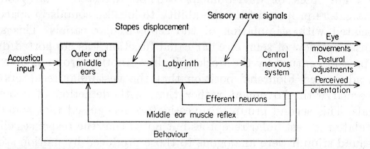

*Fig.* 1 Block diagram of acoustical vestibular stimulation, including three feedback pathways.

sound enters the body primarily at the tympanic membrane of the middle ear (due to the mechanical impedance match between body fluids and air at this point). Sound energy is transformed into tympanic membrane oscillation, and an oscillatory motion of the middle ear bones (ossicular chain) is evoked by tympanic membrane motion. The ossicular chain terminates with the footplate of the stapes at the oval window of the labyrinth.

The bony labyrinth refers to the fluid-filled cavities of the temporal bone. The membranous labyrinth is located within the bony labyrinth. The perimeter of the bony labyrinth is filled with perilymph and roughly defines the shape of the vestibule, cochlea and semi-circular canals (see Fig. 2). Figure 3 illustrates the endolymph-filled series of sacs and tubes that comprises the membranous labyrinth. The sensory receptors for the auditory system are located in the cochlea; the utricle, saccule and semi-circular canals contain the vestibular receptors.

The sensory apparatus of the vestibular system is morphologically differentiated into two types of receptors: one for detection of linear acceleration (statolith organs in the utricle and saccule) and the other

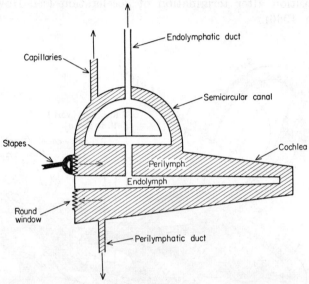

*Fig.* 2 Schematic drawing of bony labyrinth and membranous labyrinth (endolymph-filled space). Arrows indicate elastic release points for fluid displacement when stapes moves inward (modified from Békésy, 1936).

for detection of angular acceleration (crista organs in the three semi-circular canals).* Both types of receptors are activated by deformation of sensory hair cells as a result of inertial displacement of accessory components. However, the mechanism of accessory structure inertial displacement differs significantly for the two types of vestibular receptors.

Displacement of the statolith mass stimulates the sensory hair cells of the utricle and saccule. The statolith is displaced relative to the hair cells during linear acceleration exposure because the statolith has a higher specific mass than the surrounding medium. The hair cells of the

* Several recent observations indicate that the semi-circular canal receptors may be responsive to linear acceleration (Budelmann and Wolff, 1973). The function of the saccular statolith organ is uncertain (Howard and Templeton, 1966).

semi-circular canal crista organs are stimulated by displacement of a gelatinous flap (cupula) which extends into the membranous semi-circular canal. The cupula, in turn, is displaced during angular accelera-tion by inertial movement of endolymph in the membranous ring contained within the bony semi-circular canal. Both the statolith and cupula behave as though they contained a weak spring and return to a neutral position after termination of acceleration (see Howard and Templeton, 1966).

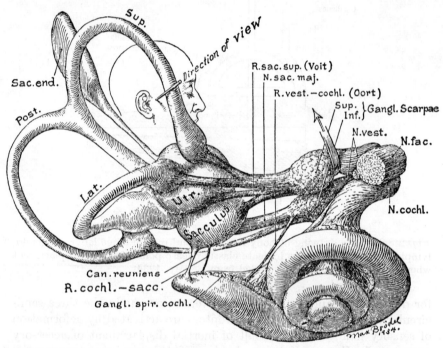

*Fig.* 3 Drawing of membranous labyrinth. Auditory receptors are located in the spiral-shaped cochlear duct at lower right. Statolith organs are located in the utricle (Utr.) and saccule (Sacculus), and crista organs are found in each of the three semi-circular canals (Lat., Sup. and Post.). The endolymphatic duct terminates in the endolymphatic sac (Sac. end.) at the upper left. The nerve supply to the auditory and vestibular receptors is also shown (from Hardy, 1934).

Differences in the nature of fluid displacement associated with stimulation of the two types of vestibular receptors may be important for our purposes. Displacement of the statolith mass is not directly dependent upon movement of labyrinth fluids; the fluid displacement resulting from a change in position of the statolith mass should be relatively small and localised. Conversely, displacement of the semi-circular canal cupula is directly dependent upon volume displacement of fluid within the membranous ring.

Ossicular chain motion results in displacement of perilymph and endolymph through the labyrinth. This labyrinth fluid displacement is dependent upon elastic "release points" in the non-elastic bony labyrinth wall. The major labyrinth release point is the round window; three additional openings in the labyrinth wall include the peri-lymphatic and endolymphatic ducts, which connect the labyrinth to the cranial cavity, and the capillaries. Labyrinth fluid displacement associated with inward (medial) displacement of the stapes is indicated by the arrows in Fig. 2.

The block diagram presented in Fig. 1 suggests that we consider sound-induced vestibular responses at three levels: *biomechanical*, *physiological* and *behavioural*. Biomechanical responses to acoustical stimulation include ossicular chain and labyrinth fluid displacement, which may result in physiological responses beginning with sensory hair cell activation. We include eye movements, postural adjustments and other reflexive (unconditioned) responses to vestibular stimulation with neural activity under the heading of physiological responses. Goal-oriented activity of an organism and stimulus-induced perceptual changes can be considered under the heading of behavioural responses. Observations from our laboratory have been primarily concerned with biomechanical and physiological responses evoked by acoustical stimulation; however, our goal is to relate these biomechanical and physiological observations to reports of other investigators regarding behavioural responses.

Three possible feedback pathways are also illustrated in Fig. 1. The pathway labelled "behaviour" indicates that an organism's overt actions can modify the acoustical stimulation that it receives. Potential physiological feedback could result from activation of the middle ear muscle (acoustic) reflex and the efferent portion of the vestibular nerve. The middle ear muscle reflex, which reduces the efficiency of sound energy transfer from air to labyrinth fluids, has a latency of 60–150 msec, and gradually adapts to continuous stimulation over a period of minutes (Weiss *et al.*, 1962; Gulick, 1971). The efferent neural fibres, which terminate on vestibular sensory hair cells, appear similar to those of the cochlea (Rasmussen, 1960; Smith and Rasmussen, 1967). Cochlear efferent neurons perform an inhibitory function (Fex, 1967; Wiederhold and Kiang, 1970); the physiological activity of the vestibular efferents has not been clearly established.

7

## II. Vestibular Responses to Acoustical Stimulation

We divide acoustical stimuli into three categories based on the temporal aspect of the pressure changes. *Pressure transients*, including pressure step functions and ramp functions, comprise one of these categories. The remaining two categories of acoustical stimulation that we employ consist of sinusoidal pressure oscillations and are defined according to oscillation frequency. *Infrasound* refers to pressure oscillation at frequencies below 20 Hz, and *audiofrequency sound* denotes oscillations in the 20–20,000 Hz frequency range. In addition to frequency, acoustical stimuli are specified by several other parameters: intensity, duration, phase and onset rate. We specify the intensity of pressure transients in centimetres of mercury (cm Hg) of over-pressure (pressure changes with respect to ambient air pressure). The intensity of oscillatory pressure is expressed in terms of the sound pressure level (spl) scale in decibels (dB) with respect to 0.0002 microbar.

### A. PRESSURE TRANSIENTS

One of our proposed mechanisms to account for acoustical vestibular stimulation is based on unidirectional (dc) flow of perilymph and endolymph through the labyrinth (see Section III.B). We postulate that a dc labyrinth fluid flow results from static displacement of the stapes. One technique for producing static stapes displacement is exposure of an animal to transient pressure changes in the outer ear canal (external auditory meatus). Therefore, we undertook a series of experiments on biomechanical and physiological responses to external auditory meatus pressure transients.

### 1. *Biomechanical Responses*

Biomechanical responses to pressure transients have been examined using two techniques: (1) direct observation of the ossicular chain and (2) labyrinth fluid pressure changes. These responses have been examined in anaesthetised guinea pigs and monkeys (*Macaca mulatta*).

Figure 4 illustrates longitudinal axis stapes displacement as a function of the intensity of a pressure step function at a guinea pig's tympanic membrane. The abscissa represents peak stimulus pressure with pressure increases to the right of the ordinate and pressure decreases to the left. Stapes displacement is indicated on the ordinate; points above the abscissa represent medial displacement (into the oval window) and points below the abscissa indicate lateral stapes displacement (out of the oval window). The stimulus source was a hypodermic syringe, which was connected to a hollow earbar with polyethylene tubing. Responses were recorded by direct observation with an operating microscope through an opening in the bulla. The curve illustrates that increased pressure at the tympanic membrane resulted in an initial medial stapes displacement. Tympanic membrane pressure decreases resulted in a lateral stapes displacement that increased

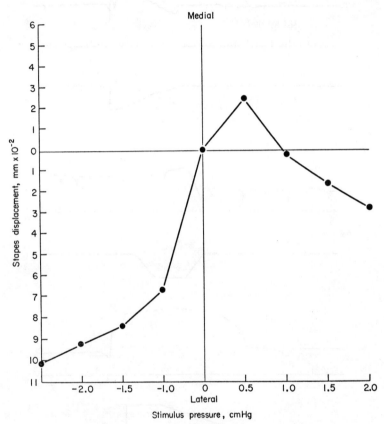

*Fig.* 4 Stapes displacement as a function of pressure change at tympanic membrane of the guinea pig. Each point represents the average of four observations. Variation was negligible. A bidirectional response to pressure increases is illustrated (from Parker and Reschke, 1972).

unidirectionally as a function of stimulus magnitude. These observations confirmed our expectations that pressure transients would produce static stapes displacements; however, the bidirectional stapes response to pressure increases was unexpected.

Variation in perilymph pressure (top trace) as a function of transient pressure change at the tympanic membrane (bottom trace) is illustrated in Fig. 5. Downward deflection for both pressure traces indicates increased pressure. The middle trace in each oscillograph record indicates time in 1 sec intervals. Records A and B illustrate responses

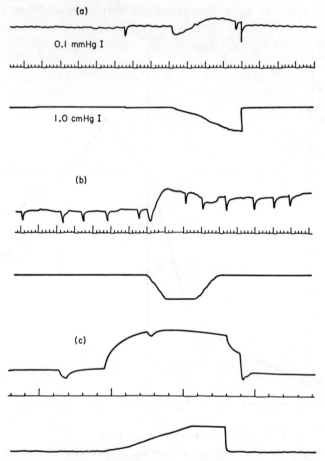

*Fig.* 5 Guinea pig perilymph pressure changes in response to increased (records A and B) and decreased (record C) pressure at the tympanic membrane. In each record the upper trace shows perilymph pressure; the lower trace, pressure change at the tympanic membrane; the middle trace, time at 1 sec per small division (from Parker and Reschke, 1972).

to ramp functions of increased pressure at the tympanic membrane; record C illustrates the response to a ramp function of decreased pressure. These responses were obtained by cementing a saline-filled glass pipette into a 1 mm hole in the superior semi-circular canal of a guinea pig and connecting the pipette to a pressure transducer. The stimulus arrangement was the same as that employed for the stapes displacement observations. The brief downward deflections in the perilymph pressure trace indicate contractions of the middle ear muscles in the lightly anaesthetised animal. The perilymph pressure recordings provide essentially the same information as the direct stapes displacement observations: transient pressure increases at the tympanic membrane elicit a bidirectional response, whereas tympanic membrane pressure decreases result in a unidirectional perilymph pressure change or stapes displacement.

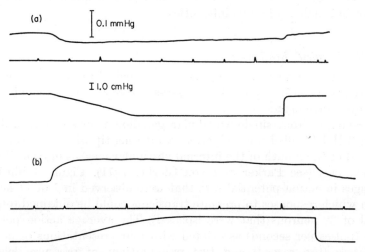

*Fig.* 6 Monkey perilymph pressure changes in response to increased (record A) and decreased (record B) pressure at the tympanic membrane. In each record the upper trace shows perilymph pressure; the lower trace, pressure change at the tympanic membrane; the middle trace, time at 1 sec per small division.

Perilymph pressure changes recorded from the horizontal semicircular canal of a monkey are presented in Fig. 6. Record A illustrates the response evoked by transient pressure increases and record B illustrates the response evoked by transient pressure decreases at the monkey's tympanic membrane.

Figures 5 and 6 essentially describe the transfer characteristics relating perilymph pressure changes to transient pressure changes at the tympanic membranes of the guinea pig and the monkey. These transfer characteristics are presented in the form of oscillograph records because repeated stimulus exposures frequently resulted in a change in the form or amplitude of the response; therefore, presentation of average response curves appears inappropriate. Figures 5 and 6 illustrate three consistent differences between guinea pigs and monkeys. First, monkeys yielded unidirectional responses to both transient pressure increases and decreases, while guinea pigs exhibited a bi-directional response to transient pressure increases at the tympanic membrane. Secondly, the maximum perilymph pressure change obtained from monkeys was invariably in the region of 0.1 mm Hg or less, whereas guinea pigs demonstrated maximum perilymph pressure changes of several times this value. Thirdly, monkey perilymph pressure changes saturated (reached maximum value) at stimulus intensities of 1.0 cm Hg or less; guinea pigs' responses saturated at somewhat higher stimulus intensities.

## 2. *Physiological Responses*

We have examined two types of physiological responses to pressure transients: (1) primary vestibular nerve activity and (2) reflexive head and eye movements.

Responses from single vestibular ganglion neurons were obtained from 3 M KCl-filled micropipettes (2 microns tip diameter) that were located at the mouth of the internal vestibular meatus in anaesthetised guinea pigs (see Parker and von Gierke, 1971). Figure 7 illustrates changes in action potential rate that were observed in 1 of 11 neurons from which responses to pressure transients could be obtained (out of a total of 32 neurons that were isolated). The average action potential rate (pulses per second) associated with four presentations of pressure increases (top record) and two presentations of pressure decreases (bottom record) is plotted in the figure. The temporal location of the stimuli is indicated by the black horizontal bars. Pressure increases of 1–2 cm Hg resulted in a decrement in neural response rate, and pressure decreases of approximately 1.5 cm Hg elicited a pulse rate increment. The response latencies indicated by the curves in Fig. 7 are relatively short (less than 1 sec); however, other neurons that were sampled exhibited response latencies of up to 5 sec. Response latencies are of interest when we compare neural pulse rate data to head and eye movement observations.

These neural response data are important because they clearly demonstrate that vestibular receptors in the guinea pig can be physiologically activated by pressure transients. The vestibular ganglion contains cells from the horizontal and superior semi-circular canals as well as the utricle and saccule. The observation that 11 of 32 isolated neurons exhibited changes in response rate to pressure transients is consistent with the suggestion that only the semi-circular canal vestibular receptors are stimulated by sound energy.

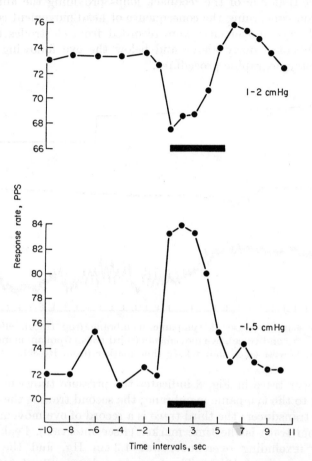

*Fig.* 7 Changes in action potential rate from a single vestibular neuron as a function of increased (top curve) or decreased (bottom curve) pressure at the tympanic membrane (guinea pig). Temporal location of the stimulus is indicated by the horizontal bar under each curve (from Parker and von Gierke, 1971).

An oscillograph record of head and eye movements elicited from an unanaesthetised guinea pig by a pressure increment step function is illustrated in Fig. 8. Head movements were recorded with a force transducer following a technique described by Parker (1970). The animal's head was restrained by a head holder that was attached to the force transducer, and the output of the force transducer indicated the attempts by the animal to change its head position in response to stimulation. Among the interesting features of this recording technique is the fact that one of the feedback loops providing the animal with information concerning the consequence of head movement commands is opened. Eye movements were recorded from electrodes that were located subcutaneously above and below the eye following ordinary electronystagmographic procedures.

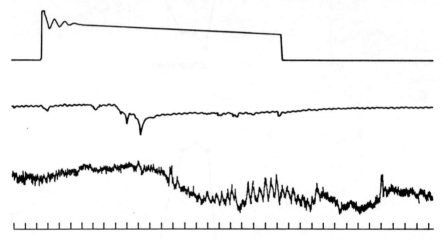

*Fig.* 8 Pressure increase at tympanic membrane (top trace), elicited head movements (second trace), eye movements (third trace) from an unanaesthetised guinea pig. Lowest trace shows 1 sec time marker (from Reschke *et al.*, 1970).

The upper trace in Fig. 8 indicates the pressure transient that was delivered to the tympanic membrane; the second trace is the output of the force transducer; the third trace is a record of eye movements; and the bottom trace is the time marker (1 sec intervals). Peak stimulus intensity (excluding overshoot) was 4.3 cm Hg, and the stimulus duration was about 19 sec. The force transducer output trace shows that the animal attempted to turn its head towards the side of stimulation about 6 sec after stimulus onset. The eye movements evoked by this stimulus were complex, and the full nature of these movements cannot be revealed by electronystagmography. Approximately 9 sec after stimulus onset, the eyeball exhibited a slow downward deflection followed by nystagmus in approximately the vertical plane, which continued beyond the termination of the stimulus.

The data presented in Fig. 8 are important because they demonstrate that responses analogous to those elicited by "normal" vestibular stimulation can be produced by stimulation with pressure transients.

The very long response latencies illustrated by these data are also of interest.

We have made numerous attempts to elicit eye movements from unanaesthetised monkeys in response to pressure transients. *We have not been able to record eye movements from monkeys in response to pressure transients up to 40 cm Hg.* Several stimulation arrangements were employed to ascertain that the stimuli were freely conducted to the tympanic membrane with the same result: no response. Rotatory nystagmus in response to intense audio-frequency sound could be elicited from the same ears with the same earbar placements as those which failed to exhibit a response to pressure transients (see Section II.C.2). The implications of this failure to replicate physiological vestibular responses to pressure transients across species are discussed in Section III.

## B. INFRASOUND

Based on our observations of responses to pressure transients, we deduced that appropriate frequencies and intensities of infrasound should elicit vestibular responses (in the guinea pig). Moreover, infrasound allowed us to estimate the frequency response of the ossicular chain–perilymph pressure system.

### 1. *Biomechanical Responses*

Pressure changes in the semi-circular canal perilymph were examined as a function of exposure to infrasound with anaesthetised guinea pigs and monkeys. A pistonphone generated acoustical stimuli at intensities from 112 dB to 150 dB spl and frequencies from 0.5 Hz to 50 Hz.

Perilymph pressure changes in response to intense infrasound are complex and difficult to interpret. Part of the difficulty results from the observation that the perilymph pressure response can exhibit at least two different response components when stimulated by infrasound; we use the labels "primary response component" and "secondary response component". Either response component may appear alone, or both may appear simultaneously, depending upon stimulus parameters. Variation in response, both within and across species, also introduces interpretation difficulties. Fortunately, differences between monkeys and guinea pigs are considerably greater than differences within either of these species.

The response of the ossicular chain–perilymph pressure system appears to be linear in the low infrasound frequency range (0.5–2 Hz) and the low audiofrequency range (50–70 Hz); that is, the perilymph pressure

output waveform nearly replicates the acoustical input waveform. At
stimulus frequencies intermediate between these values the perilymph
pressure output may be complex. Figure 9 illustrates an oscillograph

(a)

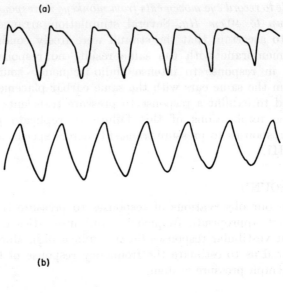

(b)

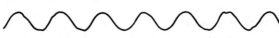

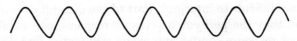

*Fig.* 9 Perilymph pressure changes in guinea pig, evoked by 150 dB spl (a) and
112 dB spl (b) stimulation at 5.7 Hz. In each record upper trace shows perilymph
pressure changes and lower trace shows pressure changes at the tympanic
membrane.

record of perilymph pressure changes evoked by 5.7 Hz infrasound at
150 dB spl (record A) and 112 dB spl (record B). The top trace in each
record illustrates perilymph pressure changes, and the bottom trace
shows the pressure changes at the tympanic membrane produced by
the infrasound stimulus. The response elicited by the high intensity
stimulus is clearly complex, whereas the response to the low intensity

stimulus approximates the input waveform. The perilymph pressure change of record B illustrates what we call the primary response component.

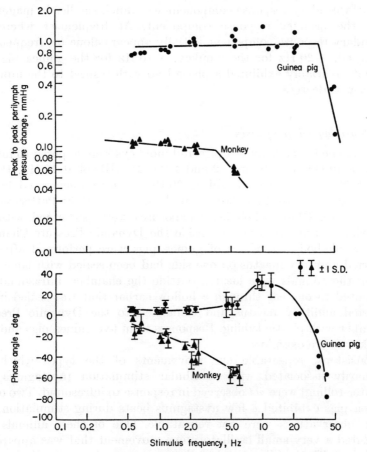

*Fig.* 10 Amplitude (top) and phase angle (bottom) of perilymph pressure response as a function of infrasound frequency.

Employing particular stimulus parameters, it was possible to determine the transfer characteristics for the primary response component of perilymph pressure change as a function of stimulus frequency. Transfer characteristics for the guinea pig and the monkey are illustrated in Fig. 10. These curves indicate two major differences between guinea pigs and monkeys. First, the amplitude of the perilymph pressure response evoked from the guinea pig was an order of magnitude greater than the perilymph pressure response evoked from the monkey by the same infrasound intensity. Second, the upper limit of the natural frequency range was greater for the guinea pig than the monkey by about three octaves.

The secondary response component was much smaller in magnitude than the primary response component. At frequencies where the secondary response component initially appears alone (as frequency is increased, $+20$ Hz for the monkey, $+40$ Hz for the guinea pig) the output invariably exhibited a phase lead with respect to the input by at least 30 degrees.

## 2. *Physiological Responses*

Restrained, awake guinea pigs and monkeys were exposed to intense infrasound (172 dB spl at 1, 2 and 4 Hz; 169 dB spl at 10 Hz; 162 dB spl at 20 Hz; and 158 dB spl at 30 Hz) that was generated by the Dynamic Pressure Chamber located at the Wright-Patterson Air Force Base, Ohio. Whole-body exposures were performed with the experimental animals located inside the Dynamic Pressure Chamber. Two whole-body exposures of guinea pigs were performed after the external auditory meatus on one side had been sealed with bone wax. When the animals were located outside the chamber, infrasound was presented to one ear through a hollow earbar that was sealed in the external auditory meatus and connected to the Dynamic Pressure Chamber with plastic tubing. Responses from five guinea pigs and four monkeys were examined.

Consistent, repeatable eye movements of the types which are ordinarily associated with vestibular stimulation (nystagmus and counter-rolling) were *not* observed in response to infrasound. Two of the guinea pigs exhibited a few nystagmus beats during stimulation, but these observations were not repeatable. One of these animals also exhibited a very small oscillatory eye movement that was apparently in phase with the stimulus, but the response was too small to record with electrophysiological techniques. None of the monkeys demonstrated any evidence of vestibular-induced eye movements.

The failure to observe physiological vestibular responses to infrasound was surprising in view of an earlier study (Parker *et al.*, 1968a) in which we demonstrated nystagmus to pressure oscillations of about 166 dB spl. In the earlier study, however, the pressure oscillation was generated by an animal respirator; the oscillations were between ambient pressure (0 cm Hg) and $+3.8$ cm Hg, rather than being symmetrical around ambient pressure, as is the case with infrasound.

## C. AUDIOFREQUENCY SOUND

The experiments presented in this section are essentially replications of the basic observations from other investigators (see Section I.C). Our variations on the theme include the use of different species, extension of the stimulus range, and examination with the perilymph pressure recording technique.

### 1. *Biomechanical Responses*

The action of the guinea pig ossicular chain was observed under stroboscopic illumination during intense audio frequency sound

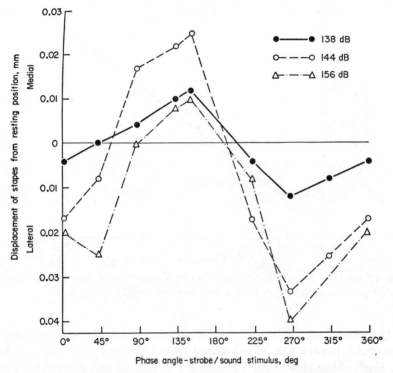

*Fig.* 11 Displacement of stapes as a function of phase of sinusoidal acoustical stimulus at three intensities (guinea pig) (from Parker and Reschke, 1972).

stimulation. This technique allowed us to determine the displacement of the stapes at various points within the stimulus sinusoid. Figure 11 indicates magnitude of stapes displacement (ordinate) as a function of the phase angle between the stroboscope flash and the stimulus sinusoid (abscissa) for three intensity levels. At the lowest stimulus intensity, the motion of the stapes was approximately symmetrical around its resting position (zero on the ordinate). At higher stimulus intensities, the motion of the stapes was increasingly asymmetrical: the stapes moved farther in the lateral direction than in the medial direction. Examination of the output of a condenser microphone or pressure transducer probe located in the external auditory meatus indicated that the response asymmetry was not a function of stimulus asymmetry. These observations, which were obtained by Reschke (1971), confirm the reports of Guinan and Peake (1967) and Kobrak (1948).

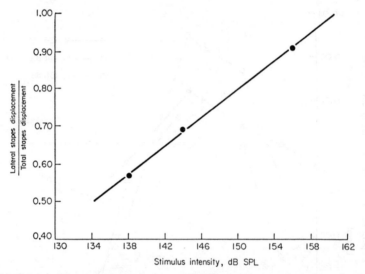

*Fig.* 12 Ratio of lateral to total stapes displacement as a function of stimulus intensity (guinea pig) (from Parker and Reschke, 1972).

The magnitude of stapes non-linear displacement as a function of stimulus intensity can be calculated from the curves presented in Fig. 11. Each of the three points illustrated in Fig. 12 was derived from one of the curves of Fig. 11 and represents the area under a particular curve indicating lateral displacement divided by the total area enclosed by the curve. If the curves of Fig. 11 were perfectly symmetrical, this calculation would yield a value of 0.5; on the other hand, if all of the stapes motion were lateral to its normal resting position, the calculation would yield a value of 1.0. Admittedly, interpretation of a function based on three points is tenuous; nevertheless, Fig. 12 suggests that the magnitude of lateral shift of stapes average position is a logarithmic function of stimulus intensity. Further, extrapolation suggests that the onset of stapes non-linearity occurs at approximately 134 dB spl and

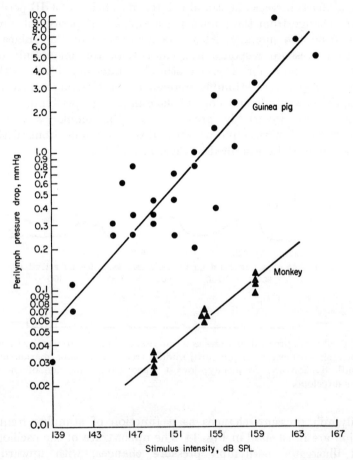

*Fig.* 13 Perilymph pressure drop as a function of intensity of 800 Hz stimulus.

that stapes oscillation completely lateral to the normal resting position would be evoked by stimulus intensities of about 160 dB spl.

Perilymph pressure change responses to intense audio-frequency sound have been recorded with the techniques previously described from anaesthetised guinea pigs and monkeys. Audio-frequency sound usually elicits a perilymph pressure drop which is similar to the drop evoked by transient pressure decreases at the tympanic membrane (see Figs. 5 and 6). Peak perilymph pressure drops evoked by stimuli of 139–163 dB spl at 800 Hz from a guinea pig and a monkey are illustrated in Fig. 13. The curves form power functions which have exponents of 1.65 for the guinea pig and 1.1 for the monkey. In other words, a 20 dB increase in stimulus intensity elicits a 33 dB perilymph pressure change from the guinea pig and a 22 dB perilymph pressure change from the monkey. Also, the magnitude of the guinea pig's perilymph pressure response is greater than the magnitude of the monkey's response for a given stimulus intensity level. Although responses vary across stimulus frequencies and among ears within a species, the magnitude and slope of the guinea pig's perilymph pressure responses were invariably greater than the monkey's responses. Observations of perilymph pressure drops are consistent with the ossicular chain data described in Figs. 11 and 12.

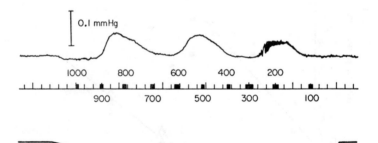

*Fig.* 14 Perilymph pressure changes as a function of stimulus frequency (monkey). Top trace shows perilymph pressure; middle trace shows time marker at 1 sec per small division *and* frequency; lowest trace shows one side of the sound stimulus envelope.

Perilymph pressure changes as a function of stimulus frequency variation are illustrated in Fig. 14. The upper trace of the oscillograph record illustrates perilymph pressure changes, with upward pen deflections indicating pressure decreases, and the lower trace shows one side of the sound stimulus envelope. The middle trace indicates time in 1 sec intervals; the marker on the time line indicates the points at which the frequency sweep reached particular values. Stimulus intensity varied irregularly from 159 dB to 168 dB spl as a function of frequency. Large perilymph pressure drops are associated with stimulus frequencies in the 200–300 Hz, 500–600 Hz and 800–900 Hz frequency ranges. Stimulation at 1000 Hz elicited a small perilymph pressure increment. The oscillation of the perilymph pressure trace in the 150–300 Hz range is an artifact. The location of the peak perilymph pressure changes varied to a small degree as a function of the direction of the frequency sweep. Examination of pressure changes in the tube connecting the speaker to the monkey's ear as well as observation of the output of a condenser microphone probe located in the hollow earbar indicated that the perilymph pressure changes illustrated in Fig. 14 were *not* a function of non-linearities in the acoustical stimulation system. The oscillograph trace presented in Fig. 14 is interesting because it suggests that considerable variation in vestibular sensitivity to acoustical stimulation as a function of frequency should be observable.

## 2. *Physiological Responses*

Eye movement responses to audio-frequency sound in the 500–2000 Hz frequency range have been examined in guinea pigs by Reschke (1971). Intensity thresholds for eliciting nystagmus from unanaesthetised guinea pigs vary as a function of stimulus frequency and duration. Stimulus durations of greater than 4 sec do not modify the intensity–frequency thresholds. Minimum threshold values which have been observed are as follows: 142 dB spl at 500 Hz; 152 dB spl at 600 Hz; 169 dB spl at 700 Hz, 800 Hz and 1000 Hz; 160 dB spl at 2000 Hz; and 162 dB spl for broad band noise. These observations are consistent with the perilymph pressure observations insofar as the 500 Hz stimuli are concerned. Unfortunately, Reschke was unable to perform eye movement threshold measures at 200 Hz and failed to do so for 900 Hz; therefore, we cannot confidently state that perilymph pressure changes are directly related to eye movement thresholds in an awake animal.

Physiological responses to intense audio-frequency stimulation have not been systematically investigated in the monkey. However, a few observations on audio-frequency effects have been made during experiments that were directed towards other goals. Audio-frequency sound at intensities between 140 dB and 145 dB spl and a frequency of 500 Hz elicits a clear, highly repeatable rotatory (corneal–retinal axis) nystagmus from the monkey. This rotatory nystagmus is difficult to record with electrodes located around the eyeball but is very distinct when the animal's eye is observed either directly or with the aid of an operating microscope. Although the monkey fails to exhibit physiological vestibular responses to pressure transients and infrasound (at the intensities that we employed), it clearly demonstrates physiological vestibular responses to audio-frequency sound at approximately the same intensity levels as required to evoke analogous responses from the guinea pig. This response discrepancy is discussed in Section III.

## D. MISCELLANEOUS ADDITIONAL EXPERIMENTS

Before performing the observations reported in the preceding sections, we undertook a series of preliminary experiments that were concerned with the effects of pressure transients in the guinea pig. We wished to ascertain that the head and eye movement responses evoked by pressure transients were a result of vestibular end-organ stimulation.

Five preliminary experiments were performed. First, we sectioned the eighth cranial nerve unilaterally in six guinea pigs. No physiological vestibular responses could be obtained from the ears on the side of the lesion. These results indicate that the transient pressure stimulus affects receptors served by the eighth nerve. Second, we subjected guinea pigs to streptomycin intoxication, which produces destruction of vestibular and cochlear sensory hair cells (see Wersäll and Hawkins, 1962). Little or no physiological vestibular response to pressure transients could be obtained from the streptomycin-intoxicated animals. The implication of these results is that physiological vestibular responses to pressure transients are mediated by membranous labyrinth sensory hair cells.

The third preliminary experiment attempted to determine whether the cochlear or vestibular hair cells are responsible for the eye movement responses to pressure transients. Stimulation deafness was produced by high intensity, long duration noise exposure. This procedure destroys the cochlear sensory hair cells (Wever and Lawrence, 1954). Nystagmus could be elicited from noise-deafened animals by pressure transient stimulation at approximately the same intensities as prior to noise exposure, indicating that the cochlear hair cells are not responsible for this response.

The fourth and fifth preliminary experiments sought to determine the vestibular receptor that mediates the eye movement responses to pressure transients. We removed the statolith mass from the statolith organs by centrifugation (see Parker et al., 1968b). Nystagmus was elicited at the usual levels of pressure transient stimulation; a subsequent experiment indicated that this procedure reduced the amplitude of head movement responses to pressure transients. Finally, we surgically blocked the semi-circular canals (see Correia and Money, 1970). Following blockage of all three canals, eye movement responses to pressure transients were eliminated. Incomplete responses were observed in those instances where only one or two of the three canals was blocked. The results of this experiment are difficult to interpret because of the high incidence of post-operative middle ear infection. The observations are consistent, however, with the hypothesis that pressure transients stimulate the semi-circular canal receptors.

## III. Discussion

The results of the experiments described in the preceding section do not provide us with clear answers to our questions concerning the biomechanical and physiological mechanisms of acoustical vestibular stimulation. A major difficulty is the failure of the monkey to exhibit physiological vestibular responses to pressure transients (at the intensities that we employed), whereas monkeys demonstrate these responses to audio-frequency sound at approximately the same intensities as the guinea pig.

In the first part of this discussion we consider differences between guinea pig and monkey ears that may help us to understand the differences in responses that we have observed. The second part of the discussion focuses on possible mechanisms of acoustical vestibular stimulation and attempts to assess our current position. Finally, we relate our observations to those which have been obtained from humans.

## A. ANATOMICAL DIFFERENCES BETWEEN GUINEA PIG AND MONKEY EARS

The ears of monkeys and guinea pigs are quite similar; however, there are a few anatomical differences between these species that may help to explain the response differences that we have observed. Three possibly important anatomical differences between the middle ears of these two species have been noted. First, the malleus and incus are fused in the adult guinea pig, whereas these two middle ear bones remain separate in the adult monkey. Second, the anterior process of the malleus is well developed in the guinea pig and severely limits medial displacement of the malleus manubrium. Our observations suggest that the guinea pig's malleus anterior process may provide a fulcrum for malleus rotation when the tympanic membrane is strongly displaced; this may account for the bidirectional stapes displacement that we have noted when the guinea pig is exposed to increased pressure transients. The anterior process of the monkey's malleus does not appear to limit medial malleus displacement. Third, the angle between the manubrium of the malleus and the long process of the incus is approximately 15° in the monkey and about 45° in the guinea pig.

Information concerning differences in the labyrinths of guinea pigs and monkeys is not readily available. For example, we do not know the relative ease of fluid flow through the perilymphatic and endolymphatic ducts in these species; we do not know if there are differences in the relative stiffness of the various labyrinth membranes. Clearly, information concerning these points is required before we can confidently account for the response differences that we have observed.

## B. MECHANISMS OF ACOUSTICAL VESTIBULAR STIMULATION

Development of a biomechanical/physiological model for vestibular stimulation by sound energy is one of the goals that has been pursued in our laboratory. Before proceeding to consideration of particular hypothetical mechanisms, we note three assumptions concerning the general nature of the system.

### 1. *Assumptions*

The following assumptions underlie our acoustical vestibular stimulation hypotheses. First, we assume that sound energy elicits vestibular responses as a result of its action upon vestibular end-organs. In other words, we do *not* believe that sound energy somehow bypasses the vestibular receptors and directly affects central nervous system nuclei. Visual, olfactory and gustatory responses would be expected if sound directly affected the central nervous system, and this is not the case (with the possible exception of focused ultrasound). This assumption is supported by the preliminary experiments that are summarised in Section II.D. Secondly, we assume that sound energy elicits vestibular responses by displacing a component of the vestibular end-organs. This assumption is based on well-established observations of vestibular physiology which indicate that vestibular end-organs are activated by the shearing force produced when accessory structures are displaced with respect to the sensory hair cells (see Section I.D). This assumption is also supported by the observation that vestibular responses evoked by particular sounds have the same form as those responses elicited by "adequate" vestibular stimulation (acceleration) and that essentially the same response can be observed across several stimulus replications. Thirdly, we assume that vestibular end-organ components are displaced as a consequence of labyrinth fluid displacement. This assumption is based on the observation that the middle ear transduces sound energy into labyrinth fluid displacement, as noted in Section I.D.

### 2. *Alternative Hypotheses*

As noted in the preceding section, we assume that sound activates vestibular receptors as a result of labyrinth fluid displacement. Alternative hypothetical mechanisms of acoustical vestibular stimulation reflect the possible types of fluid displacement in the labyrinth.

We distinguish between three main classes of sound-induced labyrinth fluid displacement: (1) ac volume displacement, (2) eddy currents and (3) dc volume displacement. Sound stimulation at ordinary intensity levels results in stapes oscillation; the stapes oscillation produces oscillation of the endolymph and perilymph (ac volume displacement) which is compensated by ac displacement of the elastic round window membrane (see Section I.D). Localised rotatory fluid motion—eddy currents—appear during high velocity fluid displacement. Deetjen (1899) and Békésy (1960) have described the appearance of eddy currents in the labyrinth during acoustical stimulation. dc volume displacement of labyrinth fluid may result from non-linear stapes displacement during high intensity sound stimulation.

High intensity sound can produce a dc labyrinth fluid volume displacement in the following manner. At appropriate intensities and frequencies of acoustical input, the stapes moves farther laterally during the rarefaction phase of the sound wave than it moves medially during the condensation phase (Kobrak, 1948; Guinan and Peake, 1967; Section II.C). Consequently, the *average* position of the stapes during stimulation differs from its resting position, and fluid must flow through the labyrinth in order to fill the volume created by this shift in average stapes position. The elastic release points discussed in Section I.D are potential sources for the required fluid. One possible dc volume displacement pathway is from the round window around the cochlear heliocotrema to the oval window; fluid displacement along this pathway would result in inward deflection of the round window membrane until the membrane reached its elastic limit. Fluid might also be displaced from the cranial cavity through the endolymphatic and perilymphatic ducts to the oval window. Finally, an increased volume of blood might flow through the labyrinth capillaries in order to compensate for a change in the average stapes position.

Two mechanisms can be proposed to account for the acoustical vestibular stimulation observations that have been described in the preceding sections. First, vestibular receptors may be activated by the dc labyrinth fluid volume displacement associated with non-linear stapes displacement. For this mechanism to be effective, fluid would have to be displaced along the endolymphatic duct and/or blood capillary pathways. It seems reasonable to suggest that fluid flow along these pathways would be opposed by a relatively high resistance; accordingly, potential vestibular stimulation as a result of this fluid flow should have a relatively long time constant (see Fig. 8). Secondly, the receptors of the vestibular apparatus could be stimulated by a combination of dc volume displacement and eddy currents in the labyrinth fluids. This second mechanism can be visualised in the following manner. Eddy currents are produced in the labyrinth fluids as a result of high velocity fluid oscillation during audio-frequency sound exposure. Normally these eddy currents remain localised in the cochlear region of the labyrinth. Increasing sound intensity has two effects. First, the strength of the eddy current may be slightly increased. Secondly, stapes non-linearity produces a dc flow of fluid through the labyrinth that displaces the eddy current from its usual location towards one of the vestibular end-organs. The manner in which this might work may be clarified if you consider the situation when a canoe paddle is passed through the water of a moving river. Passage of the paddle through the water creates small swirls or eddy currents that are carried downstream by the current of the river until they dissipate. The relatively long response time constant that was suggested for the first mechanism would also be postulated with this second mechanism.

Observations with the guinea pig support a dc fluid displacement mechanism of acoustical vestibular stimulation. Guinea pigs exhibit clear physiological vestibular responses to pressure transients. It is difficult to conceive of eddy currents being generated by pressure transient ramp functions such as those illustrated in Figs. 5 and 6; nevertheless, ramp function stimulation does elicit eye and head movement responses from guinea pigs. Consequently, the dc labyrinth fluid flow produced by static displacement of the stapes is apparently sufficient to stimulate guinea pig vestibular receptors. The experiments described in Section II.D suggest that the semi-circular canal crista organs are activated by this fluid flow.

When we examine the monkey's response to acoustical stimulation, the picture becomes confused. Part of our problem is attributable to the fact that we have been unable to obtain direct dc fluid volume displacement measurements from the labyrinths of either guinea pigs or monkeys up to the present time. In the absence of direct fluid volume displacement observations, we can suggest that perilymph pressure changes are correlated with dc volume displacements. Examination of Figs. 5, 6 and 13, keeping this assumption in mind, is instructive.

Rotatory nystagmus has been observed in the monkey following stimulation with an 800 Hz tone at 149 dB spl. Figure 13 indicates that an audio frequency stimulus of this magnitude can result in an 0.03 mm Hg perilymph pressure drop in the monkey's semi-circular canal. Figure 6 demonstrates that perilymph pressure drops of approximately 0.08 mm Hg can be elicited by pressure transients at the tympanic membrane in the monkey. If a perilymph pressure drop of 0.03 mm Hg is associated with physiological vestibular responses to audiofrequency sound, why do perilymph pressure drops of more than double this value fail to produce similar vestibular responses when pressure transients comprise the stimulus?

At least two answers can be given to the preceding question. First, our assumption regarding the correlation between perilymph pressure change and volume displacement may be incorrect; for a given perilymph pressure value, the magnitude of labyrinth fluid flow may be less in the monkey than in the guinea pig. Second, dc volume displacement alone may not be an effective vestibular stimulus for the monkey. It is quite conceivable that the various elastic release points present a different pattern of opposition to fluid flow in the monkey from that which obtains in the guinea pig. If this were the case, the pattern of dc fluid displacement resulting from stapes non-linearity in the monkey could completely bypass the vestibular receptors. Consequently, the dc displacement–eddy current mechanism of acoustical vestibular stimulation may be required to explain the results with monkeys.

The acoustical vestibular stimulation mechanisms suggested by our research differ from those proposed by previous investigators. Deetjen (1899) observed the formation of eddy currents in labyrinth fluids during intense acoustical stimulation. He hypothesised that the eddy currents stimulate the semi-circular canal crista organs because they produce endolymph displacement. We reject the hypothesis that eddy currents alone are sufficient to elicit vestibular-induced eye and head movements for the following reasons. First, several lines of evidence suggest that the mechanisms that transduce sound pressure into ac labyrinth fluid displacement saturate in the 120–140 dB spl range (Wever and Lawrence, 1954; Békésy, 1960). If eddy currents alone account for the appearance of physiological vestibular responses, we would expect to observe these responses at stimulus intensities below 135 dB spl. Secondly, Figs 11 and 12 suggest that change in the average position of the stapes first appears for stimulation in the 134–144 dB spl intensity range. The correlation between the appearance of this form of stapes non-linearity and physiological vestibular responses is consistent with the suggestion of a combination eddy current–dc fluid displacement hypothesis of acoustical vestibular stimulation (in the monkey).

In 1935, Békésy proposed that the statolith organs are stimulated by high intensity sound exposure. He suggested that eddy currents produce displacement of the statolith organ sensory epithelium. The hair cells are stimulated because the motion of the statolith mass lags behind the motion of the sensory epithelium. Our observations suggest that the semi-circular canal crista organs rather than the statolith organs are stimulated by intense sound. This conclusion is valid, however, only for the types of responses that we recorded. Other types of vestibular responses to acoustical stimulation might derive from statolith organ displacement (see Section III.C).

## C. RELATIONSHIPS TO OBSERVATIONS WITH HUMANS

In this section we note reports of vestibular responses evoked by acoustical stimulation from humans. The relationship of the human studies to our investigations on monkeys and guinea pigs is considered.

### 1. Pressure Transients

The effects of pressure transients in the 1 to 4 cm Hg intensity range on human vestibular responses have not been systematically investigated. H. Sommer (personal communication) exposed two subjects to tympanic membrane transient pressure decreases of 2.5–3.0 cm Hg. Sommer's subjects reported discomfort and crackling sounds as well as anxiety concerning potential damage. Eye movements, head movements or other indices of vestibular response were *not* observed. These observations are consistent with monkey results noted previously (Section II.A.2). On the other hand, J. H. Young (personal communication) observed eye movements in response to pressure transients at the tympanic membrane in two patients who were examined at the Kresge Hearing Research Institute. One of these patients exhibited no spontaneous or positional nystagmus but complained of pain, discharge from the ear and dizziness for 2 weeks prior to testing. Stimulus intensity was not determined. These observations indicate that pressure transients may evoke vestibular responses from abnormal ears; the implications for healthy, normal ears are unclear.

Pressure transients at the tympanic membrane analogous to those that we employ as stimuli would not ordinarily occur in the natural environment. In our situation, the stimuli are presented through an earbar that is sealed into the external auditory meatus, and a pressure differential across the tympanic membrane is maintained. Normally pressure changes at the tympanic membrane would be rapidly equalised by passage of air through the eustachian tube. If the eustachian tube is blocked, perhaps as the result of a cold, pressure differentials across the tympanic membrane may be maintained. I have experienced a eustachian tube block during the descent of an aircraft from high altitude. I did not notice any vestibular disturbance; however, the pain was intense.

### 2. Infrasound

Vestibular responses evoked by exposure to infrasound are reported elsewhere in this volume (see Chapters 5 and 6). Here we note that recent experiments employing the Dynamic Pressure Chamber at the Wright-Patterson Air Force Base have failed to produce direct evidence of vestibular stimulation by infrasound. Exposures were at intensities up to 172 dB spl for durations up to 25 sec. The failure to detect vestibular responses to infrasound with human subjects is consistent with our inability to detect eye movement responses to infrasound in guinea pigs and monkeys.

### 3. *Audiofrequency Sound*

Numerous experiments have sought to determine thresholds for acoustical vestibular stimulation in human beings (see Section I.C). Several criteria for vestibular activation have been used including subjective reports, eye movements and postural equilibrium.

Ades (1953) suggested that vestibular responses can be elicited from normal ears by stimulation at intensities of 135 dB spl in the 1000–1500 Hz frequency range. A series of later experiments employed deaf human subjects (Ades *et al.*, 1957, 1958). The lowest intensity thresholds (120–130 dB spl) were found in the 200–500 Hz frequency range; vestibular response thresholds were approximately 140 dB spl at 1000 Hz and ranged from 145 dB to 160 dB spl for 2000 Hz stimulation. The thresholds for vestibular responses in human subjects reported by Ades and his colleagues are somewhat lower than those which we observed for guinea pigs; however, the general direction of threshold change as a function of change in stimulus frequency is similar to our observations.

Harris and Sommer (1968) and Harris (1971) have performed a series of experiments concerning the effects of acoustical stimulation on human equilibrium. These experiments used the "rail test". Performance decrements were observed when the subjects were exposed to sustained audio-frequency sound of 590 Hz at 95 dB spl. The magnitude of performance decrement increased if the stimuli were asymmetrical (different intensities at the two ears) or interrupted.

The rail test studies suggest that acoustical vestibular stimulation thresholds may be significantly lower than previously reported. A question arises as to how these results should be interpreted. Two possibilities are apparent. First, the rail test may be a more sensitive technique for determining vestibular stimulation than those used in previous experiments. Secondly, the rail test may be measuring effects of acoustical stimulation in addition to those directly related to vestibular stimulation (e.g. "arousal"). The first possibility is supported by the observation that the least stimulus intensity required to elicit a detectable response from vestibular receptors in a threshold experiment is several orders of magnitude lower than the stimulus intensity necessary to evoke nystagmus.

We have not examined the biomechanical or physiological effects of interrupted audio-frequency sound with guinea pigs or monkeys.* However, these effects appear to be interpretable within a combination dc volume displacement–eddy current hypothesis. We suggest that the acoustical pulses produce labyrinthine eddy currents. The acoustical pulses should also elicit reflexive responses of the middle ear muscles, producing dc displacements of labyrinth fluids (see Fig. 5). The combination of dc fluid displacement and eddy current effects might result in vestibular receptor activation, where neither of these effects alone would elicit vestibular responses.

## IV. Summary and Conclusions

The experiments that we have undertaken are concerned with determining the mechanisms of acoustical vestibular stimulation. Two possible stimulation mechanisms are proposed: (1) a dc fluid displacement hypothesis and (2) a combination dc fluid displacement–eddy current hypothesis. Biomechanical and physiological responses to acoustical stimulation were examined in guinea pigs and monkeys. The acoustical stimuli included (1) pressure transients (step and ramp functions of pressure change at the tympanic membrane), (2) infrasound and (3) intense audiofrequency sound. Stapes displacement and perilymph pressure change were the biomechanical responses examined. Physiological responses included vestibular nerve recording, eye movements (slow rolling and nystagmus) and head movements.

The results of our experiments with acoustical pressure transients are as follows.

* Since this chapter was written, we have undertaken a series of experiments on the effects of interrupted audio-frequency sound employing guinea pigs and monkeys. Stimuli were trains of tone bursts that varied in rise time (1–50 msec), duration (10–200 msec), repetition rate (1/sec to 10/sec), frequency and intensity. These acoustical stimuli evoked transient vertical eye movements (jerks) from guinea pigs and rotatory eye jerks from monkeys. Minimum stimulus intensities required to evoke these eye jerks were 2–10 dB lower than the intensities of continuous sound required to evoke counter-rolling and nystagmus. The correspondence between the minimum stimulus intensity necessary to produce stapes non-linearity and the minimum stimulus intensity necessary to evoke eye movement jerks is notable. These data are interpreted as supporting the combination dc volume displacement–eddy current hypothesis of acoustical vestibular stimulation.

1. Longitudinal axis stapes displacement was produced by step and ramp functions of pressure in guinea pigs. Increased pressure at the tympanic membrane elicited a bidirectional stapes displacement; tympanic membrane pressure decreases resulted in unidirectionally increasing lateral stapes displacement. A transfer characteristic relating tympanic membrane pressure change to stapes displacement for the guinea pig is given in Fig. 4.

2. Perilymph pressure recordings yielded results that were essentially equivalent to the stapes displacement observations for the guinea pig. For the monkey, perilymph pressure changes were a unidirectional function of tympanic membrane pressure changes and were of smaller magnitude than those observed in the guinea pig. Transfer characteristics relating perilymph pressure changes to pressure transient stimulus intensity are given in Figs. 5 and 6 for the guinea pig and monkey, respectively.

3. Changes in rate of vestibular neuron response were elicited by pressure transients at the tympanic membrane of the guinea pig. Tympanic membrane pressure increases resulted in a decrement in neuron action potential rate and vice versa.

4. Head and eye movements were evoked from unanaesthetised guinea pigs by pressure transients. Minimum stimulus intensities required to elicit these responses were in the range of 1.5–2.0 cm Hg.

5. *No* evidence of vestibular-induced eye movements could be detected in monkeys exposed to pressure transients up to 40 cm Hg.

Stimulation with infrasound yielded the following observations:

1. Perilymph pressure changes replicated the infrasound stimulus waveform at frequencies in the low infrasonic (0.5–2 Hz) and low audio-frequency (40–50 Hz) ranges. Stimulation between these frequency ranges resulted in complex perilymph pressure changes that were composed of at least two response components. Peak-to-peak perilymph pressure changes evoked by particular stimulus intensities were lower for the monkey than for the guinea pig. The frequency response of the monkey's ear differed from the frequency response of the guinea pig's ear, when examined with infrasound.

2. Consistent vestibular-induced eye movements could *not* be detected in guinea pigs or monkeys exposed to infrasound at intensities up to 172 dB spl.

Audio-frequency sound stimulation results were as follows:

1. The average position of the guinea pig stapes during intense audio-frequency sound stimulation differed from the resting position. The magnitude of this stapes non-linearity is a logarithmic function of

stimulus intensity. The minimum stimulus intensity required to produce stapes non-linearity in the guinea pig was about 134 dB spl.

2. Intense audio-frequency stimulation produced dc perilymph pressure changes that can be related to stimulus intensity by a power function for both the guinea pig and the monkey. The magnitude of perilymph pressure response for a given stimulus intensity was greater in the guinea pig than in the monkey.

3. Both guinea pigs and monkeys exhibited nystagmus in response to audio-frequency stimulation. Minimum stimulus intensities necessary to produce nystagmus were approximately the same for both species: 140–145 dB spl.

The guinea pig observations support a dc volume displacement mechanism of acoustical vestibular stimulation. However, the monkey data indicate that a combination dc volume displacement–eddy current hypothesis may be required to account for the responses observed in this species.

## ACKNOWLEDGEMENTS

I would like to thank H. E. von Gierke and M. L. Parker for their comments and suggestions concerning this chapter. Financial support for the research reported here was derived from Contract Nos. F 33615–69C–1246 and F 33615–73C–4002 between Miami University and the Aerospace Medical Research Laboratory, Wright–Patterson Air Force Base, Ohio, and from the Miami University Faculty Research Committee.

## REFERENCES

Ades, H. W. (1953). *In*: "Benox Report: An Exploratory Study of the Biological Effects of Noise", ONR Project NR 144079. The University of Chicago, Chicago.

Ades, H. W., Graybiel, A., Morrill, S. N., Tolhurst, G. C. and Niven, J. I. (1957). "Nystagmus Elicited by High Intensity Sound", Research Project NM 13 01 99, Subtask 2, Report No. 6, Naval School of Aviation Medicine, Pensacola, Florida.

Ades, H. W., Graybiel, A., Morrill, S. N., Tolhurst, G. C. and Niven, J. I. (1958). "Non-auditory Effects of High Intensity Sound on Deaf Human Subjects", Research Project NM 001 102 503, Report No. 5, Naval School of Aviation Medicine, Pensacola, Florida.

Békésy, G. von (1935). *Pflüg. Arch. ges. Physiol.* **236**, 59.

Békésy, G. von (1936). *Akust. Zeits.* **1**, 13.

Békésy, G., von (1960). "Experiments in Hearing", McGraw-Hill, New York.

Budelmann, B.-U. and Wolff, H. G. (1973). *J. comp. Physiol.* **85**, 283.

Camis, M. (1930). "The Physiology of the Vestibular Apparatus", Clarendon Press, Oxford.

Correia, M. J. and Money, K. E. (1970). *Acta Oto-laryngol.* **69,** 7.

Deetjen, H. (1899). *Zeits. Bio.* **39,** 159.

Fex, J. (1967). *J. Acoust. Soc. Am.* **41,** 666.

Guinan, J. J. and Peake, W. T. (1967). *J. Acoust. Soc. Am.* **41,** 1237.

Gulick, W. L. (1971). "Hearing: Physiology and Psychophysics", Oxford University Press, New York.

Hardy, M. (1934). *Anat. Rec.* **59,** 403.

Harris, C. S. (1971). "Effects of Acoustical Stimuli on the Vestibular System", Technical Report 71–58, Aerospace Medical Research Laboratory, Wright–Patterson Air Force Base, Ohio.

Harris, C. S. (1972). "Effects of Increasing Intensity Levels of Intermittent and Continuous 1000 Hz Tones on Human Equilibrium", Technical Report 72–11, Aerospace Medical Research Laboratory, Wright–Patterson Air Force Base, Ohio.

Harris, C. S. and Sommer, H. C. (1968). "Human Equilibrium During Acoustical Stimulation by Discrete Frequencies", Technical Report 68–7, Aerospace Medical Research Laboratory, Wright–Patterson Air Force Base, Ohio.

Howard, I. P. and Templeton, W. B. (1966). "Human Spatial Orientation", John Wiley and Sons, London.

Kobrak, H. G. (1948). "The Middle Ear", University of Chicago Press, Chicago.

Parker, D. E. (1970). *J. Exper. Psychol.* **84,** 96.

Parker, D. E. and Reschke, M. F. (1972). *Minerva Oto-laryngol.* **11,** 111.

Parker, D. E. and von Gierke, H. E. (1971). *Acta Oto-laryng.* **71,** 456.

Parker, D. E., von Gierke, H. E. and Reschke, M. F. (1968a). *Aerospace Med.* **39,** 1321.

Parker, D. E., Covell, W. P. and von Gierke, H. E. (1968b). *Acta Oto-laryng.* Suppl. 239,

Rasmussen, G. L. (1960). *In:* "Neural Mechanisms of the Auditory and Vestibular Systems" (G. L. Rasmussen and W. F. Windle, eds.), pp. 105–115. C. C. Thomas, Springfield, Illinois.

Reschke, M. F. (1971). "High-intensity, Audio-frequency Vestibular Stimulation in the Guinea Pig", unpublished Doctoral Dissertation, Department of Psychology, Miami University, Oxford, Ohio.

Reschke, M. F., Parker, D. E. and von Gierke, H. E. (1970). *J. Acoust. Soc. Am.* **48,** 913.

Smith, C. A. and Rasmussen, G. L. (1967). *In:* "Third Symposium on the Role of the Vestibular Organs in Space Exploration", pp. 183–202, NASA SP–152, National Aeronautics and Space Administration, Washington.

Weiss, H. S., Mundie, J. R., Cashin, J. L. and Shinabarger, E. W. (1962). *Acta Oto-laryngol.* **55,** 505.

Wersäll, J. and Hawkins, J. E. (1962). *Acta Oto-laryngol.* **54,** 1.

Wever, E. G. and Lawrence, M. (1954). "Physiological Acoustics", Princeton University Press, Princeton.

Wiederhold, M. L. and Kiang, N. Y. S. (1970). *J. Acoust. Soc. Am.* **40,** 1427.

# 8. Subjective Effects of Vibration

*B. K. N. Rao* and *C. Ashley*

## I. Introduction

The aim of this chapter is to discuss, briefly, some of the best present-day knowledge available on the subjective response of human beings to low frequency vibration. For convenience, this chapter has been divided into eight sections. Section II discusses the mechanisms of human perception and the psycho-physical effects of low frequency vibrations on human beings. Section III introduces the physics of sinusoidal and random vibrational motions. Section IV discusses in general the effects of vertical, lateral, fore-and-aft, angular and combined axes vibratory motions on various performance tasks. In Section V, the effects of low frequency vibration on specific parts of the human system are discussed. Also, the effects of vibration on the postural changes of subjects are briefly covered in this section. Section VI reviews some of the physiological and pathological effects of vibration on human beings. Section VII covers the nature of vibratory forces induced by surface transport and the methods for evaluating various ride indices. Section VIII touches briefly on the measurement techniques available to evaluate the effects of vibration on human beings. Because of space limitations, additional information on each section is included in the list of references appended to this chapter.

## II. The Sensations of Vibration

### A. PERCEPTION

Human beings perceive mechanical vibrations through the system which maintains general somaesthetic sensibility. The perception of vibration is a complex physiological and psychological sensation transmitted from numerous and varied receptors by the central nervous system to the brain. These sensations are then suitably integrated in the brain to yield a subjective perception of induced vibration.

Somaethesis includes tactile, kinesthetic and internal sensitivities. Kinaesthesis is the sense arising from joints, tendons, muscles (proprioceptors) and the non-auditory labyrinth. The combination of these senses yields information about the whole-body angular and linear motion of limbs and body in space. The chief receptors of the proprioceptive sense are: (1) Pacinian corpuscles, responsive to deep pressure, (2) muscle spindles, responsive to muscle stretch, (3) Golgi tendon organs, responsive to muscle stretch.

The vestibular apparatus is housed in the non-auditory labyrinth and responds to linear and angular acceleration of the head and to whole-body vibration and also responds to position in space. The vestibular apparatus consists of three mutually perpendicular semi-circular canals and the otolith organs, utricle and saccula. There is evidence that the canals respond to linear acceleration, position and angular motion. The otolith organs control the static reflex, the position of the head and dynamic reflexes in response to movements. The threshold of the otolith organs is not known. Muscles and skin have a lower perception threshold than the vestibular apparatus. The otolith organs, utricle and saccula, are in two sacs and respond to gravity and linear acceleration. The receptors are different from the canals and are called maculae. The utricle macula lies in the horizontal plane and the saccula in the vertical plane. Certain evidence suggests that the saccula macula is a vibratory or low tone receptor.

Three frequency regions are detected by different sense organs. Frequencies from 0 Hz to 15 Hz are detected by the non-auditory labyrinth, those above 15 Hz through the skin, and for frequencies greater than 1500 Hz the vibration is sensed by the pressure receptors in the skin (Stevens, 1960).

Human response to vibration extends from below 1 Hz to at least 100 kHz. However, it is the range from 0.5 Hz to 100 Hz that concerns us most. It is also important to note that human beings are aware of vibration through a variety of sensors distributed throughout the body. Human sensitivity to vibration is not simple but changes in a complex way with (a) the intensity of vibration, (b) the spectral composition of vibration, (c) the duration of vibration, (d) the area of application and direction of transmission to the body, (e) the rate of onset/offset of stimulus, (f) presence of associated cues acting through other sense modalities, (g) physical constraints (like harness, clothing, etc.), (h) learning, (i) motivation and (j) fatigue.

The determination of the human threshold of perception for vibratory motion is a technically difficult task. Some of the factors which affect threshold determinations are (a) individual sensitivity, (b) age, (c) sex,

(d) posture, (e) activity and focus of attention at time of determination, (f) masking effect, (g) personality and (h) learning.

Some work has been done using parallel swings at low frequencies (0.1–1 Hz), and vibrating systems at other frequencies. The results of these investigations seem to indicate that the threshold for rectilinear whole-body vibration is remarkably low and of the order of 0.01 m/s² in the frequency range of 1–10 Hz; and that the threshold increases at higher frequencies. The threshold for standing subjects is lower than that for recumbent subjects. The threshold for rotational oscillations at frequencies below 1 Hz is approximately 1°/s² for motion about the z-axis (head to foot direction) (Guignard and King, 1972).

## B. DISCOMFORT

Discomfort is a subjective sensation caused by low frequency vibration resulting in physiological and psychological displeasure. Subjects usually express discomfort by various adjectives such as "disturbing", "unpleasant", "uncomfortable", "annoying", "objectionable", "alarming" and "fatiguing". The subjective judgment on discomfort is liable to wide variations due to (a) individual differences, (b) motivating factors, (c) state of health, (d) emotional factors, (e) age, sex, race, (f) time of day, (g) social factors, (h) environmental factors, (i) posture, (j) duration of exposure, (k) type of vehicle, (l) type of seat, (m) type of journey and (n) type of activity.

Some attempts have been made to relate the subjective experiences to physical characteristics of vibration, but the subjective evaluation has always been an *ad hoc* process. However, there have been few attempts to examine discomfort (or comfort) in a systematic manner. Since many of the above terms are either ambiguous or overlap in meaning, it would be worth while to reduce these terms to a smaller number of independent concepts with distinct and separate meanings. In this respect multi-dimensional analysis appears to offer an effective means of reducing a large number of possibly correlated variables to a more convenient number of orthogonal variables.

It is generally true to say that discomfort leads to fatigue. Several physiological and psychological criteria, such as electroencephalography (EEG) response, oxygen consumption, energy expenditure, heart rate, galvanic skin response (GSR), visual performance, mental performance, reaction time, critical flicker fusion and self-rating tests, have been used to measure fatigue on an objective scale. A review of literature on fatigue associated with physical tasks reveals (a) differences among physiologists with regard to the best physiological measure to use,

8

(b) a poor relationship between physiological responses and actual performance and (c) a good relationship between subjective measures of fatigue and measures of performance (Snook and Irvine, 1969).

However, in general, the following symptoms of fatigue have been observed: (a) decrease of attention, (b) slowed and impaired perception, (c) impairment of thinking, (d) decrease of motivation and (e) decrease of proficiency in mental and physical activities.

It is generally believed in ride engineering circles that vertical oscillations constitute the most important ride problem. However, at low frequencies, below 3 Hz, lateral and fore-and-aft oscillations of the seated subject are generally more disturbing than vertical oscillations of similar intensity.

Future investigations into the problems of discomfort or fatigue should therefore include the combined effects of multi-axis oscillations.

Vibrations at frequencies below 1 Hz are a special problem associated with effects such as motion sickness. Several studies are progressing into motion sickness, but little current data have been produced on sickness-inducing situations.

## C. LIMITS OF TOLERANCE

A limit of human tolerance to whole-body vibration defines in quantitative terms a level of vibration which should not be exceeded. These limits are usually related to certain criteria based on health factors, working/performance efficiency, comfort etc. A number of synonyms for "limit" exist, but an acceptable term called "boundary" has been proposed by the International Organisation for Standardisation (ISO) as recommended limits for human exposure to vibration. Tables I and II show the values of "Fatigue-decreased proficiency boundary" for x-, y- and z-axis vibration for both sinusoidal and $\frac{1}{3}$-octave band level random vibration (ISO, 1974). These levels of vibration, when exceeded, may result in a significant deterioration of mental/physical/physiological activities.

A specification for limits of exposure to vibration should include (a) physical nature and mode of vibration, (b) range of application, (c) direction of application, (d) duration of exposure, (e) intensity, (f) point of application to the body and (g) methodology of measurement.

Various national standards and codes of practice are available which specify the frequency range of exposure encountered in various fields. There is at present a draft British Standards Document DD32; 1974, entitled "Guide to the evaluation of human exposure to whole-body vibration" (BSI 1974).

The need to formulate limits below 1 Hz and above 80 Hz is recognised, and organised scientific investigations are vital to achieve valid and reliable guidelines.

TABLE I: Values of "Fatigue-decreased proficiency boundary" in m/s² (rms) acceleration for z-axis vibration. The values are defined for both sinusoidal (single frequency) vibration and ⅓-octave band level in the case of random vibration

| Frequency (or centre-frequency of ⅓-octave band) (Hz) | Effective duration | | | | | | |
|---|---|---|---|---|---|---|---|
| | 8 hr | 4 hr | 2.5 hr | 1 hr | 25 min | 16 min | 1 min |
| 1.0 | 0.63 | 1.06 | 1.40 | 2.36 | 3.55 | 4.25 | 5.60 |
| 1.25 | 0.56 | 0.95 | 1.26 | 2.12 | 3.15 | 3.75 | 5.00 |
| 1.6 | 0.50 | 0.85 | 1.12 | 1.90 | 2.80 | 3.35 | 4.50 |
| 2.0 | 0.45 | 0.75 | 1.00 | 1.70 | 2.50 | 3.00 | 4.00 |
| 2.5 | 0.40 | 0.67 | 0.90 | 1.50 | 2.24 | 2.65 | 3.55 |
| 3.15 | 0.355 | 0.60 | 0.80 | 1.32 | 2.00 | 2.35 | 3.15 |
| 4.0 | 0.315 | 0.53 | 0.71 | 1.18 | 1.80 | 2.12 | 2.80 |
| 5.0 | 0.315 | 0.53 | 0.71 | 1.18 | 1.80 | 2.12 | 2.80 |
| 6.3 | 0.315 | 0.53 | 0.71 | 1.18 | 1.80 | 2.12 | 2.80 |
| 8.0 | 0.315 | 0.53 | 0.71 | 1.18 | 1.80 | 2.12 | 2.80 |
| 10.0 | 0.40 | 0.67 | 0.90 | 1.50 | 2.24 | 2.65 | 3.55 |
| 12.5 | 0.50 | 0.85 | 1.12 | 1.90 | 2.80 | 3.35 | 4.50 |
| 16.0 | 0.63 | 1.06 | 1.40 | 2.36 | 3.55 | 4.25 | 5.60 |
| 20.0 | 0.80 | 1.32 | 1.80 | 3.00 | 4.50 | 5.30 | 7.10 |
| 25.0 | 1.00 | 1.70 | 2.24 | 3.75 | 5.60 | 6.70 | 9.00 |
| 31.5 | 1.25 | 2.12 | 2.80 | 4.75 | 7.10 | 8.50 | 11.2 |
| 40.0 | 1.60 | 2.65 | 3.55 | 6.00 | 9.00 | 10.6 | 14.0 |
| 50.0 | 2.00 | 3.35 | 4.50 | 7.50 | 11.2 | 13.2 | 18.0 |
| 63.0 | 2.50 | 4.25 | 5.60 | 9.50 | 14.0 | 17.0 | 22.4 |
| 80.0 | 3.15 | 5.30 | 7.10 | 11.8 | 18.0 | 21.2 | 28.0 |

## D. EQUAL SENSATIONS

Human judgment of whole-body vibration has been largely based on, (a) voluntary subjective tolerance levels (the approach to this has been through studies of the limits of voluntary subjective tolerance, as indicated by discomfort, pain etc.) and (b) subjective evaluation of vibration levels, by using adjectives, such as "perceptible", "unpleasant", "annoying", "alarming" etc., in conjunction with qualifiers, such as "mildly", "extremely" etc. The results obtained from these studies have shown great variations producing widely different results. Also, there is no quantitative way in which the subjective levels can be compared with one another.

TABLE II: Values of "Fatigue-decreased proficiency boundary" in m/s² (rms) acceleration for x- and y-axis vibration. The values are defined for both sinusoidal (single frequency) and ⅓-octave band level in the case of random vibration

| Frequency (or centre-frequency of ⅓-octave band) (Hz) | Effective duration | | | | | | |
|---|---|---|---|---|---|---|---|
| | 8 hr | 4 hr | 2.5 hr | 1 hr | 25 min | 16 min | 1 min |
| 1.0 | 0.224 | 0.355 | 0.50 | 0.85 | 1.25 | 1.50 | 2.00 |
| 1.25 | 0.224 | 0.355 | 0.50 | 0.85 | 1.25 | 1.50 | 2.00 |
| 1.6 | 0.224 | 0.355 | 0.50 | 0.85 | 1.25 | 1.50 | 2.00 |
| 2.0 | 0.224 | 0.355 | 0.50 | 0.85 | 1.25 | 1.50 | 2.00 |
| 2.5 | 0.280 | 0.450 | 0.63 | 1.06 | 1.60 | 1.90 | 2.50 |
| 3.15 | 0.355 | 0.560 | 0.80 | 1.32 | 2.00 | 2.36 | 3.15 |
| 4.0 | 0.450 | 0.710 | 1.00 | 1.70 | 2.50 | 3.00 | 4.00 |
| 5.0 | 0.560 | 0.900 | 1.25 | 2.12 | 3.15 | 3.75 | 5.00 |
| 6.3 | 0.710 | 1.12 | 1.60 | 2.65 | 4.00 | 4.75 | 6.30 |
| 8.0 | 0.900 | 1.40 | 2.00 | 3.35 | 5.00 | 6.00 | 8.00 |
| 10.0 | 1.12 | 1.80 | 2.50 | 4.25 | 6.30 | 7.50 | 10.0 |
| 12.5 | 1.40 | 2.24 | 3.15 | 5.30 | 8.00 | 9.50 | 12.5 |
| 16.0 | 1.80 | 2.80 | 4.00 | 6.70 | 10.0 | 11.8 | 16.0 |
| 20.0 | 2.24 | 3.55 | 5.00 | 8.50 | 12.5 | 15.0 | 20.0 |
| 25.0 | 2.80 | 4.50 | 6.30 | 10.6 | 16.0 | 19.0 | 25.0 |
| 31.5 | 3.55 | 5.60 | 8.00 | 13.2 | 20.0 | 23.6 | 31.5 |
| 40.0 | 4.50 | 7.10 | 10.0 | 17.0 | 25.0 | 30.0 | 40.0 |
| 50.0 | 5.60 | 9.00 | 12.5 | 21.2 | 31.5 | 37.5 | 50.0 |
| 63.0 | 7.10 | 11.2 | 16.0 | 26.5 | 40.0 | 45.7 | 63.0 |
| 80.0 | 9.00 | 14.0 | 20.0 | 33.5 | 50.0 | 60.0 | 80.0 |

Recently some psychological methods have been employed to establish equal sensation contours to whole-body vibration. Some of these techniques are briefly discussed below.

## 1. Magnitude Estimation Technique

This technique, which was developed by Stevens (1961), is now recognised as a very useful research tool in establishing equal sensation contours across frequency, and bearing a ratio relationship to each other. According to Stevens, the fundamental relationship between subjective magnitude of sensory qualities and the physical magnitude of stimulus is expressed by the following power function,

$$\psi = K\phi^n$$

where

$$\psi = \text{psychological magnitude}$$

$$\phi = \text{physical magnitude}$$

$$n = \text{exponent}$$

$$K = \text{constant determined by units used}$$

Using this technique Stevens has shown for more than 20 different sensory qualities that the above law holds true.

Basically, this method involves presenting a number of stimuli to subjects and requiring them to scale them, by placing them into one of a number of categories (e.g. annoying, tolerable, etc.) or, by assigning a number to each stimulus, to represent its magnitude. Using this law, Shoenberger and Harris (1971) and Shoenberger (1972) have recently demonstrated the feasibility of applying this technique to quantification of judgments of vibration intensity. This study used only z-axis vibration with the subject seated upright. However, a recent experiment by McCullogh (1972) has cast doubt on the validity of this technique. See also Miwa (1967a, 1967b, 1968, 1969), Jones (1973), and Oborne and Clarke (1974, 1975).

## 2. *Cross-matching Technique*

This technique has been adopted by Ashley (1970) using two vibrators and two different stimuli (sinusoidal and random vibration). The method required the subject (in a standing posture) to establish an equal sensation effect of a random stimulus with reference to a standard sinusoidal vibration stimulus. This technique has one advantage in that it has considerably reduced both the intra-subject and inter-subject variabilities. The direction of application of vibration was in the z-axis. At Birmingham University this technique is now being extended to the y- and x-axes. See also Ashley and Rao (1974), Dupuis, *et. al.* (1972), Griffin (1975), and Watts (1975).

## 3. *The Cross-modality Matching Technique*

This technique has been used with some success by Van Deusen (1965) and Versace (1963) for rating automobile ride vibration. The technique involved the subjects adjusting other stimuli, such as noise, light etc., to match the whole-body vibration intensity. See also Fleming and Griffin (1975), Hempstock and Saunders (1976), and Clarke and Oborne (1975).

### 4. *Fractionation and Equisection Judgment Techniques*

Miwa (1968) has developed a "Vibration greatness scale", which he contends is analogous to the sone scale in acoustics, from fractionation and equisection judgments based on a corrected ratio technique devised by Garner (1954). He used both x- and z-axes vibration.

In fractionation judgment experiments the subjects were asked to adjust the intensity of one stimulus to a given ratio of vibration level to another fixed stimulus. Reference may also be made to work carried out by Clarke and Oborne (1975).

In equisection judgments the subjects were asked to adjust a series of stimuli between two fixed end-stimuli to produce equal intervals of vibration level.

## III. Types of Motion

Since time immemorial vibration of one sort or another has always been associated with mankind. In fact, the present "civilised society" is experiencing the effects of vibration to an extent which it never even dreamt of before. Whatever the consequences of vibration on our lives may be, it poses an interesting challenge to the modern community. Control of this environment for the betterment of mankind requires an understanding of the basic causes and effects of these forces. In the present context, the term "vibration" refers to mechanically induced alternating forces (e.g. vibrations induced by motor vehicles, hovercraft, jets, helicopters, hand-operated machine tools, ships, trains, tractors, earthmoving equipment etc.).

### A. DETERMINISTIC VIBRATIONS

The simplest form of vibratory motion consists of a simple sinusoidal oscillation, that is a fundamental oscillation with no harmonics present, (see Fig. 1). Figure 2 shows the spectrum of a sinusoidal vibration consisting of a single line. In nature, pure sinusoidal vibrations rarely occur; however, they can be produced synthetically and are useful in many applications. Such a vibration can be defined by its instantaneous displacement, $x$, which is given at any instant by the peak displacement, $X$, frequency, $f$, and elapsed time, $t$, from a given datum. This is expressed mathematically as

$$x = X \sin 2\pi f t$$

By definition, velocity ($v$) is the rate of change of displacement with time. Hence

$$v = \frac{dx}{dt} = 2\pi f X \cos 2\pi f t$$

Similarly, acceleration ($a$) is the rate of change of velocity with respect to time. Therefore,

$$a = \frac{d^2 x}{dt^2} = -4\pi^2 f^2 X \sin 2\pi ft$$

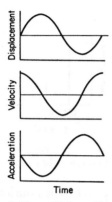

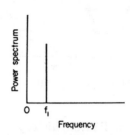

*Fig.* 1 Sinusoidal oscillations.

*Fig.* 2 Power spectrum of sinusoidal oscillation.

Vibration, therefore, may be measured in terms of displacement, velocity or acceleration. To characterise the magnitude of the vibration one could, for instance, use the peak values of the above quantities. This does, however, contain a very limited amount of information, and is normally used only in certain special cases. A more informative quantity, which gives some information about the average (or rather root-mean-square average) time history of the vibrations, is the rms-value of the displacement, velocity or acceleration. This quantity is related to the energy contained in the vibrations.

In practice, forced vibrations are far more complex. See, for example, Fig. 3. This is a periodic vibration composed of two or more super-imposed harmonic vibrations. See Fig. 4 for its spectral composition.

The following descriptive functions apply to a time history record of length $T$ seconds for which a fundamental time period $T_p$ seconds exist.

Mean value

$$\bar{x} = \frac{1}{T_p} \int_0^{T_p} x(t)\,dt$$

Variance value

$$\sigma x^2 = \frac{1}{T_p} \int_0^{T_p} [x(t) - \bar{x}]^2\,dt$$

Mean square value

$$\bar{x}^2 = \frac{1}{T_p} \int_0^{T_p} x^2(t)\, dt$$

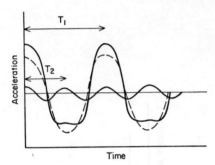

Fig. 3 Ccompex periodic vibration.    Fig. 4 Power spectrum of complex periodic vibration.

A periodic time history record may be expressed by a Fourier series. The amplitude form of the time history record $x(t)$ is here considered compounded from an amplitude component at zero frequency plus an infinitude of sinusoidal components having amplitudes $C_n$ and phase angles $\phi_n$ at frequencies $nf_1$ where $f_1$ is the fundamental frequency. Expressed mathematically,

$$x(t) = C_0 + \sum_{n=1}^{\infty} C_n \cos\left(2\pi n f_1 t + \phi_n\right)$$

## B. RANDOM VIBRATIONS

In addition to regular motions, most practical vibration problems involve random movement such as might be generated by a car wheel running over a rough surface. Under such circumstances, random vibrations cannot be described by any explicit mathematical relationships except in statistical terms. Some of the terms that are frequently encountered in this area need explanation.

### 1. *Random Vibration*

Random vibration is a signal containing no periodic components. Its instantaneous magnitude can only be described on a probability basis. This probability usually has a Gaussian or Normal distribution.

### 2. *Random (White) Vibration*

This may be defined as vibration having equal power per cycle of band-width. In other words, if the spectral energy is approximately uniform in distribution, the vibration is sometimes called "white" vibration. See Figs. 5 and 6.

## 3. *Composite Vibration*

If one or more discrete frequency components are superimposed upon a random motion the spectrum of such vibration, although continuous, contains distinct peaks. See Figs. 7 and 8.

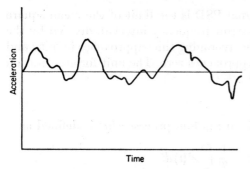

*Fig.* 5 Random vibration (white).

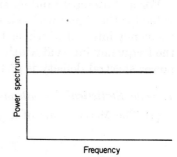

*Fig.* 6 Power spectrum of (white) random vibration.

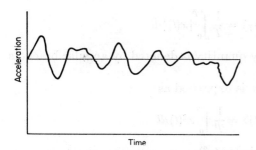

*Fig.* 7 Composite vibration.

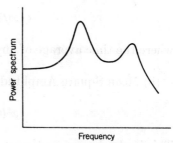

*Fig.* 8 Power spectrum of composite vibration.

## 4. *Normal or Gaussian Distribution*

The natural probability distribution valid for the majority of uncertain and unordered occurrences whose value can only be determined on a probability basis, such as the throw of a dice or the instantaneous value of a random process.

## 5. *Stationary and Non-stationary Vibrations*

Random data generated in everyday life situations will be either stationary or non-stationary. By stationary, we mean that the statistical properties (mean square value) do not vary with time. It is necessary to assume stationarity for the purposes of analysis but it is frequently untrue. This, in practice, means that considerable care must be taken in the selection of samples for analysis to ensure they are reasonably constant within themselves. Standard methods exist to test for stationarity.

## 6. *Power Spectral Density (PSD)*

For a stationary random signal PSD is the limit of the mean square value for the signal within a narrow frequency interval, divided by the frequency interval width, as the averaging time approaches infinity and the frequency interval width approaches zero. The unit for acceleration power spectral density is $g^2/Hz$.

## 7. *Some Statistical Definitions*

(a) The Mean Value of a given random process $x^1(t)$ is defined as

$$\bar{x}'(t) = \frac{1}{T} \int_0^T x^1(t)\, dt$$

and the mean amplitude of the new random variable $x(t)$ is given by

$$\langle |x(t)| \rangle = \frac{1}{T} \int_0^T |x(t)|\, dt$$

where the time average of any quantity is denoted by angular brackets $\langle\ \rangle$.

(b) Mean Square Amplitude is expressed as

$$\langle x^2(t) \rangle = \frac{1}{T} \int_0^T x^2(t)\, dt$$

This is also known as the variance ($\sigma^2$).

(c) The Root Mean Square Amplitude is

$$\sqrt{[\langle x^2(t) \rangle]} = \sqrt{\left[ \frac{1}{T} \int_0^T x^2(t)\, dt \right]}$$

(d) The Probability Density Function is a curve showing the times during which the random process lies in a narrow band about any value $x$. These times can then be divided by the sample time $T$, giving the probability density distribution for the random process as shown in Fig. 9.

(e) A means of describing a random process in terms of frequency content as a continuous curve can also be established by using Fourier transforms.

A thorough treatment of random process analysis is beyond the scope of this section. Interested readers are however, advised to consult the references appended to this chapter, especially Bendat (1958), Blackmann and Tukey (1958), Crandall (1963), Robson (1963) and Bendat and Piersol (1964, 1965).

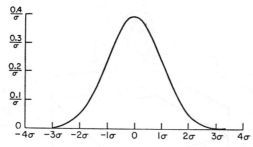

*Fig.* 9 The normalized gaussian probability density curve.

## IV. Effects of Directional Vibration on Performance

### A. INTRODUCTION

The direction of vibratory motion greatly affects the transmission of vibration and the frequency characteristics of body resonances. Direction of motion is defined according to an orthogonal system centred in the heart, with the body (or the head and torso when the person is seated) in the normal anatomical position as shown in Fig. 10. The effects of directional vibration are therefore discussed with reference to this system.

### B. EFFECTS OF z-AXIS VIBRATION ON PERFORMANCE

Guignard and Irving (1960) have found the greatest decrements on a visual search task between 3 Hz and 5 Hz. Dennis' (1960) number reading task has showed the most errors at 5 Hz and 14 Hz when the input acceleration was $\pm 0.25$ g, and at 7 Hz and 14 Hz with an input of $\pm 0.5$ g. Hornick (1962a) reports an increase in response time during a post-vibration test. Lovesay (1971) reports that 2 Hz and 2.7 Hz vibration degrades subjects' ability to maintain a target spot at the centre of a collimated head-up display in azimuth and in elevation (see also Chapter 9). It appears that when human beings are exposed to z-axis vibration in an upright seated position there are primarily three frequency-related factors that appear to have a bearing on visual decrements. These are (a) compensatory tracking movements of the eye at very low frequencies, (b) amplification or attenuation of vibration from seat to head and (c) resonance associated with the eyeball and/or

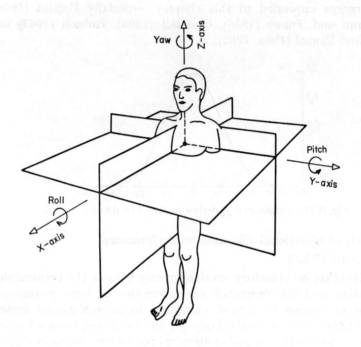

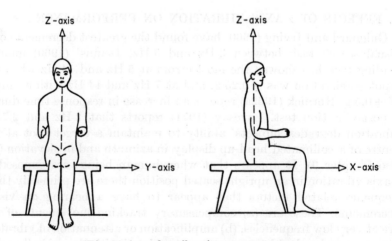

*Fig.* 10 Axes for vibration measurement.

its supporting structures at high frequencies. Rao and Ashley (1974) have shown that a 30 min duration z-axis narrow band random vertical vibrational stress of 0.23 rms g at a peak frequency of 2.5 Hz significantly reduces proficiency at a simple vigilance task for seated subjects. Bulger (1972) has shown that random vibration stress reduces subjects' sensitivity to peripherally occurring stimuli such that there is a decline in percentage correct detections.

Very few studies appear to have been performed on the effects of z-axis vibration on intellectual tasks. In general, these results seem to indicate that intellectual tasks can be affected by certain vibration conditions, but the effect does not appear to be a mechanical one.

## C. EFFECTS OF x- AND y-AXIS VIBRATION ON PERFORMANCE

Hornick (1962a) reports an increase in response time during post-vibration testing after vibration in the y-axis. It has been demonstrated by Rubenstein and Kaplan (1968) that great losses in visual acuity between 22 Hz and 34 Hz have resulted when subjects were vibrated in the y-axis. In a testing situation which included both choice response time and two-dimensional compensatory tracking in the x-axis and y-axis, Shoenberger (1970) has shown significant increases in response time to green and red lights in the frequency range 1–8 Hz. Tracking decrements in the frequency range 1–3 Hz have been reported.

## D. EFFECTS OF ANGULAR OSCILLATIONS

Very little is known about the effects of angular oscillations (roll, pitch and yaw motions) on human performance.

In a study by Coermann et al. (1962), blindfolded subjects, restrained by a standard harness, sat on a modified Air Force chair, which was programmed to move in random patterns in pitch and roll, and counteracted these motions by using a control stick. The whole device was mounted on a vibration table producing vertical sinusoidal motion in the frequency range 2–20 Hz and at amplitudes corresponding to one-third of the subjective tolerance limits. The angular deviations from the upright position were evaluated relative to the disturbing input for both pitch and roll for 1 min during the vibration and for 1 min after cessation of the vibration. Some individual subjects were not influenced by the vibrations, others showed performance decrements. In the main, these measures of performance reflected the mechanical resonances within the body previously established by other methods. The frequencies which most affected performance were found to be between 3 Hz and 12 Hz. Residual affects were detected by the measurements after vibration.

The effect of angular oscillation in yaw on vision has been studied by Benson (1972). It was previously thought that the frequency response of the vestibulo-ocular reflex was comparable to that of the pursuit reflex; Benson has demonstrated that the response of the vestibulo-ocular system extends to a frequency a decade higher than that of the pursuit reflex. Refer also to investigations carried out by Rance and Barnes (1973), Rance (1975), and Barnes and Rance (1975).

## E. EFFECTS OF COMBINED-AXES VIBRATIONS

Most of the studies concerned with vibration have been confined to a single axis, but in practice this situation rarely occurs. Measurements of the vibrations in modern transportation have shown appreciable quantities of vibration along the three axes. Lovesay (1972) and others have confirmed the following:

(a) Combined 2 Hz heave and $3\frac{1}{2}$ Hz sway vibrations contribute to significant degradation in tracking performance.

(b) Instrument reading becomes more difficult to combined dual-axis heave and sway vibrations.

(c) Difficulty in aircraft control tasks is often experienced when small quantities of low frequency sway vibrations are added to the heave.

(d) Dual-axis vibration has a particularly adverse effect upon a pilot's ability to transfer suddenly from a "head-up" to "head-down" task.

(e) Manual positioning errors are greatly increased when dual-axis heave and sway vibrations are present.

(f) Loss in tracking performance can occur with severe multi-axis heave, roll and pitch motions, or heave and sway vibrations.

Walsh's (1966) investigations into the head movements during rail travel have shown that the head oscillates in the z- and x-axes, and in the y-axis the head oscillates in the region of 0.5–1.5 Hz.

A recent study by Rance and Barnes (1973), concerning head movements which occurred when an unrestrained seated subject was oscillated in yaw, revealed that head movements occur in all three rotational axes. Movement in pitch showed frequency doubling when the yaw input was in the frequency range of 2–4 Hz.

The effect of combined-axes vibration on human judgments is a function of relative intensities and the phase relationship of component vibrations.

The survey of available literature on human response to vibration indicates that research is particularly needed to establish criteria and limits on the effects of prolonged and multi-axis vibrations on human health, comfort and performance.

# V. Vibration of Specific Parts of the Body and Effects of Posture

## A. HAND VIBRATION

Raynaud's phenomenon, resulting from the handling of vibrating tools, has been recognised since 1911. This phenomenon has been observed in grinders and other workers exposed to vibration (e.g. chain-saw operators) in this country (Keighley, 1970). Operation of the following tools is considered responsible for this phenomenon (Pelmear 1972a):

(a) riveting hammers and "holding up" tools
(b) pneumatic chisels, chipping hammers
(c) portable rotary tools
(d) large grindstones against which small castings are being ground.

Intense vibration can be transmitted to the fingers, hands and arms of the operator from these tools. A detailed study of portable vibrating tools in relation to the clinical effects which they produce has been reported by Agate and Druett (1946).

The evidence, in general, suggests that if a tool produces high amplitudes (0.1 mm or more) in the low frequency range of 40–125 Hz, it is likely to produce Raynaud's phenomenon, particularly if it is in continuous use (Guignard and King, 1972).

A working group of ISO is currently considering methods of evaluating hand-transmitted vibration in the frequency range of 2–1400 Hz.

The best known proposal for hand tool vibration is based on a Russian standard and was submitted to ISO by Czechoslovakia (ISO, 1969). This is written in terms of exposure limits for vibration transmitted to the hands from the point of view of health protection. The recommended limits are specified in terms of rms acceleration measured by octave filters centred on seven frequencies. They apply to both sinusoidal and random vibration and to all directions of vibration which are considered independently. The maximum admissible values of vibration transmitted to the hands for an 8 hr exposure are reproduced from this document and are shown in Table III. Miwa (1967a) has measured the hand sensation both in the vertical and the horizontal directions in postures similar to those used when handling tools, using his "Vibration Greatness Level" (VGL) corresponding to loudness level (Phon) and "Vibration Greatness (VG) corresponding to loudness (Sone). The vibration affecting the hand is analysed by an octave band filter in the frequency range 0.5–300 Hz using 20 Hz as reference. Using this technique Miwa has produced a set of equal sensation contours for various VGL's.

For additional information on this subject, readers are referred to the list of references appended to this chapter, especially Hempstock

(1972), Keighley (1972), Walton (1972), Pelmear (1972b), James (1972), Angelova (1972), Reynolds (1972), Suggs (1972), O'Connor and Hempstock (1973), Thompson (1973) and BSI DD43 (1975).

TABLE III: Maximum admissible values of vibration transmitted to the hands for an 8 hr duration of vibration

| Octave centre frequency (Hz) | Maximum rms acceleration for 8 hr exposure (m/s$^2$) |
|---|---|
| 8 | 1.0 |
| 16 | 1.0 |
| 31.5 | 1.0 |
| 63 | 3.16 |
| 125 | 5.63 |
| 250 | 5.63 |
| 500 | 5.63 |

## B. FOOT AND STANDING VIBRATION

Hornick (1962b) conducted experiments to determine the effectiveness of human legs as low frequency vibration isolators over a 2 min time period. Six subjects stood on a vibration platform. Each subject experienced vertical vibration of 2–5 Hz at 2.54 cm peak-to-peak amplitude $\pm 0.21$ g and $\pm 1.3$ g peak accelerations. Results revealed that during the 2 min, the legs gradually lost their ability to isolate and increasing intensities of motion were found at head level.

In work by Ashley and Rao (1974) on an equal sensation study of differential vibration between feet and seat, five subjects were seated in a car seat without any restraints, and narrow band low frequency random body vibration was used as a reference to yield equal sensation contours for sinusoidal foot vibration in the frequency range of 2–20 Hz. The results of these experiments have shown that the equal sensation curve rises with frequency at an overall slope of 3 dB/octave. Another experiment using the same number of subjects was carried out in which the same random vibration level was applied as a reference to the feet and an equal sensation contour for sinusoidal body vibration was obtained. The data revealed that the judgment mechanisms of vibration sensation by the feet and the body are entirely different, particularly at high frequencies.

Miwa (1967b), using the method of paired comparisons to measure the threshold and equal sensation contours for whole-body vertical and horizontal vibrations on standing subjects, has constructed equal sensation curves over the frequency range 0.5–300 Hz, using 20 Hz as the standard vibration frequency. He found that the sensation for vertical vibration above 5 Hz was stronger than that for horizontal vibration by 13 dB.

Ashley (1970), using a narrow band random vibration stimulus as a reference, and sinusoidal vibrations for comparison, has shown that standing subjects exhibit a minimum sensitivity at 1.7 Hz with increased sensitivity towards 0.7 Hz. Maximum sensitivity occurred between 6 Hz and 15 Hz.

McKay (1971) has investigated the threshold of perception for whole-body vertical sinusoidal vibration in the frequency range of 1.5–100 Hz. He used both men and women subjects in the standing posture. He observed at 1.5 Hz, 2.5 Hz and 15 Hz significant differences between standing and sitting subjects, and at 6.5 Hz and 15 Hz between male and female subjects, males being generally more sensitive at these frequencies.

Jones and Saunders (1972), using the method of adjustment, whereby standing subjects equate two stimuli by active adjustment of one to match the other, have constructed equal comfort curves for men in the frequency range of 4–80 Hz. They used 20 Hz as a reference vibration frequency. They found good agreement with Ashley's results for frequencies below 10 Hz, but poor agreement for frequencies above 10 Hz.

The ISO standard is concerned with horizontal and vertical vibrations transmitted to the whole body through the feet of a standing man.

## C. SEATED VIBRATION

Clarke *et al.* (1962) have investigated the effects of forced sinusoidal vibration above 2 Hz, and at vector accelerations below 1 g, upon the human in the form of circumferential strain of chest, abdomen, pelvis and thigh, in the sitting erect and sitting relaxed positions.

The maximum body strain in the sitting positions occurred between 4 Hz and 6 Hz. The mean strains of chest and abdomen at resonance were found to be 0.02 in./in./g and 0.026 in./in./g respectively when standardised to a table acceleration of 1 g. The strain on the pelvis was 0.032 in./in./g in the sitting position.

Levels of threshold and equal sensation for both vertical and horizontal whole-body vibrations have been measured by Miwa (1967b) on seated subjects in erect and relaxed postures. He covered a frequency range of 0.5–300 Hz and up to 60 VAL (Vibration Acceleration Level, expressed in dB), using a reference frequency of 20 Hz. The curves of threshold for vertical and horizontal vibrations consist of four or five straight lines with varying slopes, respresenting jerk, acceleration, velocity and displacement. Also a difference of 10 dB in the vibration acceleration level between the vertical and horizontal thresholds has been reported. The contours of equal sensations for both vibrations above 5 Hz are composed of three lines with slope of acceleration, velocity and displacement with bending points at 5 Hz and 60 Hz. Below 5 Hz the equal sensation contours for horizontal vibration show considerably lower values than those for vertical vibration. The same studies were then extended to random vibrations of $\frac{1}{1}$ or $\frac{1}{3}$-octave bands in the frequency range of 2–250 Hz (Miwa, 1969). The difference in sensation between the vertical and horizontal whole-body vibration with $\frac{1}{1}$-octave band stimulation was examined and it was revealed that the sensation of the vertical vibration was equal to that of the horizontal vibration at frequencies above 16 Hz when the horizontal level was 10 dB higher.

The determination of the threshold of perception on male and female subjects, while sitting and standing, has been investigated by McKay (1971) in the frequency range of 1.5–100 Hz. His findings revealed that subjects were generally more sensitive while seated, and the result was statistically significant at the lowest vibration frequencies. In the region of 15–25 Hz subjects showed increased sensitivity while standing, and the result revealed a statistically significant difference at 15 Hz. The threshold of perception had a median of $\pm 0.003 \, A_z$ and interquartile range of $\pm 0.002$ to $\pm 0.004 A_z$ ($A_z$ being the acceleration in g experienced in the z-axis). The median was dependent on the frequency of vibration, there being statistically significant differences between ten frequency points within the range of 1.5–100 Hz.

The ISO standard (1974) is concerned with both vertical and horizontal vibrations transmitted to the body as a whole through the buttocks of a seated human. For vibration along the z-axis, it is suggested that the body, while standing or sitting, is most sensitive in acceleration terms to vibration in the frequency range 4–8 Hz, with a tolerance increasing at 3 dB/octave for lower frequencies and increasing by 6 dB/octave at higher frequencies. For the frequency range 8–80 Hz the standard is really one of constant sensitivity to root mean square velocity.

For vibration perpendicular to the body axis, the standard has a peak sensitivity in the frequency range 1–2 Hz. At higher frequencies constant sensitivity to velocity is again suggested. Comparison between horizontal and vertical vibration curves shows that the tolerance to horizontal vibration is lower below 5 Hz, but greater at higher frequencies.

Jones and Saunders (1972) employing a method of adjustment have derived equal comfort curves for whole-body vertical vibration in the frequency range 4–80 Hz for both men and women in an unrestrained sitting position. Significant differences were shown to exist between the response of male and female subjects at some of the vibration frequencies employed. At low frequencies and at low levels of vibration, women appear to be more sensitive than men. Above 30 Hz, women appear to be more sensitive than men. The effects on equal comfort contours of postural change between standing and sitting male subjects have resulted in the change of shape primarily at the lower frequencies. The subjects in the standing posture found they required a higher vibration level at frequencies below 10 Hz for equality of sensation of comfort with a 20 Hz refreence than did their seated counterparts.

Simić (1970) investigated the reaction of some ten seated male subjects to vertical sinusoidal vibration, using a Daimler–Benz car seat with an electrohydraulic vibrator covering a frequency range between 0.1 Hz and 50 Hz. His studies covered thresholds of perception and curves of "equal perception strength". The latter were obtained by subjective judgment of acceptable exposure durations from 10 min to 8 hr, and the results showed an increase in g from 0.2 Hz to 1 Hz, then levelled to 2.5 Hz, falling to a trough between 5 Hz and 25 Hz.

## D. HEAD VIBRATION

The human head is a vital member of our system. It not only incorporates very delicate and highly sensitive sensors but, also, in it is located the unique and unparalleled dynamic information centre, the brain, which receives, stores, retrieves, processes and controls all the information quickly and efficiently.

The head is considered as a very unstable member, possessing six degrees of freedom. A constant effort is therefore exerted by the vestibular system and certain other sections of the brain to stabilise its position while walking or riding in vehicles. Any impairment in this function due to any external disturbances may lead to undesirable effects.

In the transportation field it is now realised that the transmission of vibration to the head over a long period is a major disturbing factor. It reduces the driver's or pilot's dynamic visual acuity, which results in "tunnelling", and sometimes blurring, of vision. It also impairs short and long term memories, and affects both simple and complex reaction times. These are obviously undesirable effects while driving a car or piloting a helicopter.

Coermann (1962) has demonstrated the transmission of vibration from the seat to head of one subject over a frequency range of 1–20 Hz. His results show that the motions of the head are not the same as those of the effective mass of the body. The head resonates at around 5 Hz in the seated erect position. In the sitting relaxed posture the peak occurs at a lower frequency of 4.5 Hz and the damping for the transmission of vibrations to the head decreases. Above the main resonance the vibrations to the head are attenuated at a much faster rate. This, therefore, shows that in order to protect the head against vibrations at frequencies below 5 Hz it is better to assume the erect posture, and at frequencies above 5 Hz to relax the muscles and to bend the spine.

The transmission factor in the standing erect posture is very similar to the sitting erect posture, which proves that the stiff legs have no damping effect in the frequency range up to 20 Hz.

Studies by Von Gierke (1968) on a mechanical model of the human response to z-axis vibration have shown that the resonant frequency of the head lies around 25–30 Hz and resonant frequencies of the eyeball and intra-ocular structures lie in the region 30–90 Hz. Between 10 Hz and 30 Hz, numerous minor resonances of superficial body structures including the scalp and soft tissues of the face have been observed by Snyder et al. (1968).

When the seated subject is vibrated in y- or x-axis at frequencies in the region of 2 Hz, nodding of the head is reported by Hornick et al. (1961).

On a train, vertical vibrations of 3–4 Hz and lateral vibrations of 0.5–1.5 Hz at passengers' head level have been reported by Begbie et al. (1963).

In an experiment designed to determine the triaxial vibrations experienced by pilots in the scout helicopter, Griffin (1972) reports the following:

(a) The level of head vibration at a single frequency did not exceed 0.03 g rms in any axis.

(b) Lateral head vibration is less than vertical and horizontal vibration at almost all frequencies.

(c) Fore-and-aft head motions are of a similar magnitude to vertical motions.

(d) Vertical head vibration is greater than vertical seat vibration at frequencies between 2 Hz and 10 Hz.

(e) Anatomical differences between subjects have a significant influence on vibration transmission to the head.

In an experiment conducted by Rao et al. (1975) to investigate the effects of postural changes (standing erect and standing with knees bent) on the head response of eight standing subjects to low frequency "constant velocity" spectral inputs, in the frequency range 0.5–40 Hz, the following provisional conclusions were deduced:

(a) Irrespective of the posture adopted by the subjects, the spectra revealed the basic characteristics of a second-order mechanical system, with the first peak occurring in the region of 2–5.5 Hz and the second peak occurring in the region of 10–15 Hz.

(b) Transmissibility spectra showed non-linear trends for higher input levels, shifting the peaks towards higher frequencies.

(c) In the knees-bent posture, the resonant peaks seemed to drift towards the lower end of the frequency scale.

(d) In the knees-bent posture, human legs seemed to offer good vibration isolation of the head. However, at low inputs, human legs seemed to lose much of their isolation properties.

(e) Within the exposure duration considered (i.e. 1 min 30 sec) in this investigation, the vibration isolation properties of human legs appeared not to deteriorate with time.

The reaction of the human body to extremes of vibration has been studied by Magid and Coermann (1963). They revealed that the head sensations were first experienced at approximately 9 Hz and the sensations appeared to increase in violence up to 13 Hz after which they subsided considerably.

## E. EFFECTS AND CHARACTERISTICS OF SEATS

The seat is an important link between man and his machine. It is the opinion of many medical doctors and specialists that drivers of tractors, trucks and earth-moving equipment are exposed to excessive health hazards from the levels of shock and vibration. Seat design is therefore an important aspect of vehicle design. Its sole purpose is to improve the ride characteristics of the vehicle, thus affording better health, safety and efficiency to the occupants of the vehicle. The factors influencing the optimum vehicular seat design are: (a) shock and vibration, (b) static posture support, (c) static pressure distribution, (d) adequate seat adjustability and (e) seat ventilation.

Vehicle ride problems exist because of the different spring rates of the vehicles. Many vehicle-springs have natural frequencies in the range of 2–6 Hz. Unfortunately, the natural frequency of a driver on a conventional seat cushion occurs between 2.5–5 Hz. This resonance between the vehicle and seat cushion results in the occupants being subjected to greater vibration than occurs on the vehicle floor. This amplified rough ride imposes a limiting factor on the occupant, and may be felt as "fatigue" resulting in deterioration of task performance.

The transmission of vibration to the drivers of vehicles through the seats can be reduced. There are simple physical laws governing the behaviour of vibrating systems. They stipulate that the vehicle seat must have a natural frequency (with driver) below the disturbing frequency of the vehicle. The measure for vibration isolation is "transmissibility" and its relationship with the seat and vehicle natural frequencies is shown in Fig. 11. This indicates that vibration and shock

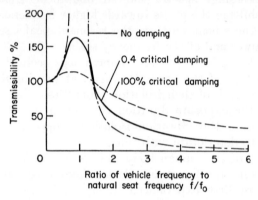

*Fig.* 11 Vibration transmissibility curves.

isolation can only be achieved if the natural frequency of the mass on the seat is lower than the exciting frequency by at least a factor of 2. This figure also shows the effect of viscous damping on transmissibility. Obviously damping is desirable only near resonances. For predominant vehicle frequencies of 2–5 Hz a seat frequency of 1 Hz would theoretically provide good isolation for the driver. Typical response curves for conventional and suspension seats are shown in Fig. 12. These curves reveal that the vehicle vibration may be amplified or attenuated at critical frequencies by the seat. As shown, foam and spring cushions tend to amplify the input motion at the low frequencies where man is most sensitive and where the vehicle vibration tends to be concentrated. Good suspension seats are designed to overcome this problem by elastically coupling the cushion to the vehicle by means of mechanical, pneumatic or hydro-pneumatic springs incorporating viscous damping.

This arrangement effectively lowers the resonant frequency of the seating system so that significant isolation is achieved at the predominant frequencies in the vehicle vibration spectrum. The subjective studies confirm that the human body can tolerate the highest amplitude in the 1–1.5 Hz frequency range of heart beat and walking frequencies and these are desirable seat frequencies for improving the vehicle ride.

Additional references on this subject include Clayberg (1949), Poulson and Elmer (1949), Fishbein and Salter (1950), McFarland and Strondt (1955), Haack (1956), Radke (1956), Simons *et al.* (1956), Chisholm (1968) and Stikeleather *et al.* (1972).

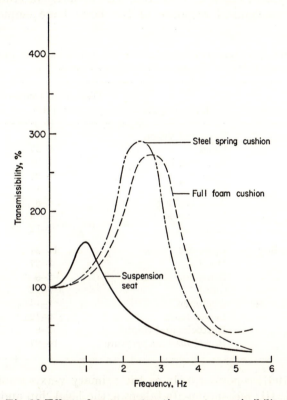

*Fig.* 12 Effect of seat construction on transmissibility.

## VI. Physiological Effects of Vibration

### A. NATURAL FREQUENCIES OF BODY ORGANS

The first modes of human body resonance in the z-axis occur at approximately 5 Hz and 12 Hz. The anatomical bases for these resonances are not yet clearly known. It has been concluded from transmissibility measurements that the 5 Hz resonance is due largely to the upper torso and the shoulder girdle. Using the impedance method and measurement of internal pressures in the lungs and abdomen, it has been demonstrated that at 4 Hz a major resonance of the thoraco-abdominal viscera occurs. It has been argued that this system is one of the most important resonant systems limiting the human tolerance to vibration. A third resonance has been reported as occurring in the range of 17–25 Hz, and attributed to resonant oscillation of the head with respect to the trunk. In the region of 30–40 Hz a resonance of the hand–arm system has been observed. The majority of studies investigating the mechanical response of the body have employed z-axis vibration.

TABLE IV: Concentration of disturbing sensations and ranges of frequencies for sitting and standing subjects

| Posture | Body organs | Disturbing frequencies (Hz) |
|---------|-------------|------------------------------|
| Sitting | Eyes and vision | 12–27 |
|         | Head | 8–27 |
|         | Face and jowl | 4–27 |
|         | Throat | 6–27 |
|         | Chest | 2–12 |
|         | Arms and legs | 2–8 |
|         | Lower back | 4–14 |
|         | Abdomen | 4–12 |
| Standing | Eyes and vision | 12–27 |
|         | Head | 8–27 |
|         | Arms and shoulders | 2–8 |
|         | Chest | 2–12 |
|         | Abdomen | 2–14 |
|         | Lower back | 6–12 |
|         | Buttocks and thighs | 2–8 |
|         | Bowel bladder pressure | 10–27 |

Woods (1967) reports 1.5 Hz as the primary y-axis resonance for a seated man. His measurements taken at the head, hip and knee show the greatest transmissibility for all three locations at this frequency.

In the x-axis, for seated subjects, Goldman and Von Gierke (1961) report that there are resonances at 1.5 Hz at the hip and 2 Hz at the head.

Since all critical resonant frequencies appear to be between 1 Hz and 3 Hz, the tolerances in the x- and y-axes should be based on this information.

Parks and Snyder (1960) and Chaney (1964) have developed extensive catalogues of the bodily resonances reported by seated subjects. Chaney (1965) has reported similar information for the standing subjects undergoing whole-body vibration. Table IV covers a brief summary of the findings of Parks and Snyder (1960) and Chaney (1964).

Von Gierke (1964) and Payne and Band (1971) have produced mechanical analogues of the human body based on physical measurements. The model presents the human body as a lumped parameter system composed of masses, springs and dampers. Such mathematical models and mechanical analogues describe the essential characteristics of the observations and allow insight into the reasons behind them.

## B. IMPEDANCE OF THE HUMAN BODY

Impedance techniques have been in use for many years in solving electrical network problems, and recently their application has been extended to study mechanical structures. Impedance measurements are also extremely important for the synthesis of human analogues.

Measurements of the body's mechanical impedance help in describing mechanical energy transmission to a complex bio-mechanical system.

When an alternating force is applied to the body, the mechanical impedance is defined as the ratio of the transmitted force to the velocity of the point at which the force is applied.

The general impedance concept is ordinarily used in conditions where the motion is linear but applies equally well for angular motions or combinations of linear and angular motions.

For the steady-state sinusoidal input vibration

$$\text{Impedance} = \frac{\text{force}}{\text{velocity}} = Z(\omega)$$

and

$$Z(\omega) = \frac{F(\omega)}{V(\omega)} = \frac{F \sin(\omega t + p_f)}{V \sin(\omega t + p_v)}$$

or

$$Z(\omega) = \frac{(R_f(\omega) + jI_f(\omega))}{(R_v(\omega) + jI_v(\omega))}$$

where

$$\omega = 2\pi f$$

and

$p_v$ = phase reference for velocity

$p_f$ = phase reference for force

$R_f$ = real part of complex representation of force

$R_v$ = real part of complex representation of velocity

$I_f$ = imaginary part of complex representation of force

$I_v$ = imaginary part of complex representation of velocity

$F$ = peak value of force

$V$ = peak value of velocity

In the case of the steady-state non-sinusoidal excitation it is necessary to resolve the force and velocity waveforms into a finite series (Fourier) of sinusoidal components in order to solve the above equations.

$$F(n\omega_f) = \frac{1}{T} \int_{-\frac{1}{2}T}^{+\frac{1}{2}T} f(t) \exp(-jn\omega_f t)\, dt$$

$$V(n\omega_f) = \frac{1}{T} \int_{-\frac{1}{2}T}^{+\frac{1}{2}T} v(t) \exp(-jn\omega_f t)\, dt$$

where

    $n$ = number of harmonic

    $T$ = period, in sec

    $\omega_f$ = fundamental angular frequency, in radians/sec

In the case of random excitation, it is still possible to calculate the impedance by dealing with auto and cross-correlation functions of force and velocity. These functions are actually definitions of the average characteristics of the signals and are indicated below.

$$\phi_{fv}(T) = \frac{1}{A} \int_0^A f(t)\, v(t+T)\, dt$$

$$\phi_{vv}(T) = \frac{1}{A} \int_0^A v(t)\, v(t+T)\, dt$$

$$\phi_{fv}(\omega) = \tfrac{1}{2}\pi \int_{-B}^{+B} \phi_{fv}(T) \exp(-j\omega T)\, dT$$

$$\phi_{vv}(\omega) = \tfrac{1}{2}\pi \int_{-B}^{+B} \phi_{vv}(T) \exp(-j\omega T)\, dT$$

$$Z(\omega) = \frac{\phi_{fv}(\omega)}{\phi_{vv}(\omega)} = \frac{F(\omega)\,\overline{V(\omega)}}{V(\omega)\,\overline{V(\omega)}} = \frac{F(\omega)}{V(\omega)}$$

where

  $\phi_{fv}(T)$ = cross-correlation between force and velocity

  $\phi_{vv}(T)$ = auto-correlation function of velocity

  $\phi_{fv}(\omega)$ = cross-power density spectrum between force and velocity

  $\phi_{vv}(\omega)$ = power density spectrum of velocity

    $A$ = length (in time) of the record of force and velocity and must be sufficient to provide a significant estimate

    $B$ = maximum value of $T$

  $\overline{V(\omega)}$ = complex conjugate of $V(\omega)$

Since the human body reacts like a complex mass–spring–damper system, it shows two resonant peaks at 5 Hz and 11 Hz. From these peaks the effective masses, elasticities and damping factors at these

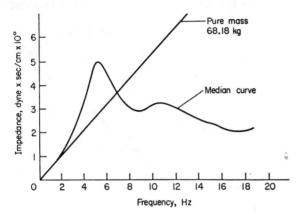

*Fig.* 13 A typical human impedance curve.

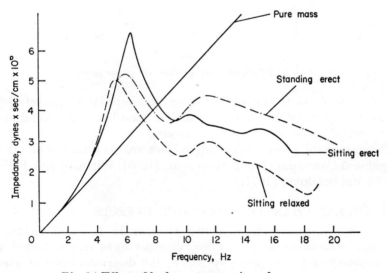

*Fig.* 14 Effect of body posture on impedance curve.

frequencies can be calculated. A typical human impedance curve is shown in Fig. 13. The impedance curve changes significantly for different postures as shown in Fig. 14. The phase between the translated force and the velocity of the vibrating table similarly undergoes changes with posture as shown in Fig. 15 (Coermann, 1962).

Edwards and Lange (1964) have investigated the impedances of the supine, lateral and standing positions of humans. They have also illustrated the manner in which impedance varies with muscle tone. Non-linearity of the human body has been shown to exist.

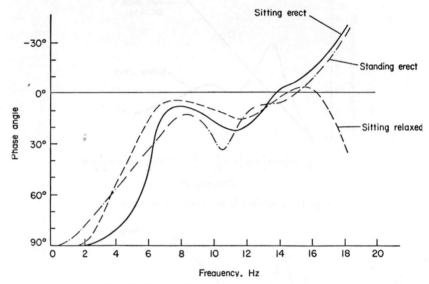

*Fig.* 15 Effect of body posture on phase angle.

Using steady-state sinusoidal testing, the impedance characteristics of the human hand in a working configuration have been determined by Suggs (1972) for the translatory modes.

Further useful references on this subject are Coermann *et al.* (1960), Magid and Coermann (1960), Weis *et al.* (1966), Wittman and Phillips (1969) and Sandover (1971).

## C. VASCULAR CHANGES AND OTHER EFFECTS

Histological studies have shown changes in the architecture of vascular connective tissues. These changes have demonstrated the vulnerability of the vascular system to the destructiveness of whole-body vibrations. It has also been recently suggested that direct mechanical excitation is only part of the pathogenesis of the trauma and that other factors such as hormonal imbalance resulting from vibration also play a part.

The pathological consequences of vibration on vegetative functions have been well documented (Clayberg, 1949; Paulson and Elmer, 1949; Fishbein and Salter, 1950; Rosseger and Rosseger, 1960).

Berthoz (1972) has investigated the activity induced by low frequency vibration (0–20 Nz) in striated and smooth muscle. Some of his main findings are noted below:

(a) The electromyographic (EMG) rhythmic activity of the para-vertebral and neck musculature are closely related to the occurrence of the mechanical resonance of the body (4–5 Hz).

(b) There exists a relationship between EMG activity and head movement.

(c) A study of the behaviour of normal and pathological (cerebellar, parkinsonian) subjects revealed that the resonance observed at 4–5 Hz was dependent on central nervous mechanisms as well as peripheral mechanical factors.

(d) It was demonstrated in a cat that low frequency vibration (10 Hz) could act on the peristaltic activity of the ureter (smooth muscle).

Curister and Harding (1973) have recently carried out some physiological measurements of muscle responses to whole-body vertical vibration.

Preliminary investigations into the effects of vibration and other stresses on human steroid excretion have been carried out by Cole (1973). He has offered some suggestions as to how the results obtained from this study might be applied to help evaluate the effects of these stresses on humans.

Hoover and Ashe (1962) have studied respiratory function during extended vibration exposures in the z-axis. Their results indicate that respiratory minute volume changes observed in subjects are a function of both respiratory rate and tidal volume.

Nerem (1973) has investigated the fluid dynamic aspects of cardio-vascular behaviour during low frequency whole-body vibration. The results are included of studies of the effects of vibration on the work done by the heart on pulsatile flow in blood vessels. It is shown that important changes in pulse velocity, the instantaneous velocity profile, mass flow rate and wall shear stress may occur in pulsatile flow due to the presence of vibration.

Supine whole-body x-axis sinusoidal vibration in humans was found to produce increases in mean arterial blood pressure, heart rate, cardiac output, oxygen consumption and minute volume of ventilation. These physiological effects were more marked at 1.2 Hz peak acceleration than at 0.6 g and at 8 Hz and 10 Hz than at frequencies to either side of this range (Hood et al., 1966). However, no drop in arterial pressure was found in seated (restrained) subjects when vibrated in the x-axis (Clark et al., 1967).

## VII. Ride Indices and Vibration in Transport

Passenger comfort during ride situations is mainly influenced by (a) the nature of the medium on which, or through which, the vehicle travels, (b) the nature of the propulsion system, (c) the environmental factors, such as heat, noise, humidity, dynamic forces resulting from starting, stopping and steering the vehicle, (d) psychological and physiological factors and (e) many other factors discussed earlier in this chapter. On account of these multi-dimensional effects, the problem of evaluating ride comfort has become extremely complex and an optimum solution could only be achieved through multi-disciplinary co-operation and effort. In the past, various criteria have been established and new criteria are being proposed in the light of improved methodology and techniques. It is the aim of this section to cover some of these aspects in brief.

### A. MEDIUM-INDUCED VIBRATION

The effects of road surface roughness on the design and operation of road-using vehicles have been evaluated for quite some time. Early attempts were made in the motor industry to study this problem and consisted of subjecting mathematical models to deterministic inputs. Later on, better methods of measuring and recording actual surface profiles were developed mainly by the aircraft industry in an attempt to classify runway profiles. At the same time the U.S. Army were developing statistical techniques to classify surface roughness of different terrains. The statistical determination of surface roughness appears to be very promising in the study of the behaviour of humans and vehicles while traversing road surfaces.

Data on road surface measurements are to be found in Walls *et al.* (1954), Craggs and Colledge (1964), Pevzner and Tikhonov (1964), Braun (1966), Loebich (1967), Van Deusen (1967), Parkhilovski (1968), Dodds (1969), Kanashige (1969) and Dodds and Robson (1970, 1972, 1973). A review of the existing literature on surface roughness measurements suggests that roads can be described in terms of their vertical amplitude power spectral density. Studies of a large number of power spectra for different roads reveal that the majority of roads can be approximated by a simple power law, namely,

$$S(n) = S(n_0) \left(\frac{n}{n_0}\right)^{-w}$$

where

$S(n)$ = power spectral density (psd) at a frequency $n$

$S(n_0)$ = power spectral density (psd) at a frequency $n_0$

$n_0$ = fixed datum frequency, in cycles/m

$n$ = variable frequency, in cycles/m

$w$ = integer exponent

Investigations at the Motor Industries Research Association, Nuneaton (La Barre *et al.*, 1970), have revealed that a road could better be described by its power spectrum at a particular frequency by exponents of slope. Based on this the BSI panel has recently put forward a proposal for "Generalised Terrain Inputs to Vehicles (BSI, 1972).

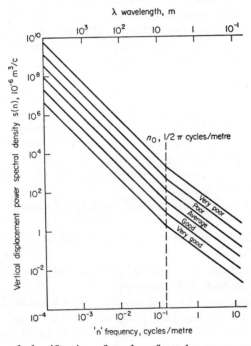

*Fig.* 16 Proposed classification of road surfaces by power spectral density.

Figure 16 is the proposed classification of road surfaces by the BSI panel MEE/158/3/1. As can be seen from this figure

$$n_0 = \frac{1}{2\pi} \text{ cycles/m}$$

Also,

$$S(n) = S(n_0) \left(\frac{n}{n_0}\right)^{-w_1} \quad \text{for } n \leqslant n_0$$

and

$$S(n) = S(n_0) \left(\frac{n}{n_0}\right)^{-w_2} \quad \text{for } n \geqslant n_0$$

$S(n)$ is the basic roughness exponent and is measured in units of $10^{-6}\ \mathrm{m^3/cycle}$. The values of $w_1$ and $w_2$ are fixed at 2 and 1.5 respectively. The figure also shows the completely contradictory significance of $w_1$ and $w_2$.

Looking at Fig. 16 it is clear that for this part of the spectrum the amplitude squared is proportional to the wavelength. This is because wavelength is inversely proportional to frequency, and, for a given vehicle velocity, the average road is approximated by an amplitude spectral density inversely proportional to frequency. This is an important concept which means that the vertical velocity input power spectral density to a vehicle traversing a road is "white". Hence the usage of the term "constant velocity" inputs.

The following assumptions have been made by various authors during the evaluation of road surface roughness:

(a) The road profile $y(x)$ is assumed to be a member-function of a stationary ergodic random process $\{y(x)\}$. However, there is limited evidence which points to the fact that the vehicle vibration environment generated by travelling over a section of motorway is non-stationary and non-ergodic.

(b) The amplitude distribution of road undulations is assumed to be Gaussian.

(c) The vehicle is assumed to have travelled at constant velocity and in a straight line.

(d) The effects of any obstacles (e.g. potholes), cornering and accelerating loads have been ignored.

In spite of the above limitations, the proposed classification of road surface roughness by the BSI panel does seem to offer some useful guidelines for conducting meaningful evaluations of human response to vibration in transportation.

## B. RIDE INDICES

### 1. *Road Vehicles*

One of the first attempts to tackle the problem of human comfort was by Reiher and Meister (1931), followed in 1935 by Meister alone. In the final test programme Meister tested 15 subjects by exposing them for 15 min to various sinusoidal frequencies and amplitudes. At the end of the test periods the subjects were asked to classify their reaction in one of a number of categories, ranging from "not perceptible" to "very unpleasant". The one conclusion stated was that the dividing lines between the categories was drawn on the basis of mean velocity of vibration, $V = 2df$, where $d =$ the total amplitude of vibration and $f =$ the frequency.

Lemair, of the University of Lyons, France, made some progress along the above lines by setting up a seat on a vibrator platform which was driven sinusoidally in the vertical direction. His conclusion was that the feeling of comfort or discomfort depended upon the time rate of variation of acceleration called "jerk".

Investigations were carried out by Jacklin and Liddell (1933) who observed the reactions of subjects to vibration when sitting on a controlled vibrating seat, and in moving vehicles. The subjective sensations were categorised as "perceptible", "disturbing" and "uncomfortable". The results of the tests carried out with subjects seated on hard seats was then represented by the equation

$$K = A \exp(0.6f)$$

where

$$K = \text{constant called "comfort index"}$$

$$A = \text{maximum acceleration, m/sec}^2$$

$$e = \text{basis of natural logarithms}$$

$$f = \text{frequency of vibration, Hz}$$

When dealing with vertical, longitudinal and horizontal vibration, the maximum $K_c$ value is given by the vector sum

$$K_c = \sqrt{(K_v{}^2 + K_L{}^2 + K_T{}^2)}$$

Jacklin (1936) used a "control group" comprising about 35 people in test rides in a dozen different automobiles on various types of roads. A Purdue accelerometer mounted on a dummy was used to measure vibration. With the "control" subject seated beside the dummy, the car speed was increased on a selected road until the subject observed the "disturbing" reaction. Accelerometer records obtained in the three directions (x-, y- and z-axes) were analysed for maximum acceleration ($A$) and calculations were made involving the waveforms and time record for frequency ($f$). Using this technique they evaluated an index $D$ which is expressed as

$$D = 4.5 = A \exp(0.045f) - 0.9 \cos 1.57f$$

If $D > 4.5$, the ride was considered to be "disturbing".

9

Janeway (1950) reviewed the available data on this subject. After studying them, he proposed an empirical curve to fit one of Meister's bands, above which vibrations caused undue discomfort and fatigue. In producing this curve, Janeway divided the curve into three sections, covering frequency bands in the region of 1–6 Hz, 6–20 Hz and 20–60 Hz. He further stated that, for the lowest band, the jerk value was the criterion, for the middle band, the acceleration and, for the upper band, the criterion was the velocity.

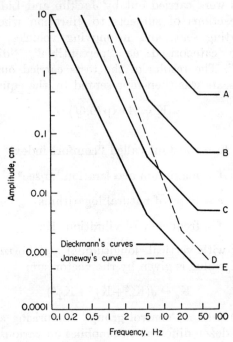

*Fig.* 17 Dieckmann's and Janeway's comfort curves: A, not admissible; B, tolerable for short periods; C, acceptable level; D, Janeway's limit curve; E, threshold level.

Dieckmann (1958) conducted a similar series of tests to Meister. Like Janeway, he also proposed an empirical method of assessing the degree of comfort, and broke the curve into three frequency bands 0–5 Hz, 5–40 Hz and 40–100 Hz. He suggested that, for the lowest band, the acceleration was the criterion, for the middle band, the velocity and, for the upper band, the displacement. Both the Janeway curve and the Dieckmann comfort criterion are shown in Fig. 17.

Ranking and rating scale techniques of measurement have been applied to the vehicle ride problem by Aspinall (1960) and Aspinall and Oliver (1964) of MIRA with some success. The same authors carried out some work on the effects of roll and pitch judgment (Aspinall and Oliver, 1967). They found some correlation between these two at frequencies below 7 Hz, when displacement amplitude would be large. Refer also to Cooper (1973). Jensen (see Versace, 1962) made the first attempt to scale ride intensity along the dimension of amplitude level. In this study, two subjects made cross-modality matchings of noise to sine wave vertical vibration of a vibrator while seated on it. This technique was extended by Versace (1962). His findings revealed that

$$\text{Ride sensation} = CA^q$$

where

$C$ = scale factor

$A$ = acceleration in g units

$q = 3.7$ at 2 Hz;   10 at 5 Hz;   3.3 at 10 Hz

This technique was also used by Van Deusen (1968).

Fine (1964) reported a correlation between comfort and vehicle acceleration on the road. He measured the slope of the acceleration versus time plot and correlated this with subjective judgments. He concluded that an accurate correlation could be found between acceleration slope and observed ride differences.

Pradko and Lee (1966) developed a new criterion called "absorbed power" based on the application of transfer functions applied to randomly varying vibration conditions. This is defined mathematically as

$$\text{Averaged ``absorbed power''} = \lim_{t \to \infty} \frac{1}{t} \int_0^t F(t)\, V(t)\, dt$$

where

$F(t)$ = input force

$V(t)$ = input velocity

The authors claim that the subjective human response may be accurately described by this technique. Also "absorbed power" describes human response quantitatively in stationary random environments. Kawai and Morisaki (1965) adopted the power spectral density (psd) technique to examine the road vibration and ride comfort of cars. They related the ride comfort $C(f)$ due to vertical vibration of cars to road surface, car, seat and human being and exposed $C(f)$ as

$$C(f) = |A_H(f)|^2 |A_s(f)|^2 |A(f)|^2 P_x(f)$$

where $A_H(f)$, $A_s(f)$ and $A(f)$ represent the frequency response functions of human being, seat and the vehicle respectively, and $P_x(f)$ is the psd of road roughness.

Butkunas (1968) proposed that the concepts of psd and transfer functions be applied to random vibrations. The two main advantages of this method are (a) it gives a single number representation of the comfort achieved and (b) it gives a detailed comfort picture.

Tokuda et al. (1972) have evaluated harshness (which is a typical transient interdisciplinary phenomenon of noise and vibration) and shake, which are considered as non-stationary vibrations, using a paired comparison method and linear regression analysis. They have shown that harshness could approximately be determined by knowing the characteristics of tyre and suspension fore-and-aft compliance.

## 2. Rail Studies

Helberg and Sperling (1941) evaluated the riding quality of railcars on some 25 experienced subjects. The tests lasted from 2 min to 10 min, after which they assessed the discomfort they experienced. From the results the comfort index $W_z$ was derived, using the formula

$$W_z = 0.896 \sqrt[10]{\frac{A^3}{f}}$$

where

$A$ = peak of amplitude acceleration, m/sec²

$f$ = frequency, Hz

Sperling and Betzholt (1957) introduced a correction factor into the above formula to account for human reactions. The corrected formula is

$$W_z = 2.7 \sqrt[10]{[A^3 f^5 F(f)]}$$

where

$F(f)$ = correction factor as a function of frequency

Since the riding quality is not uniform over a long distance, even if the speed remains constant, it was considered necessary to evaluate the mean value, $W_{z_m}$, as the ride index.

$$W_{z_m} = \sqrt[10]{\left(\frac{L_1 W_{z_1}{}^{10} + L_2 W_{z_2}{}^{10} + L_3 W_{z_3}{}^{10} + \dots}{L_1 + L_2 + L_3}\right)}$$

where

$L_1, L_2, \dots$ = lengths of different sections of test run

$W_{z_1}, W_{z_2}, \dots$ = comfort indices

Mauzin and Sperling (1951) evolved curves of equal comfort and equal fatigue from which it is possible to convert acceleration data into the amount of time after which an "average" passenger will feel a definite sense of fatigue.

Under varying conditions, but at constant speed, the average overall fatigue time $T$ is calculated as shown by

$$T = \frac{t_1 + t_2 + t_3 + \dots}{(t_1/T_1) + (t_2/T_2) + (t_3/T_3) + \dots} = \frac{l_1 + l_2 + l_3 + \dots}{(l_1/T_1) + (l_2/T_2) + (l_3/T_3) + \dots}$$

where $t_1$, $t_2$ etc. are the durations of time of the measurements during which the fatigue times $T_1$, $T_2$ etc. were recorded. Since the runs were made at constant speed the distances $l_1$, $l_2$ etc. are proportional to $t_1$, $t_2$ etc. The above technique was later adapted by Loach (1958) for the assessment of passenger vehicles.

In conclusion, it could be said that up to now no foolproof method of evaluating riding comfort has been established.

## VIII. Measurement Techniques

Measuring, recording, analysing and controlling physical, physiological and psychological variables are basic essentials in the study of the overall behaviour of man–machine systems. This is particularly so in the field of human response to shock and vibration. As a result of this, measurement techniques in existence are so varied and sophisticated that, as yet, there have been no attempts to bring out any agreed national or international standards. Doubtless such a standard is, however, desirable as it would offer a solution to the difficulty of providing a homogeneous body of information which would be acceptable for collective study and analyses.

Measurement systems, in general, comprise the following:
(a) signal generators
(b) signal shapers
(c) power amplifiers

(d) vibration exciters

(e) sensing devices

(f) matching devices and amplifiers

(g) signal processors.

An overall system description is shown in Fig. 18. Using the facilities shown in this figure it should be possible to measure and carry out the following:

(a) displacement, velocity and acceleration

(b) mobility, impedance, transmissibility

(c) power spectral density measurements and random process analyses

(d) statistical analyses

(e) ride comfort

(f) physiological measurements and analyses

(g) reaction times.

The choice of a measuring system depends upon ones particular needs. Factors affecting the choice of instrumentation are:

(a) the dynamic range of vibrations encountered

(b) the nature and number of parameters to be measured

(c) the location from which the measurements are taken

(d) compatibility, operational adaptability and reliability

(e) weight and size.

Before setting up a particular measuring system, it would be advisable to give further consideration to the following:

(a) analytical capabilities of the system of interest

(b) degree of flexibility in computation

(c) means available for the control of measurement resolution and statistical uncertainty.

It should be mentioned at this stage that a "Working Group" representing Universities and State and Private research bodies who are interested in the field of human response to vibration has recently prepared a draft guide to the safety aspects of human vibration experiments, which is being issued as BSI DD23 (BSI, 1973). This guide is divided into four main sections. Section 1 considers the general ethical and medical aspects of this type of experimental work. Section 2 deals with vibration-generating equipment and recommends certain minimum safeguards that should be applied. Section 3 deals with the restrictions which should be placed on the choice of subject, depending upon the degree of vibration being used. Section 4 sets out experimental procedures so that the subject and other personnel are not exposed to unnecessary risk.

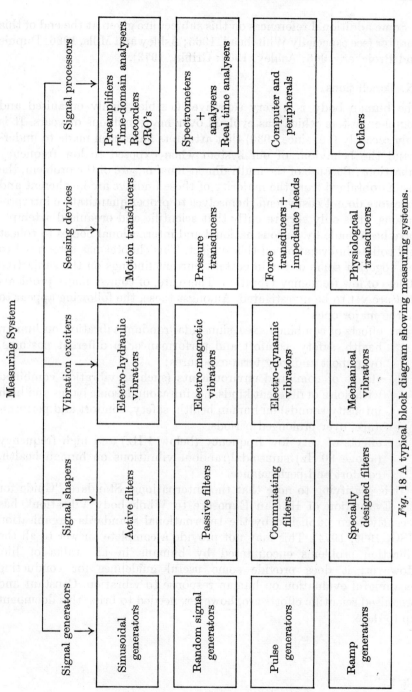

*Fig.* 18 A typical block diagram showing measuring systems.

Some additional references on this subject are given at the end of this chapter (see especially Whitehead, 1965; Ashley and Mills, 1966; Dupuis and Broicher, 1966; Ashley, 1969; Griffin, 1973).

## IX. Conclusions

The human body is a very sensitive, flexible, highly organised and complex system which has evolved over many millions of years. It is only recently (i.e. since 1930) that attempts have been made to understand the behaviour of our system when exposed to low frequency vibrations. Because of the multi-dimensional nature of the problem, the results obtained from the majority of these findings are incoherent and therefore do not easily lend themselves to proper quantitative interpretations. It is only very recently that scientific and organised attempts have been made by various national and international bodies to collect and collate information on this subject. This chapter has attempted to put together some of the important current findings on the subjective effects of low frequency vibration. There are, of course, many problems that are yet to be investigated. Amongst these, the following appear to be the major ones:

(a) effects of combined axes, sinusoidal/random vibration on human health, safety, comfort and performance, in different postures, over short and long term exposures;

(b) effects of combined environments (such as vibration combined with noise of different kinds, i.e. infrasound, sonic bangs and high intensity sounds) on human health, safety, comfort and performance, over prolonged periods.

(c) effects of very low frequency (below 1 Hz) and high frequency (above 80 Hz) sinusoidal/random vibrations on human health, comfort and performance.

It is gratifying to note that the International Standard "Guide for the Evaluation of Human Exposure to Whole-body Vibration" has recently been published by the International Standards Organisation (ISO, 1969, 1974). This may not provide a complete answer to all the vibration problems encountered by humans in all walks of life. However, it does provide some useful guidelines for conducting meaningful evaluation on human response to vibration. Constant and organised scientific efforts are, however, needed to bring this document up to date.

REFERENCES

Agate, J. N. and Druett, H. A. (1946). *British Journal of Industrial Medicine* **3**, 159–166.

Angelova, M. (1972). "General Review of Latest Research on Vibration Induced Occupational Diseases at the Institute of Hygiene, Sofia, Bulgaria", Paper presented at the International Conference on Hand-Arm Vibration, University of Dundee, July.

Ashley, C. (1969). "Simulation of the Vehicle Ride Environment in the Laboratory", Paper presented at Transpo' 69, Symposium of Society of Environmental Engineers, London, May.

Ashley, C. (1970). "Equal Annoyance Contours for the effect of Sinusoidal Vibration on Man", Paper presented at the Human Response to Vibration Conference, Loughborough University, September.

Ashley, C. and Mills, B. (1966). *Journal of Mechanical Engineering Science* **8** (1), 27–35.

Ashley, C. and Rao, B. K. N. (1974). *Ergonomics* **17** (3), 331–342.

Aspinall, D. T. (1960). Motor Industries Research Association, U.K., Report No. 1960/4.

Aspinall, D. T. and Oliver, R. J. (1964). Motor Industries Research Association, U.K., Report No. 1964/10.

Aspinall, D. T. and Oliver, R. J. (1967). "The Correlation between Subjective Assessments of Vehicle Ride and Handling", *I. Mech. E. and A.S.A.E. Symposium*, July.

Barnes, G. R. and Rance, B. H. (1975). "Head Movement induced by Angular Oscillation of the Human Body in the Pitch and Roll Axes". U.K. Group Meeting on Human Response to Vibration. Southampton.

Begbie, G. H., Gainford, J., Mansfield, P., Stirling, J. M. M. and Walsh, E. G. (1963). *Journal of Physiology* **165**, 72–73.

Bendat, J. S. (1958). "Principles and Applications of Random Noise Theory", John Wiley and Sons, New York.

Bendat, J. S. and Piersol, A. G. (1964). "Design Considerations and Use of Analogue Power Spectral Density Analysers", Honeywell, Denver Division.

Bendat, J. S. and Piersol, A. G. (1965). "Measurement and Analysis of Random Data", John Wiley and Sons, New York.

Benson, A. J. (1972). "Effect of Angular Oscillation in Yaw on Vision". Paper presented at the Human Response to Vibration Conference, University of Sheffield, September.

Berthoz, A. (1972). "Striated and Smooth Muscle Activity during Low Frequency Vibration", Paper presented at the Human Response to Vibration Conference, University of Sheffield, September.

Blackman, R. B. and Tukey, J. W. (1958). "Measurement of Power Spectra", Dover Publication, New York.

Braun, H. (1966). Untersuchungen über *Fahrbahnuneben Heiten. Deut. Kraft.* No. 186.

British Standards Institution (1972). "Generalised Terrain Inputs to Vehicles", Proposal of BSI Panel MEE/158/3/1, Document 72/34562.

British Standards Institution (1973). "Guide to the Safety Aspects of Human Vibration Experiments", BSI DD 23; 1973.

British Standards Institution (1974). "Guide to the Evaluation of Human Exposure to Whole-body Vibration", BSI DD 32; 1974.

British Standards Institution (1975). "Guide to the Evaluation of Exposure of the Human Hand–Arm System to Vibration", BSI DD 43; 1975.

Bulger, P. M. J. (1972). "The Effects of Random Vibration on the 'Tunnel Vision' Phenomenon", Paper presented at the Human Response to Vibration Conference, University of Sheffield, September.

Butkunas, A. A. (1968). "Power Spectral Density and Ride Evaluation", Society of Automotive Engineers Report No. 660139, January, U.S.A.

Chaney, R. E. (1964). "Subjective Reaction to Whole-body Vibration", The Boeing Co. Wichita, Kansas, Document D3-6474, September.

Chaney, R. E. (1965). "Whole-body Vibration of Standing Subjects", The Boeing Co. Wichita, Kansas, Document D3-6779, August.

Chisholm C. J. (1968). *Design and Components in Engineering*, September.

Clark, W. S., Lange, R. O. and Coermann, R. R. (1962). *Human Factors* **4** (5), 255–274.

Clark, J. G., Williams, J. D., Hood, W. B. (Jr.) and Murray, R. H. (1967). *Aerospace Medicine* **38**, 464–467.

Clarke, M. J. and Oborne, D. J. (1975). 1975 Ride Quality Symposium. NASA TM X-3295, 267–286.

Clayberg, H. D. (1949). *Military Surgeon*, October 299–311.

Coermann, R. R. (1962). *Human Factors* **4** (5), 227–253.

Coermann, R. R., Magid, E. B. and Lange, K. O. (1962). *Human Factors* **4** (5), 315–324.

Coermann, R. R., Ziegenruecker, G. H., Wittwer, A. L. and von Gierke, H. E. (1960). *Aerospace Medicine* **31**, 443–455.

Cole, S. H. (1973). "A Preliminary Study into the Effects of Abnormal Environments on Human Steroid Excretion", Paper presented at the Human Response to Vibration Conference. University of Salford, September.

Cooper, D. R. (1973). M.Phil. Thesis, London University.

Craggs, A. and Colledge, R. B. (1964). Motor Research Association, U.K., Report No. 1964/9.

Crandall, S. H. (1963). "Random Vibration", Technology Press and John Wiley and Sons, New York.

Curister, M. C. and Harding, R. H. (1973). "Some Physiological Measurements of the Human Response to Vertical Vibration", Paper presented at the Human Response to Vibration Conference, University of Salford, September.

Dennis, J. P. (1960). "The Effect of Whole-body Vibration on a Visual Performance Task", Directorate of Physiological and Biological Research, Report No. 104, C.E.P.R.E. (U.K.), AD 247, 249.

Dieckmann, D. (1958). *Ergonomics* **1** (4), 347–355.

Dodds, C. J. (1969). "The Laboratory Simulation of Vehicle Service Stress", Department of Mechanical Engineering Report, University of Glasgow.

Dodds, C. J. and Robson, J. D. (1970). "The Response of Vehicle Components to Random Road-surface Undulations", FISITA Paper 17.2.D, Brussels.

Dodds, C. J. and Robson, J. D. (1972). *Journal of Automotive Engineering*, April 17–19.

Dodds, C. J. and Robson, J. D. (1973). *Journal of Sound and Vibration* **31** (2), 175–183.

Dupuis, H. and Broicher, H. A. (1966). *A.T.Z.* **68** (2), 41–44.

Dupuis, H., Hartung, E. and Louda, L. (1972). RAE Library Translation No. 1603.

Edwards, R. G. and Lange, K. O. (1964). Aeromedical Research Laboratory, Report AMRL–TR–64–91.

Fine, R. (1964). *Society of Automotive Engineers Journal* **72**, 101–103.

Fishbein, W. I. and Salter, L. C. (1950). *Industrial Medicine and Surgery* **19** (9), 444–445.

Fleming, D. B. and Griffin, M. J. (1975). *Journal of Sound and Vibration* **42** (4), 453–461.

Garner, W. R. (1954). *Journal of the Acoustical Society of America* **26**, 73.

Goldman, D. E. and Von Gierke, H. R. (1961). *In*: "Shock and Vibration Handbook" (C. M. Harris and C. E. Crede, eds.), Vol. 3, Chapter 44, McGraw-Hill Book Co., New York.

Griffin, M. J. (1972). Institute of Sound and Vibration Research, Report No. 58, University of Southampton, August.

Griffin, M. J. (1973). Institute of Sound and Vibration Research, Report No. 60, University of Southampton, March.

Griffin, M. J. (1975). "A Study of the Subjective Equivalence of Sinusoidal and Random Whole-body Vibration". U.K. Group Meeting on Human Response to Vibration. Southampton.

Guignard, J. C. and Irving, A. (1960). *Engineering* **190**, 364–367.

Guignard, J. C. and King, P. F. (1972). AGARDograph No. 151, November, NATO.

Haack, M. (1956). *Agricultural Engineering* **37** (4), 253–257.

Helberg, W. and Sperling, E. (1941). *Organ für die Fortschritte des Eisenbahnwagen* **96**, 177–187.

Hempstock, T. I. (1972). "The Vibration Characteristics of Several Engineering Processes Producing White Fingers", Paper presented at the International Conference on Hand–Arm Vibration. University of Dundee, July.

Hempstock, T. I. and Saunders, D. J. (1976). *Journal of Sound and Vibration* **46** (2), 279–284.

Hood, W. B. (Jr.), Murray, R. H., Urschel, C. W., Bowers, J. A. and Clark, J. C. (1966). *Journal of Applied Physiology* **21** (6), 1725–1731.

Hoover, G. N. and Ashe, W. F. (1962). *Aerospace Medicine* **33**, 980–984.

Hornick, R. J. (1962a). *Journal of Engineering Psychology* **1**, 93–101.

Hornick, R. J. (1962b). *Human Factors* **4** (5), 301–304.

Hornick, R. J., Boettcher, C. A. and Simons, A. K. (1961). Bostram Research Laboratories Final Report, Ordnance Project TE–1000.

International Organisation for Standardisation (1969). ISO Document ISO/TC 108/WG 7 (CSSR–4) 26.

International Organisation for Standardisation (1974). ISO Standard 2631, "Guide for the Evaluation of Human Exposure to Whole-body Vibration".

Jacklin, H. M. (1936). *SAE Transactions* **39**, 401–407.

Jacklin, H. M. and Liddel, G. J. (1933). *Engineering Bulletin*. Research Series No. 44, Purdue University.

James, P. B. (1972). "Arteriography and the Vibration Syndrome", Paper presented at the International Conference on Hand–Arm Vibration, University of Dundee, July.

Janeway, R. N. (1950). "Ride and Vibration Data", SAE Publication, 2nd edn. Society of Automotive Engineers, U.S.A.

Jones, A. J. and Saunders, D. J. (1972). *Applied Acoustics* **5** (4), 279–300.

Jones, A. J. (1973). Ph.D. Thesis, University of Salford.

Kanashige, I. (1969). Society of Automotive Engineers, Paper No. 690111, U.S.A.

Kawai, H. and Morisaki, K. (1965). *Technical Review* 58–67, May.

Keighley, G. D. (1970). "Vibration Effects on Chain Saw Operators—Remedial Measures adopted by the Forestry Commission", Paper presented at the Human Response to Vibration Conference, Loughborough University, September.

Keighley, G. D. (1972). "Vibration Measurements in Chain Saws and Acceptable Vibration Standards", Paper presented at the International Conference on Hand–Arm Vibration, University of Dundee, July.

LaBarro, R. P., Forbes, R. T. and Andrew, S. (1970). Motor Industries Research Association, U.K., Report No. 1970/5.

Loach, J. C. (1958). *The Institution of Locomotive Engineers*, 48 (2), 183–208.

Loebich, R. (1967). *Deaut Kraft. Strass Verk* No. 189.

Lovesay, E. J. (1971). "Effects of Dual Axis Vibration and other Factors upon Human Performance", Paper presented to the Human Response to Vibration Conference. University of Swansea, September.

Lovesay, E. J. (1972). *Shock and Vibration Digest* 4 (12), 3–6.

Magid, E. B. and Coermann, R. R. (1960). *Proceedings of the Institute of Environmental Sciences* 135–153.

Magid, E. B. and Coermann, R. R. (1963). Chapter 5: Human Response to Vibration. *In*: "Human Factors Technology" (Bennett, E. *et al.*, ed.). McGraw-Hill.

Mauzin, H. and Sperling, E. (1951). Un Appareil de Contrôle de la Qualité de Circulation du Matériel roulant. *Revue générale des Chemin de Fer*.

McCullogh, M. L. (1972). "Towards the Development of a Ratio Scale", Paper presented at the Human Response to Vibration Conference. University of Sheffield, September.

McFarland, R. A. and Strondt, H. W. (1955). "Physical Variables influencing Driver Comfort, Efficiency and Safety", Harvard School of Public Health Report, March.

McKay, J. R. (1971). Institute of Sound and Vibration Research, Report No. 435, University of Southampton, September.

Meister, F. J. (1935). *Forschung auf dem Gebiete des Ingenieurswensens* 6, 116–120.

Miwa, T. (1967a). *Industrial Health* 5, 213–219.

Miwa, T. (1967b). *Industrial Health* 5, 183–205.

Miwa, T. (1968). *Industrial Health* 6, 1–10.

Miwa, T. (1969). *Industrial Health* 7, 89–115.

Nerem, R. M. (1973). "Fluid Dynamic Aspects of Cardiovascular Behaviour during Low Frequency Whole-body Vibration", Final Report, Department of Aeronautical and Astronautical Engineering, Ohio State University, Research Foundation, Columbus.

O'Conner, D. E. and Hempstock, T. I. (1973). "The Parameters of Hand–Arm Vibration and their Measurement", Paper presented at the Human Response to Vibration Conference, University of Salford, September.

Oborne, D. J. and Clarke, M. J. (1974). *Ergonomics* 17 (6), 769–782.

Oborne, D. J. and Clarke, M. J. (1975). *Ergonomics* 18 (1), 67–79.

Parkhilovski, I. G. (1968). *Avtom. Prom.* 8, 18–22.

Parks, D. L. and Snyder, F. W. (1960). "Human Reaction to Low Frequency Vibration", The Boeing Co. Wichita, Kansas, Document D3–3512–1, July.

Payne, P. R. and Band, E. G. U. (1971). Aeromedical Research Laboratory, Report AMRL–TR–70–35, January.

Pelmear, P. L. (1972a). *Journal of the Society of Environmental Engineers* **54**, 27–28.

Pelmear, P. L. (1972b). "Raynaud's Phenomenon in Pedestal Grinders", Paper presented at the International Conference on Hand–Arm Vibration, University of Dundee, July.

Pevzner, Y. M. and Tikhonov, A. A. (1964). *Avtom. Prom.* **1**, 15–18.

Poulson E. C. and Elmer, C. (1949). *Minnesota Medicine* **32** (4), 386–387.

Pradko, F. and Lee, R. A. (1966). Society of Automotive Engineers, Report No. 660139, U.S.A., January.

Radke, A. O. (1956). Bostrom Research Laboratories, Report No. 117.

Rance, B. H. and Barnes, G. R. (1973). "Transmission of Angular Acceleration to the Head", Paper presented at the Human Response to Vibration Conference, University of Salford, September.

Rance, B. H. (1975). "Angular Head Motion produced by Linear Vertical (Giz) Vibration of Seated Subjects". U.K. Group Meeting on Human Response to Vibration. Southampton.

Rao, B. K. N. and Ashley, C. (1974). *Journal of Sound and Vibration* **33** (2), 119–125.

Rao, B. K. N., Ashley, C. and Jones, B. (1975). *Journal of Society of Environmental Engineers* **14**, (1), 27–30.

Reiher, H. and Meister, F. J. (1931). *Forschung auf dem Gebiete des Ingenieurswesens* **2**, 381–386.

Reynolds, D. D. (1972). "Dynamic Response of the Hand–Arm System to a Sinusoidal Input", Paper presented at the International Conference on Hand–Arm Vibration, University of Dundee, July.

Robson, J. D. (1963). "An Introduction to Random Vibration", Edinburgh University Press.

Robson, J. D. (1968). *Journal of Sound and Vibration* **7** (2), 156–158.

Rosseger, R. and Rosseger, E. (1960). *Journal of Agricultural Engineering Research* **5** (3), 241–275.

Rubenstein, L. and Kaplan, R. (1968). Aerospace Medical Research Laboratories, Technical Report No. AMRL–68–19.

Sandover, J. (1971). "Study of Human Analogues. Part 1. A Survey of the Literature", Department of Cybernetics and Ergonomics, Loughborough University of Technology, April.

Shoenberger, R. W. (1970). Aerospace Medical Research Laboratory, Report 70–7.

Shoenberger, R. W. (1972). *Perceptual and Motor Skills*, Monograph Supplement 1, **34**, 127–160.

Shoenberger, R. W. and Harris, C. S. (1971). *Human Factors* **13** (1), 41–50.

Simić, D. (1970). RAE Library Translation, No. 1707, February 1974.

Simons, A. K., Radke, A. O. and Oswald, W. C. (1956). Bostrom Research Laboratory, Report No. 118.

Snook, S. H. and Irvine, C. H. (1969). *Human Factors* **11** (3), 291–300.

Snyder, F. W., Beaupeurt, J. E., Brumaghim, S. H. and Knapp, R. K. (1968). "Ten Years of Vibration Research and Beyond", Paper presented at the 15th Annual ONR Research Seminar, Seattle, Washington, June.

Sperling, E. and Betzholt, C. (1957). *Monthly Bulletin of the International Railway Congress Association* (Belgium) **34**, 672–678.

Stevens, S. S. (1960). "Handbook of Experimental Psychology", John Wiley and Sons, New York.

Stevens, S. S. (1961). "Sensory Communication" (W. A. Rosenblith ed.), M.I.T. Press, Boston.

Stikeleather, L. F., Hall, G. O. and Radke, A. O. (1972). Society of Automotive Engineers, U.S.A., Report No. 720001.

Suggs, C. W. (1972). "Modelling of the Dynamic Characteristics of the Hand–Arm System", Paper presented at the International Conference on Hand–Arm Vibration, University of Dundee, July.

Thompson, S. E. (1973). Society of Automotive Engineers, U.S.A., Paper No. 730702.

Tokuda, T., Hiruma, M. and Fukiage, K. (1972). *Bulletin of Journal of Society of Automotive Engineers* 26, 91–100, U.S.A.

Van Deusen, B. D. (1965). U.S. Army Corp. of Engineers Contract, Report No. 3–104.

Van Deusen, B. D. (1967). NASA Contractor Report NASA–CR–659.

Van Deusen, B. D. (1968). Society of Automotive Engineers, U.S.A., Paper No. 680090.

Versace, J. (1962). "Scaling of Ride", Chrysler Corporation Report, July.

Versace, J. (1963). Society of Automotive Engineers, U.S.A., Paper No. 638 E.

Von Gierke, H. E. (1964). *Applied Mechanics Review* 17, 951–958.

Von Gierke, H. E. (1968). *Annals of the New York Academy of Sciences* 152, Article 2, 172–186.

Walls, J. H., Houboult, J. C. and Press, H. (1954). NACA Technical Note 3305.

Walsh, E. G. (1966). *Bio-medical Engineering* 1, 402–407.

Walton, K. W. (1972). "The Pathology of Raynaud's Phenomenon", Paper presented at the International Conference on Hand–Arm Vibration, University of Dundee, July.

Watts, N. H. (1975). "The Evaluation of the Effect of Random Vibration on the Human Body". U.K. Group Meeting on Human Response to Vibration. Southampton.

Weis, E. B. (Jr.), Clarke, N. P. and von Gierke, H. E. (1966). Aerospace Medical Research Laboratories, Report No. AMRL–TR–66–84.

Whitehead, G. D. (1965). "A Review of Data Analysis Systems", Advanced School of Automobile Engineering Memo, No. 76, September.

Wittmann, T. J. and Phillips, N. S. (1969). *Journal of Biomechanics* 2, 281–288.

Woods, A. G. (1967). *Aircraft Engineering* 39, (7,) 6–14.

# 9. The Occurrence and Effects upon Performance of Low Frequency Vibration

*E. J. Lovesey*

## I. Introduction

There is no simple relationship between the level of vibration to which a person is exposed and the resulting level of task performance. This chapter will discuss some of the more important factors which determine performance under whole-body vibration, together with some typical vibration levels at which tasks are performed with varying difficulty in actual vehicles.

Most performance data have been obtained from tests performed in the vibration laboratory, generally using sinusoidal or near sinusoidal motions to vibrate a seated man. Tests to determine operator performance in the field have yielded little usable data since the number of unknown or uncontrolled variables have made detailed analysis of the results almost impossible.

Since the title of this publication links infrasound with low frequency vibration, it must be emphasised that the task performance changes which are discussed in this chapter have been produced by low frequency whole-body vibration and not by the effects of infrasound. Although vibration rigs used in experiments may vibrate at or below 20 Hz, measurements by the author have shown that the quantity of infrasound generated is negligible and can be assumed to have no influence upon the vibrating subject.

### A. RELEVANT FACTORS

Even where tests have been carried out under controlled conditions, the number of differences between separate test series are often considerable. For example, some of the more important parameters which might, and generally do, affect human performance are listed below:

(1) Direction and number of axes of vibration
(2) Acceleration level of the vibration
(3) Frequency content of the vibration
(4) Seat geometry and dynamics including seat cushion and restraining harness characteristics etc.
(5) Task difficulty
(6) Subject skills and training
(7) Subject population
(8) Subject motivation
(9) Subject clothing, e.g. protective headgear
(10) Duration of vibration test.

## 1. *Vibration Characteristics*

In most laboratory tests, the vibration frequencies and/or acceleration levels have been varied in some predetermined order to demonstrate the relative effects of vibration upon the ability of subjects to perform a particular task. In the majority of experiments, only linear single axis vertical (heave) vibrations have been used. A small number of experiments have employed single axis lateral (sway), longitudinal (shunt) or the rotational vibrations of roll, pitch or yaw. Very few experimental investigations into the effects of vibration upon human performance have used combinations of vibration in different axes. However, as can be seen from Table VI (p. 258), in real vehicles, vibration is rarely confined to a single axis but is usually to be found simultaneously in all three linear axes. The reasons for this restriction of interest and lack of realism in the laboratory are unclear but thought to be due to an absence of dual or multi-axis vibration facilities coupled with a certain traditionalism of experimenters to be preoccupied with heave vibrations.

## 2. *Vibration Input to Subject*

In both laboratory and vehicle situations, the effects of the vibration upon human comfort and performance can be influenced radically by simple changes in seat geometry, cushion or harness design. For example, if a thick sponge rubber cushion is added to a rigid seat it might absorb almost all of the low amplitude seat vibrations above 20 Hz. Paradoxically, the same cushion could amplify low frequency 2 Hz heave vibrations by a factor of 2 or more (Lovesey, 1971).

Similarly, although it has usually been assumed that the addition of a tight restraining harness will attenuate the effects of vibration, there is evidence to show that at, or near, the body resonance condition, a harness will reduce both task performance and comfort (Lovesey, 1968). However, in most vibration investigations the seat characteristics are kept constant for the duration of the test programme but do, of course, vary from test series to series and from vibration rig to rig. Fortunately, there is a trend towards the use of simple rigid seats mounted directly upon a vibration rig. This reduces at least one unknown—that of the cushion characteristics.

## 3. *Task Difficulty*

Task difficulty is one of the factors which has perhaps the greatest effect upon the performance of a task under stress. Whilst being an important factor, task difficulty is almost impossible to quantify. The purpose of performing a task under vibration is either (i) to illustrate the relative severity of different vibrations or (ii) to demonstrate in the laboratory that a task, such as flying an aircraft, can be performed efficiently or safely.

Frequently, vibration experiments use a task which is also performed outside the laboratory. This has the advantage that the experimental findings of this *ad hoc* test can be applied directly to the specific situation, but the disadvantage of having limited application to other situations. Additionally, this type of task is often so easy that it can be performed at quite severe vibration levels without any loss of performance. In fact, the stress of vibration has often motivated subjects to improve their performance above that achieved under the static control conditions.

Alternatively, if a performance task of a more basic nature is used, the task difficulty can be designed so that large errors are produced by small increases in vibration level. This type of task has the advantage that it illustrates the relative effects of vibration severity without being tied to any specific real-life situation which might prevent more general conclusions from being drawn from the results. Some assessment of the level of task difficulty must therefore be made when evaluating the effects of vibration upon operator performance.

## 4. *Subject Population and Design of Test*

There are several factors which are linked inseparably with task difficulty. Of these, subject population, skills and training are, perhaps, the most important. For example, one would expect subjects from a test pilot population to perform a compensatory tracking task under vibration with less difficulty than subjects drawn from a middle-aged female non-car driving population. At first, this example may seem to be absurd, yet several vibration experiments have been conducted using test pilots. The results from these tests have later been applied directly to predict the effects of vibration upon the general public.

Whenever performing or applying the findings from vibration tests, it is important to note the subject's age, sex, body build, occupation and acquired skills etc. It is also necessary to record factors which may affect performance such as eyesight, the wearing of clothing such as protective helmets, or even gloves which might reduce the ability to manipulate a control.

Obviously, if some form of tracking task is used to assess the effects of vibration upon human performance, the subjects must be given a task with which they are familiar and for which they have already acquired the appropriate skills. If this is not the case, then the subjects must be taught and must practise the task until they have reached a steady-performance level. Since Hornby and Wilson (1967) have shown that performance at certain tracking tasks may still be improving after 1500 practice runs, then, depending upon the type of task, it is sometimes preferable to select subjects who have already acquired the necessary task skills.

A compromise solution is often adopted when selecting subjects and task. Instead of choosing a very difficult task requiring specialist subjects or subjects who have had a lengthy training time, it is better to choose a less severe task. This task will be still difficult enough to be affected by vibration but will require less specialised subjects. The subjects will still require some training but should reach an adequate level of skill after only a few practice runs. Even if the subjects have still not reached the highest level of performance, the learning effects can be minimised by using a Latin square experimental design. This design should randomise the order of presentation of experimental conditions such that both learning and also fatigue effects tend to be cancelled out.

A typical Latin square test design for four subjects (Messrs. Brown, Black, Grey and White) and four vibration conditions (1–4) is shown in Table I. It can be seen that an additional test condition has been added at the beginning and end of each subject's set of vibration conditions. This is a control test without vibration and will help to indicate if any gross learning or fatigue effects are still present.

This particular square is designed so that each interaction between pairs of conditions is unique (vibration condition 1 precedes condition 2 only once in the square), yet every combination of two conditions is represented. Although each set of conditions is unique, the combination is repeated in reverse order by another subject. For example, Mr.

Brown's order of 012430 is the reverse of Mr. Grey's order of 034210. Thus the order of presentation of conditions is optimally randomised such that unwanted interactions are minimised between subjects and conditions.

TABLE I: Latin square test design for four subjects and four vibration conditions

| Subjects | Test order | | | | | |
|----------|---|---|---|---|---|---|
| Mr. Brown | 0 | 1 | 2 | 4 | 3 | 0 |
| Mr. Black | 0 | 2 | 3 | 1 | 4 | 0 |
| Mr. Grey  | 0 | 3 | 4 | 2 | 1 | 0 |
| Mr. White | 0 | 4 | 1 | 3 | 2 | 0 |

## 5. Subject Motivation and Duration of Tests

Although the influence of learning and fatigue can largely be designed out of a test by using the Latin square method, the effects of subject motivation may still affect the results. In most experiments, subjects are well motivated, but occasionally a subject may not attempt to perform the test as is required. Usually, this can be spotted by greatly fluctuating task performance or very poor performance when compared with other subjects. Sometimes this lack of motivation is due to poor initial test instructions or lack of communication between experimenter and subject. At other times it may be that the duration of the vibration test is too long and that the subject is becoming bored or fatigued. Very often the situation can be remedied by suitable action from the experimenter.

Returning to the subject of duration of tests, care must be taken when applying test findings to real-life situations. Most tests to investigate the effects of vibration upon performance have been from 5 min to 15 min duration. Most real-life situations in which vibration is present last for far longer periods, sometimes hours. Whereas a subject may be able to perform difficult tasks quite well in a vibration simulator for a few minutes, there is little evidence to show how well tasks are completed at the end of several hours of vibration.

## 6. Interpretation and Application of Vibration Data

The foregoing sections illustrate that it is essential to take account of task difficulty, subject population characteristics, training, motivation, duration of tests etc. whenever experimental results are interpreted and when the findings are applied to other situations. Thus, although the following sections may provide some idea of the effects of low frequency vibration upon man's performance, they should be used with care and extrapolations made only with extreme caution.

As an example, one simple but recurring misuse of vibration data is that of the extrapolation of the ISO (1974) fatigue decreased proficiency boundaries. For heave vibration, these boundaries start at 1 Hz and continue up to 100 Hz. This frequency range excludes the motion sickness range which extends approximately from 0.1 Hz to 0.7 Hz. Unfortunately many users of the ISO boundaries extend the 1–4 Hz lines below 1 Hz to include this low frequency region. This results in the extrapolated negative slope lines being far too lenient. Although human response data for frequencies below 1 Hz are sparse, there is some evidence to show that the curve should have a positive slope from 0.4 Hz to 1 Hz parallel to the 8–100 Hz line rather than the negative slope which is produced by the usual extrapolation (Lovesey, 1972).

## II. Performance Effects

Because of the many factors which influence human performance under vibration, it is not feasible to construct simple curves relating performance decrement to vibration level. It is possible, however, to illustrate with examples, some of the relative effects of vibration upon performances and the methods by which performance is degraded.

There are several ways in which vibration can affect task performance, of which the most important are (a) by reducing visual acuity (b) by mechanically interfering with control manipulation and (c) by creating general discomfort which causes fatigue and which reduces motivation. Other ways in which vibration may influence performance are by its direct effects upon the central nervous system and its effects upon physiological processes such as heart rate or respiratory rate. There is little conclusive evidence of this at normal transport vibration levels and these physiological effects are considered to be of much lesser importance than the three primary methods mentioned above.

## A. EXPERIMENTAL EVIDENCE

### 1. *Visual Acuity*

This topic is dealt with at some length in Chapter 10, and will only be briefly discussed here.

Many vibration experiments have been performed to investigate the effects of vibration upon visual acuity. In some of these, the man has been vibrated and asked to interpret statically displayed information. In other tests the man has remained static while the display has been vibrated. In the remainder of tests, both the man and the information display have been vibrated together. In all three types of tests, visual acuity and consequently performance have been degraded whenever there has been relative angular motion between the subject's eyes and the display. Figure 1 illustrates the effects of vibration frequency and

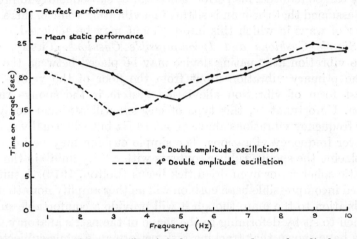

*Fig.* 1 The effect of heave vibration frequency and angular displacement of display upon tracking performance.

angular movement of a tracking task display upon visual performance as demonstrated by Huddleston (1967). Although Huddleston vibrated the display while the subject remained stationary, the curves reflect the relative trends due to the vibration, whether the man or the display or both are vibrated.

The mechanism by which visual acuity is degraded may be explained as follows. Up to about 2 Hz, the human eye can follow the movement of a display oscillating sinusoidally. In fact the pursuit movements of the eye are almost compulsive at these low frequencies. Above 2 Hz, the eye gets out of phase with the motion and can no longer follow the display movement. Eventually, if the frequency is increased above 5 Hz, the display will appear as two nodal images. If the relative motion is sufficiently great, as shown by the 4° double amplitude line in Fig. 1, the nodal images will be quite separate and, thus, will become readable again.

In another experiment to detect the gap direction of vibrating Landolt C's, O'Hanlon and Griffin (1971) noted similar low frequency effects. However, it was found that in the 5–30 Hz range at constant vibration amplitude, errors increased with advancing frequency. Above 30 Hz errors were more frequent still when the nodal images of the Landolt C's fused and were seen only as a blur.

## 2. *Vibration Alleviation*

Obviously if, the relative angular motion between the man and the display can be reduced, his performance will be subsequently improved. If it is assumed that the man is sitting in a vibrating vehicle, there are a number of ways in which this improvement may be achieved.

(a) *Simple Cushions and Incompressible Cushions.* Firstly, some passive vibration attenuating device may be placed between the man and the primary vibration input from the floor of the vehicle. The simplest form of vibration alleviation system is the sponge rubber cushion. Unfortunately, this type of cushion will attenuate only the higher frequency vibrations above about 10 Hz but will usually amplify the lower frequency vibrations. The simple cushion may be improved by replacing the sponge rubber contents with a "dry fluid" in the form of plastic spheres—or even dried tick beans (Bolton, 1972). A suitably designed incompressible bean cushion will neither amplify nor attenuate the vibration to the man, though it will provide a comfortable surface on which to sit by deforming to the shape of the user's anatomy. Pilot studies have shown that tracking task performance while subjected to low frequency multi axis vibrations is reduced significantly less when the operator is seated on an incompressible bean cushion than when seated on a conventional sponge rubber cushion (Lovesey, 1972).

(b) *The Sprung Seat.* An improvement upon the simple cushion is the anti-vibration or sprung seat. This seat consists of springs and dampers which will effectively isolate the man from 4 Hz to 5 Hz heave vibrations. This is the frequency at which the human torso exhibits a major resonance in heave. At this frequency the corresponding head and eye motions are largest. Although this type of seat can be extremely beneficial in some vehicles, which vibrate predominantly in heave at frequencies above 2 Hz, it can reduce human comfort and performance if used incorrectly. For example, the seat also has a natural heave resonance. This is usually at about 1 Hz. Thus, if this seat is installed in a vehicle which also has a significant proportion of 1 Hz heave vibration, the seat will amplify the input motion to the man, with the result that his visual acuity will be degraded.

(c) *Active Anti-vibration Seat.* A recent development of the sprung seat is the active anti-vibration seat. With this seat, the onset of an acceleration is sensed and the signal is amplified to drive the seat and occupant such that they remain at a constant level in space, irrespective of the vehicle motion. This is an effective solution to the problem of vibration protection for the human operator. The complexity and cost of this type of system are great and there are other shortcomings. Its amplitude is limited to a stroke of a few inches whereas the vehicle, in which the seat is fitted, might vibrate with amplitudes of several feet at low frequencies. Existing active seats tend to be single axis devices that remove only heave motions, although the vehicles for which the seats have been designed vibrate along all three linear axes. However, even if the active anti-vibration seat does manage to maintain a driver at a constant level, there will still be some relative movement remaining between the operator and both his controls and his instrument display.

(d) *The Collimated Display.* Perhaps the most promising method, by which the effects of vibration upon visual acuity may be minimised, is that of the collimated display. This is usually in the form of a Head Up Display (HUD) which presents information focused at infinite distance in front of the operator. The vehicle operator looks ahead, through the windscreen, and can see his speed indicator etc. superimposed upon the real visual field outside. Since the display image is seen at infinity, if the operator's head vibrates in heave, sway or shunt, the angular movement of the image upon the operator's retina is effectively zero. The display can therefore be seen clearly and without difficulty even though the operator's head and eyes might be vibrating with appreciable amplitude.

Few things are ever perfect, and so it is with the collimated display. The collimated display will only improve the operator's vision and will not reduce the vibration affects upon the rest of the body. Neither will it remove all of the effects due to linear motions if these vibrations produce angular movements of the operator's head, when angular movements of the display image will be produced at the retina. Fortunately, these head-nodding movements are not usually great in current vehicle vibration environments and the collimated display can be used to great advantage.

In a recent flight simulation of a large jet transport aircraft performed under severe vibration conditions (Lovesey, 1972) a collimated HUD was compared with the equivalent conventional head down (HDD) instrument. Take-offs and climbs were performed by five pilots under the four conditions of: (i) no vibrations, (ii) modulated 2 Hz heave vibration at 0.25 g rms (H), this heave coupled with modulated (iii) $3\frac{1}{2}$ Hz sway at 0.07 g rms (H + S1) and (iv) at 0.15 g rms (H + S2). Under these four conditions, performances using HUD and HDD instruments were assessed by deviation from the optimum flight path.

Table II shows the average performance scores under the three vibration conditions. These scores have been normalised through division by the no-vibration datum score.

TABLE II: Experimental data showing the effects of vibration and collimation upon control performance in the form of percentage time on target scores divided by the no-vibration score and averaged for five subjects

| Instrument | Vibration[a] | | | |
|---|---|---|---|---|
| | None | H | H + S1 | H + S2 |
| Conventional head down display | 100 | 96 | 89 | 80 |
| Collimated head up display | 100 | 110 | 112 | 112 |

[a] H = 2 Hz heave vibration at 0.25 g rms.
S1 = $3\frac{1}{2}$ Hz sway vibration at 0.07 g rms.
S2 = $3\frac{1}{2}$ Hz sway vibration at 0.15 g rms.

This table illustrates the beneficial effects of the collimated display upon performance when subjected to vibration. Without vibration, both instruments produced similar performances. When heave vibration was introduced the average performance deteriorated slightly while using the conventional instrument but the performance actually improved with the collimated display. As vibration severity was increased by the addition of increasing amounts of sway, the performance using the easily seen collimated HUD remained improved over the static case. This experiment serves to demonstrate the effects of vibration both of motivating the subjects to perform better and of degrading performances by reducing their visual acuity.

## B. VIBRATION EFFECTS UPON CONTROL MANIPULATION

### 1. *Introduction*

Several experiments have been conducted to investigate the effects of heave and sway vibrations upon the ability of the human operator to perform compensatory tracking and other manipulative tasks (Shurmer, 1967). But, as has been suggested earlier, it is often difficult to draw general conclusions from the results of specific tests, due to the many variables present. A basic experiment investigating the interacting effects of vibration, restraining harness, control force and subject-induced errors due to over-correction was performed to help to clarify the situation (Lovesey, 1971). A summary of this experiment is given as an example to demonstrate how various parameters can combine with vibration to influence human performance.

## 2. Experimental Details

(a) *The Task.* A manipulative task was chosen which required no additional training, yet which was fairly difficult to perform under moderate levels of vibration. This task was installed in a vehicle simulator that could vibrate simultaneously in heave and sway at low frequencies.

The task required a seated subject to maintain a target spot at the mid-position of a two-dimensional collimated display by keeping an aircraft control stick in its mid-position throughout a 40 sec test period. Subjects were instructed that, if the spot moved from the mid-position, it was to be returned by the relevant control movement. Any deviation of the spot from the centre was produced by a control movement that was itself caused voluntarily or involuntarily by the subject. This task required no additional learning from the subjects who, though technical staff and not pilots, had been given previous experience of vibration in the simulator.

The control-display (CD) ratios between the controls and the collimated target spot were 1 : 7 in elevation and 1 : 4 in azimuth and had no lag. Thus a control movement of 1° forward in pitch produced an instantaneous increase in spot elevation of 7° subtended at the subject's eye. These CD ratios are more sensitive than those used in most vehicles and were chosen to produce an adequate level of task difficulty, rather than to reproduce an actual vehicle's control characteristics.

A control force bias was applied during half of the tests to investigate the effects of vibration upon maintaining a steady force. When this bias was applied, the stick was trimmed such that a push forward of 11·4 kg and a push to the left sideways of 4·5 kg were required to maintain it, and therefore the spot, in their mid-positions. Half of the tests were performed with the subject sitting unrestrained in the simulator's aircraft seat, and half with them wearing the seat's five-point harness. This enabled the harness-vibration interactions to be studied.

Similarly, for an assessment of subject-induced errors to be made, half of the tests were carried out with visual and kinesthetic feedback information from the collimated display. The remainder were performed with the subject's eyes shut and thus with only kinesthetic information of the control position. Altogether, some 48 different combinations of vibration, control force, harness and feedback served to illustrate the various effects which might influence performance at manual positioning tasks.

(b) *Vibration Conditions*. The fundamental heave and sway vibration frequencies that were used in the tests were 2 Hz and 2.7 Hz. These frequencies were applied as both single and dual axis heave and sway vibrations. These vibrations were chosen since they are typical of the frequencies to be found in existing forms of transport.

All of the vibrations at the floor of the simulator were nominally sinusoidal at $\pm 0.25$ g in heave and $\pm 0.14$ g in sway, but they contained some degree of harmonic distortion. The seat structure and cushion amplified the heave vibrations by a factor of approximately 1.5 and reduced the sway by a factor of 3. Thus the primary vibration input to the subjects through the seat produced heave and sway levels of about $\pm 0.38$ g and $\pm 0.05$ g respectively.

(c) *Test Procedure*. The 48 combinations of vibration (6), harness (2), spot-control position feedback (2) and control force (2) were presented randomly to reduce order- and time-dependent effects.

Most vibration tests lasted for about 40 sec. When the subject was ready, with harness tight or stowed, the vibration was increased to the appropriate level. The subject then tried to keep the spot at the centre of the display for the next 35 sec. For half of this period the subject viewed the collimated display and could see any spot deviations from the centre. For the other half his eyes were closed. This was the easiest way of removing visual feedback and restricted the positioning of the spot to kinesthetic feedback alone.

(d) *Results and Analysis*. Each test performance was recorded in the form of continuous traces of control position in elevation and azimuth. Two nominal measures of error were made for each trace. The first was the sum of the maximum deviations either side of the control's correct position. These are given on the left-hand side of Table III. The second quantity to be noted was the number of peaks greater than a nominal 1 mm in height. These results are given on the right-hand side of Table III and are presented as a measure of subject-induced errors, rather than errors due to vibration exciting the control itself. The latter were less than 1 mm in height.

## 3. *Discussion*

The effects of the different variables upon manual positioning can be seen by comparing the totals for each matched pair of variables given in Table III. Wilcoxon's signed Rank Test was also used on the data to determine if there are any statistically significant differences between performance under different conditions. Both the measures of maximum peak deviation (MPD) and the number of peaks (NP), used in assessing the results, were degraded by all of the test vibrations. It

TABLE III: Experimental data showing the effects of heave and/or sway vibration, harness and feedback upon manual control in the form of averages of manipulated control errors

**Elevation scores**

| Vibration[a] | Average of maximum peak deviations | | | | | | Average of number of peaks | | | | | |
|---|---|---|---|---|---|---|---|---|---|---|---|---|
| | 2H | 2.7S | 2H + 2.7S | 2.7H | 2S | 2.7H + 2S | 2H | 2.7S | 2H + 2.7S | 2.7H | 2S | 2.7H + 2S |
| No control force | 2.6 | 1.6 | 3.7 | 1.9 | 2.5 | 4.1 | 0.9 | 0.4 | 3.8 | 1.3 | 0.8 | 3.0 |
| With control force | 4.1 | 2.9 | 7.1 | 4.9 | 4.1 | 8.4 | 8.0 | 1.3 | 12.3 | 8.5 | 3.0 | 11.3 |
| No harness | 3.0 | 1.9 | 5.0 | 3.6 | 2.8 | 5.7 | 3.4 | 0.5 | 7.2 | 4.1 | 1.9 | 7.2 |
| With harness | 3.7 | 2.6 | 5.8 | 3.2 | 3.8 | 6.8 | 5.5 | 1.2 | 8.9 | 5.7 | 1.9 | 7.1 |
| With visual feedback | 2.6 | 1.5 | 4.3 | 2.5 | 2.2 | 4.5 | 5.3 | 1.2 | 8.8 | 6.2 | 2.1 | 7.9 |
| No visual feedback | 4.1 | 3.0 | 6.5 | 4.3 | 4.4 | 8.0 | 3.6 | 0.5 | 7.3 | 3.6 | 1.7 | 6.4 |

**Azimuth scores**

| Vibration[a] | Average of maximum peak deviations | | | | | | Average of number of peaks | | | | | |
|---|---|---|---|---|---|---|---|---|---|---|---|---|
| | 2H | 2.7S | 2H + 2.7S | 2.7H | 2S | 2.7H + 2S | 2H | 2.7S | 2H + 2.7S | 2.7H | 2S | 2.7H + 2S |
| No control force | 2.1 | 3.0 | 5.5 | 2.3 | 3.6 | 4.3 | 0.8 | 5.0 | 10.9 | 0.8 | 6.3 | 12.7 |
| With control force | 4.5 | 14.4 | 34.6 | 6.4 | 19.4 | 43.8 | 1.4 | 5.5 | 11.9 | 1.4 | 9.9 | 16.1 |
| No harness | 2.5 | 8.3 | 18.7 | 3.9 | 10.5 | 22.5 | 0.9 | 5.7 | 12.3 | 1.1 | 7.2 | 13.8 |
| With harness | 4.1 | 9.1 | 21.4 | 4.8 | 12.5 | 25.6 | 1.3 | 4.8 | 10.5 | 1.1 | 9.0 | 15.0 |
| With visual feedback | 3.0 | 6.1 | 19.8 | 3.8 | 11.0 | 20.1 | 1.6 | 5.9 | 10.3 | 1.5 | 9.5 | 14.9 |
| No visual feedback | 3.6 | 11.3 | 20.3 | 4.9 | 12.0 | 28.0 | 0.6 | 4.6 | 12.5 | 0.7 | 6.7 | 13.9 |

Note: All values are the average of six test subject results.

[a] 2H = 2 Hz heave vibration at ± 0.38 g.

2.7H = 2.7 Hz heave vibration at ± 0.38 g.

2S = 2 Hz sway vibration at ± 0.05 g.

2.7S = 2.7 Hz sway vibration at ± 0.05 g.

These are approximate values of the vibration input to the subject through the seat, see text for further details.

should be noted that, without vibration, all subjects were able to hold the control stationary at all times and no position errors were then recorded.

(a) *Vibration Effects.* Although the effects of combining vibration axes will be discussed in more detail later, the results of the single and dual axis scores obtained during this experiment will be briefly summarised here.

The 2.7 Hz sway vibration had the least effect upon elevation position score, while the 2 Hz heave had the least effect upon azimuth control. Sway of 2 Hz, followed by 2 Hz heave and 2.7 Hz heave, had increasingly greater effects upon elevation control. Azimuth control was increasingly reduced by 2.7 Hz heave, 2.7 Hz sway and 2 Hz sway. The dual axis vibrations of 2 Hz heave combined with 2.7 Hz sway and the 2.7 Hz heave combined with 2 Hz sway had the greatest adverse effects upon control both in azimuth and elevation.

Combined or dual axis vibration errors were greater than those of the sum of the individual single axis vibration errors. The errors recorded due to the dual axis were significantly different ($P = 1\%$) from those produced when only single vibrations were applied.

(b) *Control force Effects.* The MPD and the NP elevation scores obtained with control force bias are between 1.5 and 6 times the value of those with no control force under vibration conditions. Thus the control force bias significantly ($P = 1\%$) degraded positional control in elevation. Similarly, the MPD and NP scores for azimuth control obtained with the control force bias are between 2 and 10 times greater than those resulting from no control bias. Positional control in azimuth is thus significantly ($P = 1\%$) degraded by control force bias under the vibration conditions etc. used in the tests.

(c) *Harness Effects.* Elevation scores, with the exception of the 2.7 Hz heave are significantly greater ($P = 1\%$) when a harness was worn under these low frequency vibrations than when no harness was used. Azimuth error scores are just significantly greater ($P = 5\%$) when a harness was worn. Two exceptions to this trend were observed in the NP scores with vibrations of 2.7 Hz sway and the 2 Hz heave combined with the 2.7 Hz sway.

(d) *Position Feedback Effects.* At no time did subjects experience difficulty in seeing the collimated display during the visual feedback phase of each test. All of the elevation and azimuth MPD scores under vibration with no vision are greater than those obtained with visual feedback of spot position. Conversely all elevation and all but one azimuth NP scores obtained under vibration without vision are less than those resulting from visual feedback. This can be explained as follows. Potentially large deviations of the target spot from the centre of the display can be spotted quickly visually and corrected before they become very great. Without visual information, they go uncorrected until the control movement becomes large enough to be noticed kinesthetically by hand or arm position. The differences between position scores with and without visual information are significantly different ($P = 1\%$) in both azimuth and elevation.

The reduction in the NP scores when visual feedback was removed indicates that subjects tend to overcorrect small deviations which are sensed visually and consequently increase their control movements and errors. Without vision, these small fluctuations are not noticed and tend to decay naturally.

It should be noted that the control display ratios used in these tests were, perhaps, an order greater than would be obtained on, say, an attitude indicator in a typical aircraft. In addition, the response was immediate. In a real aircraft the response to such small rapidly fluctuating control inputs would be very small and would probably be damped out before the pilot could take any correcting action.

## 4. Concluding Remarks

The vibration experiment, which has been described briefly above, serves to illustrate several points. Firstly, although the vibrations chosen were typical of the level to be found in several types of vehicle, the task was not meant to represent the control characteristics of any of those particular vehicles. The task was selected for its level of difficulty and the requirement for minimum training of semi-skilled subjects. This enabled the relative effects of vibration and other factors to be clearly and quickly observable. The test summary also mentions the fact that the seat and its soft cushion amplify the heave and attenuate the sway input vibrations to the subjects. Without this knowledge, any user of the resulting data could be in error by factors of 2/3 to 3.

The tests were designed to investigate the effects of combining two separate axes of low frequency vibrations and also the effects of both these vibrations together with the factors of harness, control force bias and visual feedback. The tests go some way in achieving their original purpose, but, as in all vibration studies, they require to be expanded still further. For example, only the frequencies of 2 Hz and 2.7 Hz were used at constant g levels, and then only in heave and sway. Future experiments will be required to expand the frequency range, the acceleration range and the number of axes of vibration.

## C. VIBRATION AXIS COMBINATION

### 1. *Dual Axis Vibrations*

Some effects of combined or dual axis vibrations upon man's performance have already been mentioned, while the occurrence of multi-axis vibrations will be discussed in detail in Section D of this chapter. However, since it will be shown that multi-axis vibrations exist in most vehicles, it is surprising to learn that more than 99% of all human vibration experiments have been restricted to the use of single axis vibrations. Of these, the majority of tests have employed heave as the sole vibration stress. A smaller number of tests have used sway while only a few have embodied shunt as the axis of vibration. As stated earlier, in Section I.A.1, the reasons for this restriction of interest and lack of realism in the past are unclear, but increasing interest in multi-axis vibrations is now becoming apparent both in the U.S.A. and the U.K.

Some further experimental evidence is available which demonstrates the effects of combining vibration axes upon human performance. An experiment that was performed to investigate the relative influence of single and dual axis heave and sway vibrations upon tracking performance is described below. The investigations are reported in some detail to enable potential users of the information to assess the effects of the various vibrations and other factors upon task performance.

### 2. *Experimental Details of a Tracking Investigation*

To investigate the relative effects of heave and sway vibrations upon human performance, an experiment was devised around a small dual axis vibration rig and a two-dimensional compensatory tracking task. Eighteen male subjects were exposed to 12 heave and/or sway vibration conditions at frequencies and g levels typical of those measured in existing vehicles. Elevation and azimuth tracking performance under the different vibration conditions were used to assess the relative severities of the vibrations.

(a) *Design of Experiment*. (i) The Compensatory Tracking Task: A two-dimensional zero-order (displacement) tracking task was set up on a computer to produce an apparently random movement of a spot on a fixed base oscilloscope. This display was positioned approximately 80 cm in front of the subject's eyes. The movement of the spot was not, in fact, random, but consisted of a combination of two sine waves whose frequencies were 3 cycles/min and 11 cycles/min. Spot movements were required to be nulled out, returning the spot to the crosswire centre by movement of a miniature control stick. This stick was 5.4 cm from rotational axis to the 1 cm diameter knurled top. The stick was situated on the right-hand arm-rest of the vibration seat since all subjects were right-handed. The control display ratio was 1 : 1 so that the total movement of ± 3 cm at the top of the stick produced a ± 3 cm movement of the spot on the 8 cm diameter oscilloscope. The control–display relationship was compatible and was the same as that of modern anti-tank missile controls. The spot motion, if unaltered by stick movement, repeated after 1 min.

The tracking task was originally devised by Shurmer (1967) as a performance measure to assess the effects of vibration upon missile aimers. The task was adopted by the author as it was thought to be similar to many real-life operations. Secondly, it was decided that it would be useful for a common task to be used in different experiments. This would reduce the number of parameters and might make the comparisons of different experiments slightly simpler.

(ii) The Vibration Rig: All tests were performed while subjects were seated on a two-axis vibration rig. This consisted of a tubular magnesium alloy seat frame with a plywood backrest inclined at 103° to a 5 cm thick rigid horizontal wooden seat, the whole of which could be vibrated simultaneously in heave and sway by two hydraulic jacks.

(iii) Test Procedure: Eighteen physically fit male technical staff, whose ages ranged from 22 to 55, were asked to take part in the tests under various vibration conditions. It was explained to each subject that he would be given a number of 1 min two-dimensional compensatory tracking tasks under static conditions. When judged to be proficient by the experimenter (which was usually when error scores had dropped to an almost steady level) the subject would be exposed to heave and/or sway vibrations for 1 min periods. It was made clear to the subject that if at any time he felt unwell or wished to discontinue the test he had only to notify the rig controller who would stop the rig immediately.

A 12 × 12 Latin square was devised in order to present each subject with a different sequence of vibration conditions. In fact, 18 subjects finally completed the tests, which required half of the vibration sequences to be repeated. Three no-vibration periods were also incorporated into the test at the first, middle and last runs to provide a static tracking error datum. These scores also enabled a rough check on learning or fatigue effects to be made.

The vibration frequencies and levels which were used in the tests were 2 Hz, 5 Hz and 7 Hz at ± 0.2 g in heave (H) and ± 0.1 g in sway (S). These frequencies and levels were also used in combination at 2H + 5S, 2H + 7S, 5H + 7S, 7H + 2S and 7H + 5S. The frequencies were chosen for the tests since they coincide with major body resonances and are also to be found in existing forms of transport.

(iv) Test Environment: The environmental conditions in the room in which the tests were conducted remained essentially constant. An overall noise level of 62 dB(A) was measured at the subject's head position. This level remained constant throughout all tests, including the no-vibration datum condition.

The dry bulb temperature also remained approximately constant at $20 \pm 1$ °C. The illumination was maintained at a constant level by the use of artificial fluorescent lighting. Using an exposure photometer the luminance of the 8 cm diameter display was found to be 8.5 cd/m², with an actual target spot illumination of 51.5 cd/m². The display was set at the centre of a 40 cm square matt black panel whose luminance was 4.5 cd/m². The luminance of the surrounding room was approximately 17 cd/m².

(b) *Results and Analysis.* Azimuth and elevation error scores were recorded at the end of each 1 min tracking period. Due to the large variations in tracking ability between subjects the scores of each subject were normalised by dividing each subject's score under vibration by the average of his three scores obtained in the no-vibration tests.

(i) Tracking Errors: These errors, averaged for 18 unharnessed subjects, show that $\pm 0.2$ g heave at 2 Hz, 5 Hz and 7 Hz produces greater tracking decrements than $\pm 0.1$ g sway. (See Tables IV and V.) Dual axis vibration combined from the same heave and sway conditions generally show even greater decrements than those produced by either condition alone. Only in the case of 5 Hz heave and 7 Hz sway vibration on azimuth tracking was tracking ability impaired less by the multi-axis combination. The standard deviation tends to increase with tracking error.

At the start of the tests it was hypothesised that errors produced by combined heave and sway vibrations would be equal to the product of errors produced by each vibration acting alone. Results show that this is approximately the case.

(ii) Significance of Results: Student's $t$-test was used to compare the results obtained under vibration with those of the no-vibration datum condition.

In azimuth tracking, all of the sway and the combined 5 Hz heave + 7 Hz sway conditions were found to produce results just significantly different $(P = 5\%)$ from the datum condition. Heave results of 2 Hz and 7 Hz were significantly different $(P = 1\%)$ while all of the remaining vibration conditions were highly significantly different $(P = 0.2\%)$ from the no-vibration datum.

TABLE IV: Experimental data showing the effects of heave and/or sway vibration upon a tracking task in the form of normalised elevation compensatory tracking error scores for 18 unharnessed subjects

| Subject No. | First no vib. | Vibration[a] | | | | | | | | | | | | Mid no vib. | Last no vib. |
|---|---|---|---|---|---|---|---|---|---|---|---|---|---|---|---|
| | | 2H | 5H | 7H | 2S | 5S | 7S | 2H+5S | 2H+7S | 5H+2S | 5H+7S | 7H+2S | 7H+5S | | |
| 1 | 1.14 | 1.67 | 1.31 | 1.70 | 1.04 | 1.35 | 0.94 | 1.65 | 1.06 | 1.47 | 2.00 | 1.36 | 1.30 | 0.90 | 0.95 |
| 2 | 1.53 | 1.43 | 1.47 | 1.04 | 1.24 | 0.89 | 1.25 | 1.10 | 0.99 | 1.00 | 1.08 | 1.05 | 1.30 | 0.70 | 0.77 |
| 3 | 0.86 | 1.20 | 0.54 | 1.63 | 1.21 | 1.30 | 0.63 | 0.62 | 1.51 | 1.81 | 1.12 | 1.93 | 1.97 | 1.13 | 1.01 |
| 4 | 1.25 | 1.25 | 1.05 | 1.36 | 0.81 | 0.98 | 0.95 | 1.38 | 1.65 | 1.11 | 1.23 | 1.73 | 1.71 | 0.81 | 0.93 |
| 5 | 1.54 | 1.21 | 1.12 | 1.30 | 1.41 | 0.90 | 0.88 | 1.25 | 1.02 | 1.59 | 1.13 | 1.69 | 0.95 | 0.72 | 0.75 |
| 6 | 1.18 | 0.86 | 1.35 | 1.12 | 0.59 | 1.08 | 0.95 | 0.92 | 0.99 | 0.74 | 1.31 | 0.89 | 0.77 | 0.98 | 0.84 |
| 7 | 0.94 | 1.28 | 1.10 | 1.49 | 1.23 | 1.20 | 1.25 | 1.43 | 1.28 | 1.24 | 1.54 | 1.28 | 1.34 | 0.96 | 1.10 |
| 8 | 1.26 | 1.00 | 1.36 | 1.20 | 1.08 | 1.29 | 1.14 | 1.70 | 1.13 | 1.08 | 1.28 | 1.49 | 1.30 | 0.88 | 0.85 |
| 9 | 1.00 | 2.24 | 1.57 | 1.68 | 1.47 | 1.54 | 0.88 | 1.97 | 3.12 | 2.23 | 2.98 | 1.56 | 2.12 | 1.13 | 0.87 |
| 10 | 0.99 | 1.34 | 1.29 | 1.06 | 1.21 | 1.12 | 1.17 | 1.42 | 1.62 | 1.49 | 1.58 | 1.25 | 1.50 | 1.13 | 0.88 |
| 11 | 1.27 | 0.85 | 1.09 | 0.94 | 1.03 | 0.94 | 0.97 | 1.34 | 1.07 | 1.04 | 0.98 | 1.52 | 0.98 | 0.83 | 0.90 |
| 12 | 1.04 | 1.10 | 1.44 | 0.98 | 1.56 | 0.91 | 1.26 | 1.96 | 1.18 | 1.40 | 1.33 | 1.49 | 1.51 | 1.07 | 0.90 |
| 13 | 1.10 | 1.22 | 1.26 | 1.28 | 1.12 | 1.14 | 1.34 | 1.24 | 1.28 | 1.30 | 1.36 | 1.03 | 1.34 | 0.91 | 0.99 |
| 14 | 0.94 | 1.34 | 1.09 | 1.20 | 1.51 | 0.87 | 1.17 | 1.37 | 1.33 | 1.27 | 1.38 | 1.22 | 1.23 | 0.89 | 1.17 |
| 15 | 1.03 | 1.05 | 1.34 | 1.22 | 1.26 | 1.28 | 0.97 | 1.14 | 1.25 | 1.34 | 1.14 | 1.75 | 1.26 | 1.05 | 0.91 |
| 16 | 1.17 | 1.10 | 1.22 | 1.24 | 0.97 | 0.96 | 1.07 | 1.05 | 1.53 | 1.98 | 1.94 | 1.48 | 1.30 | 0.95 | 0.87 |
| 17 | 1.08 | 1.40 | 1.47 | 1.31 | 0.86 | 0.92 | 1.12 | 1.10 | 1.17 | 1.15 | 1.08 | 1.54 | 1.42 | 1.05 | 0.88 |
| 18 | 1.27 | 1.13 | 1.49 | 1.23 | 0.82 | 0.98 | 0.88 | 1.23 | 1.08 | 0.99 | 0.81 | 1.07 | 1.28 | 0.75 | 0.98 |
| Ave. | 1.14 | 1.27 | 1.24 | 1.28 | 1.15 | 1.10 | 1.05 | 1.33 | 1.36 | 1.37 | 1.39 | 1.43 | 1.37 | 0.95 | 0.92 |
| Std dev. | 0.19 | 0.32 | 0.23 | 0.23 | 0.25 | 0.19 | 0.18 | 0.34 | 0.48 | 0.36 | 0.47 | 0.27 | 0.32 | 0.13 | 0.09 |

[a] 2H = 2 Hz heave vibration at ± 0.2 g.    2S = 2 Hz sway vibration at ± 0.1 g.
5H = 5 Hz heave vibration at ± 0.2 g.    5S = 5 Hz sway vibration at ± 0.1 g.
7H = 7 Hz heave vibration at ± 0.2 g.    7S = 7 Hz sway vibration at ± 0.1 g.

TABLE V: Experimental data showing the effects of heave and/or sway vibration upon a tracking task in the form of normalised azimuth compensatory tracking error scores for 18 unharnessed subjects

| Subject No. | First no vib. | 2H | 5H | 7H | 2S | 5S | 7S | 2H+5S | 2H+7S | 5H+2S | 5H+7S | 7H+2S | 7H+5S | Mid no vib. | Last no vib. |
|---|---|---|---|---|---|---|---|---|---|---|---|---|---|---|---|
| | | | | | | | Vibration[a] | | | | | | | | |
| 1 | 1.13 | 1.02 | 1.57 | 1.13 | 1.05 | 1.04 | 1.08 | 1.48 | 1.38 | 1.82 | 1.46 | 1.43 | 1.30 | 0.90 | 0.97 |
| 2 | 0.98 | 1.54 | 1.19 | 1.12 | 1.22 | 1.30 | 1.23 | 1.16 | 1.59 | 1.32 | 0.93 | 0.97 | 0.99 | 1.12 | 0.90 |
| 3 | 1.02 | 0.94 | 0.73 | 0.80 | 0.82 | 1.62 | 0.87 | 0.82 | 1.12 | 1.27 | 0.93 | 1.20 | 1.17 | 1.17 | 0.91 |
| 4 | 1.07 | 0.86 | 0.99 | 0.89 | 0.81 | 0.92 | 0.89 | 0.89 | 1.24 | 1.20 | 0.95 | 1.36 | 1.68 | 1.07 | 0.86 |
| 5 | 1.23 | 1.04 | 1.16 | 1.80 | 1.04 | 0.97 | 0.86 | 1.16 | 1.17 | 1.81 | 1.15 | 1.64 | 1.07 | 0.84 | 0.93 |
| 6 | 0.92 | 1.14 | 1.20 | 1.41 | 1.31 | 1.20 | 1.70 | 1.54 | 1.07 | 1.04 | 1.62 | 1.72 | 1.31 | 1.15 | 0.93 |
| 7 | 0.87 | 1.15 | 1.41 | 1.06 | 1.17 | 1.41 | 1.08 | 1.08 | 1.42 | 1.02 | 1.12 | 1.50 | 1.50 | 0.85 | 1.27 |
| 8 | 0.89 | 1.31 | 1.16 | 1.40 | 1.24 | 1.45 | 1.21 | 1.38 | 1.65 | 0.98 | 1.47 | 1.10 | 1.29 | 1.16 | 1.26 |
| 9 | 0.84 | 2.34 | 2.26 | 1.80 | 1.60 | 2.22 | 1.29 | 1.89 | 3.48 | 2.58 | 2.78 | 1.63 | 2.67 | 0.85 | 1.00 |
| 10 | 1.17 | 1.70 | 1.44 | 1.44 | 1.52 | 1.18 | 1.18 | 2.15 | 1.60 | 2.06 | 1.61 | 1.47 | 1.64 | 0.88 | 0.96 |
| 11 | 1.36 | 1.20 | 1.33 | 1.09 | 1.02 | 0.92 | 1.00 | 1.64 | 1.33 | 1.15 | 0.97 | 1.93 | 0.83 | 0.90 | 0.74 |
| 12 | 0.98 | 1.36 | 1.57 | 2.93 | 1.24 | 1.07 | 1.08 | 2.18 | 1.36 | 1.29 | 1.14 | 1.78 | 2.24 | 1.03 | 0.98 |
| 13 | 0.96 | 1.06 | 1.38 | 0.92 | 0.61 | 1.12 | 0.89 | 1.15 | 1.47 | 1.12 | 1.06 | 1.19 | 1.03 | 1.29 | 0.75 |
| 14 | 1.20 | 1.05 | 1.16 | 1.23 | 1.50 | 1.32 | 1.55 | 1.62 | 1.50 | 1.15 | 1.06 | 1.13 | 1.65 | 0.94 | 0.86 |
| 15 | 1.10 | 1.32 | 1.52 | 1.16 | 0.93 | 1.16 | 1.28 | 1.26 | 1.14 | 1.32 | 1.08 | 1.40 | 1.64 | 1.01 | 0.89 |
| 16 | 1.25 | 1.41 | 1.96 | 1.22 | 1.57 | 0.93 | 0.79 | 0.98 | 1.56 | 2.12 | 1.28 | 1.08 | 2.42 | 0.85 | 0.90 |
| 17 | 1.14 | 1.18 | 1.42 | 1.41 | 0.80 | 0.79 | 1.14 | 1.06 | 1.62 | 0.84 | 1.09 | 0.92 | 0.97 | 0.98 | 0.88 |
| 18 | 1.44 | 1.35 | 1.73 | 1.50 | 0.46 | 1.16 | 1.32 | 1.71 | 1.12 | 1.42 | 0.72 | 0.76 | 1.43 | 0.87 | 0.69 |
| Ave | 1.07 | 1.27 | 1.38 | 1.34 | 1.14 | 1.21 | 1.13 | 1.38 | 1.51 | 1.42 | 1.28 | 1.38 | 1.49 | 1.00 | 0.94 |
| Std dev. | 0.14 | 0.34 | 0.35 | 0.48 | 0.29 | 0.33 | 0.24 | 0.40 | 0.52 | 0.47 | 0.44 | 0.29 | 0.50 | 0.14 | 0.14 |

[a] 2H = 2 Hz heave vibration at ±0.2 g.   2S = 2 Hz sway vibration at ±0.2 g.
5H = 5 Hz heave vibration at ±0.2 g.   5S = 5 Hz sway vibration at ±0.1 g.
7H = 7 Hz heave vibration at ±0.2 g.   7S = 7 Hz sway vibration at ±0.1 g.

In elevation tracking, the 7 Hz sway result was not found to be significantly different from the no-vibration datum although the 2 Hz and 5 Hz sway results were just significantly different ($P = 5\%$). The 2 Hz heave, 2 Hz heave + 7 Hz sway and 5 Hz heave + 7 Hz sway results were calculated to be significantly different ($P = 1\%$) from the no-vibration result while all of the remaining results were found to have highly significant differences ($P = 0.2\%$) from the datum.

## 3. *Conclusions from Dual Axis Vibration Tests*

The tests described above indicate that performance of a zero-order two-dimensional compensatory tracking task of moderate difficulty is degraded by single axis 2 Hz, 5 Hz and 7 Hz single axis heave vibration at $\pm 0.2$ g and sway at $\pm 0.1$ g. When these heave and sway vibrations are combined together, tracking performance tends to be degraded by an amount equal to the product of the tracking decrements produced by the component single axes alone.

Thus, we have a method of predicting tracking performance decrement for dual axis heave and sway ($e_{hs}$) from the tracking decrements obtained from the single axis vibration test results, ($e_h$ and $e_s$), such that

$$\frac{\text{Predicted dual axis score}}{\text{No-vibration score}} = \frac{\text{Heave score}}{\text{No-vibration score}} \times \frac{\text{Sway score}}{\text{No-vibration score}}$$

or

$$e_{hs} = e_h \times e_s \tag{1}$$

This equation is also supported by the results from two other dual axis vibration experiments, reported in detail elsewhere (Lovesey, 1972). Tracking performance data from all three experiments have been incorporated in Fig. 2.

Figure 2 shows the actual dual axis performance decrements plotted against the predicted decrements that have been calculated from the component single axis scores. The above equation would appear to hold for most cases when the task difficulty is great enough to be adversely affected by single axis heave and sway vibrations. If the task difficulty is such that performance is actually improved by the vibration, then this equation no longer holds good. This is shown in Fig. 2 by the crosses which lie at or above unity and depart from the line $e_{hs} = e_h \times e_s$. These crosses represent the results from a HUD tracking test where vibration very often resulted in improved performance by one subject.

When no errors are produced during the static control conditions, as in the manual positioning task of Section II.B, the effects of dual axis vibration cannot be predicted by the above method. This is because any performance reduction is infinitely worse than the zero error performance achieved with no vibration. However, an approximate prediction

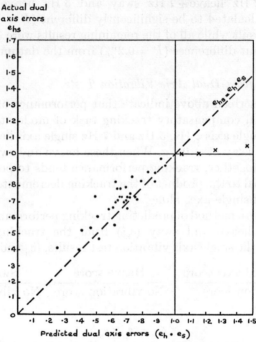

Fig. 2 Comparison of actual with predicted dual axis compensatory tracking errors. Dots represent tests where vibration degraded performance; crosses represent tests where single axis vibration actually improved performance.

of dual axis performance may still be obtained by simply adding the single axis error scores. Such as

$$e_{hs} = e_h + e_s \qquad (2)$$

The two performance prediction equations (1) and (2) are simple in form and therefore simple to apply. No doubt more sophisticated equations could be produced; however, further mathematical processing of the underlying experimental data is thought to be unjustified because of the many factors that are difficult to quantify which subtly influence the experimental results. The studies of single and dual axis vibration upon performance described in this chapter are necessarily limited and are only a small step towards fully understanding the effects of vibration upon man. If laboratory vibration tests are to be useful to others such as vehicle designers etc., they must simulate the most important factors which influence man. The work summarised here attempts to simulate the most frequently occurring vibrations of heave and sway. Future tests must include shunt vibrations and also the rotational vibrations of roll, pitch and yaw. Further research is also required into seat design, cushion dynamics and information presentation, when vibration is present.

## III. The Occurrence of Vibrations in Vehicles
### A. FIELD MEASUREMENTS OF VIBRATIONS
#### 1. *Introduction to Multi-axis Measurements*

Until recently, both vibration measurements and investigations into vibration effects upon man have been limited mainly to the heave axis. The investigations reported in Section II have shown that sway vibrations have a significant effect upon man's performance, especially when combined with heave. However, little information is available concerning the frequency of occurrence or magnitude of sway or shunt vibrations for existing transport systems. To help to further our knowledge of the occurrence of low frequency vibrations, a portable tape recorder system was assembled to record the output signals from three accelerometers mounted mutually perpendicular to each other. This vibration-recording equipment was then used to obtain three axis acceleration traces from the floors of several different types of vehicle while operating under typical conditions. The resulting accelerometer records gave an indication of the frequency, magnitude and phase relationships of the vibrations to be found in the vehicles and are summarised in Table VI. These data are relatively crude but should give the reader an idea of the nature of the multi-axis vibration to be found in existing forms of air and surface transport.

#### 2. *Analysis of Records*

The three axis vibration records were recorded on magnetic tape. This was replayed on separate equipment and reproduced on ultra-violet (UV) light-sensitive paper as continuous acceleration-time traces. Initially, it was intended that the magnetic tapes should be analysed automatically to produce Power Spectral Density plots and cross-correlations between axes. Due to equipment incompatibilities this was not achieved. The quality of the UV records was also too poor to warrant the use of an automatic data-processing system and the UV traces were eventually analysed manually.

Each of the traces was examined for predominant or recurring vibrations. The frequencies, average amplitudes, duration and,

TABLE VI: Typical predominant three axis vibration frequencies and g levels at vehicles floors

| Vehicle | Heave | | Sway | | Shunt | | Vibration duration | Estimated speed km/hr | Notes | Comments |
|---|---|---|---|---|---|---|---|---|---|---|
| | f(Hz) | ±g | f(Hz) | ±g | f(Hz) | ±g | | | | |
| **Helicopters** | | | | | | | | | | |
| Sioux | 11.5 | 0.06 | 11.5 | 0.05 | 24 | 0.05 | 5 min | 130 | Cruise, 305 m agl[a] | Smooth ride but noisy |
| Scout | 27 | 0.07 | 27 | 0.05 | 27 | 0.05 | 5 min | 185 | Cruise, 305 m agl | Smooth ride |
| **Fixed wing aircraft** | | | | | | | | | | |
| Dove | 0.25 | +0.5 / −0.25 | 1 | 0.03 | 1 | 0.03 | 10 sec | 204 | Cruise, 460 m agl | Bumpy ride through mild turbulence |
| HS 748 | 0.5 | 0.2 | 1.2 | 0.03 | 1.2 | 0.03 | 1 min | 204 | Cruise, 460 m agl | Passengers sick |
| | 0.9 | 0.12 | 0.9 | 0.05 | 0.9 | 0.05 | 1 min | 204 | Cruise, 460 m agl | Axes in phase |
| | 12.2 | 0.04 | 12.2 | 0.04 | 12.2 | 0.02 | 6 min | 278 | Cruise, 400 m agl | Axes in phase. |
| | 80 | 0.08 | 80 | 0.08 | 80 | 0.04 | 6 min | 278 | Cruise, 400 m agl | Axes in phase. |
| Beverley | 0.5 | 0.10 | 0.5 | 0.05 | 0.5 | 0.05 | 1 min | 297 | Cruise, 610 m agl | Axes in phase. |
| | 65.5 | 0.16 | 65.5 | 0.13 | 40.5 | 0.06 | 1 min | 297 | Cruise, 610 m agl | High frequency due to engine revs |
| | 40.5 | 0.25 | 40.5 | 0.15 | 40.5 | 0.10 | 1 min | 297 | Finals | |
| **Hovercraft** | | | | | | | | | | |
| SR-N4 | 0.3 | 0.20 | 0.18 | 0.10 | 3 | 0.05 | 1 min | 46 | 2–3 m waves | Unpleasant ride |
| | 0.9 | 0.07 | 28 | 0.03 | 8 | 0.03 | 1 min | 111 | 60 m waves | Smooth ride |
| | 7.5 | 0.25 | 11.5 | 0.05 | 7.5 | 0.02 | 10 min | 83 | 90–120 cm waves | Unpleasant ride |
| SR-N5 | 0.9 | 0.25 | 12.5 | 0.05 | 18 | 0.05 | 10 min | 28 | 90–150 cm waves | Rough ride in gale |
| | 1.3 | 0.3 | 2.6 | 0.04 | 3.2 | 0.05 | 10 min | 28 | White horses | Rough ride in gale |
| | 4.7 | 0.14 | 12.5 | 0.05 | 4.7 | 0.06 | 1 min | 83 | 30 cm waves | Slightly bumpy ride |
| HM-2 | 1.3 | 0.05 | 43 | 0.05 | 43 | 0.05 | 7 min | 56 | 0–30 cm waves | Smooth but noisy |
| | 2.5 | 0.12 | 44 | 0.08 | 44 | 0.05 | 10 sec | 56 | 0–30 cm waves | Smooth but noisy |
| **Boat** | | | | | | | | | | |
| Hydrofoil, 18 m | 0.9 | 0.10 | 0.9 | 0.10 | 0.9 | 0.05 | 1 min | 65 | Flat calm sea | Smooth ride |
| | 22 | 0.10 | 34 | 0.10 | 34 | 0.07 | 1 min | 65 | Flat calm sea | Smooth ride |
| Launch, 8·5 m | 1.3 | ±1.4 | 1.3 | 0.15 | 1.3 | 0.10 | 30 sec | 52 | 30–45 cm waves | Accelerations 1·8 m from stem |
| | 37.5 | 0.15 | 37.5 | 0.10 | 37.5 | 0.07 | 10 min | 52 | 30–45 cm waves | Violent and uncomfortable |
| **Trains** | | | | | | | | | | |
| Electric train | 1.8 | 0.10 | 1.8 | 0.05 | — | — | 1 min | 56 | Between Brookwood and Woking | Slightly bumpy |
| | 12 | 0.06 | 12 | 0.05 | 12 | 0.02 | 1 min | 56 | | |
| **Cars** | | | | | | | | | | |
| Morris 1300 | 1.8 | 0.15 | 1.5 | 0.07 | 1.8 | 0.08 | 1 min | 111 | Smooth A class road | Very smooth ride |
| | 19 | 0.25 | 19 | 0.20 | 19 | 0.25 | 1 min | 111 | Smooth A class road | 19 Hz at floor only |
| Minx Estate | 1.6 | 0.10 | 1.5 | 0.02 | 2 | 0.02 | 4 min | 28–46 | Medium/rough B class road | Smooth ride |
| | 19 | 0.02 | 25 | 0.01 | 25 | 0.01 | 4 min | 28–46 | Medium/rough B class road | Smooth ride |
| **Buses** | | | | | | | | | | |
| Double-decker bus | 2.8 | 0.12 | 22 | 0.11 | 22 | 0.10 | 1 min | 19–37 | Aldershot, side-roads | Slightly bumpy ride |
| | 11 | 0.40 | 14 | 0.20 | 40 | 0.20 | 1½ min | 19–37 | Aldershot, side-roads | Slightly bumpy ride |
| Single-decker bus | 2.5 | 0.80 | 20 | 0.10 | 30 | 0.10 | 1 min | 19–37 | Farnborough, side-roads | Slightly bumpy ride |
| | 3.0 | 0.10 | 12 | 0.10 | 13 | 0.10 | 1 min | 19–37 | Farnborough, side-roads | Slightly bumpy ride |

[a] agl—above ground level.

sometimes, phase relationships between axes of vibration were noted. Generally, one or more high frequency vibrations appeared as a ripple on top of a much lower frequency. Details of these are shown by rows bracketed together in Table VI.

Sometimes, the traces were of such random appearance that it was impossible to determine any basic frequency. In such cases, analysis was postponed until the trace became more cyclical in nature and a predominant frequency could be ascertained. Usually, however, analysis of only a few sections of each trace were required as the vibration conditions varied little throughout the sortie.

### 3. *Discussion of Vehicle Vibrations*

The results from the UV trace analysis are summarised in Table VI for each of the 15 vehicles investigated. The average peak g levels, which were measured at the vehicle's floor, are given for the corresponding predominant heave, sway and shunt vibration frequencies. An indication of the duration of the vibration is given, together with vehicle speed, environmental conditions and a subjective assessment of the ride.

Predominant vibration frequencies are plotted against $\pm g$ levels (half peak to peak values) for each vehicle in Fig. 3. In all vehicles listed in Table VI, the heave acceleration levels were generally the greatest. However in the two helicopters, the HM-2 sidewall hovercraft and the double-decker bus, the acceleration levels were approximately the same along all three axes for some of the runs. In the HS 748, the 18 m hydrofoil and the electric train, the heave and sway levels both tied for the axes with the greatest acceleration levels.

In the Beverley, the hydrofoil, the launch, the double- and single-decker buses, where the sway and shunt g levels reached or exceeded $\pm 0.1$, the corresponding frequencies were usually relatively high and above the 0–20 Hz range. This range, for a given g level, causes the greatest discomfort to the seated man. Alternatively, on some of the runs, sway and shunt g levels reached $\pm 0.1$ g in this critical 0–20 Hz range, e.g., in the SR-N4, the hydrofoil, Morris 1300 and in both buses. Thus, there is evidence that significant levels of horizontal vibration exist at frequencies which might affect human comfort and performance.

It is important to note that all frequencies and g levels, given in Table VI and shown in Fig. 3, relate to the vibrations measured at the floors of the vehicles. Seat dynamics may have amplified or attenuated the vibrations reaching the vehicle's occupants. This table gives an indication only of the subjective comfort of the ride in the vehicles and should therefore be used with caution.

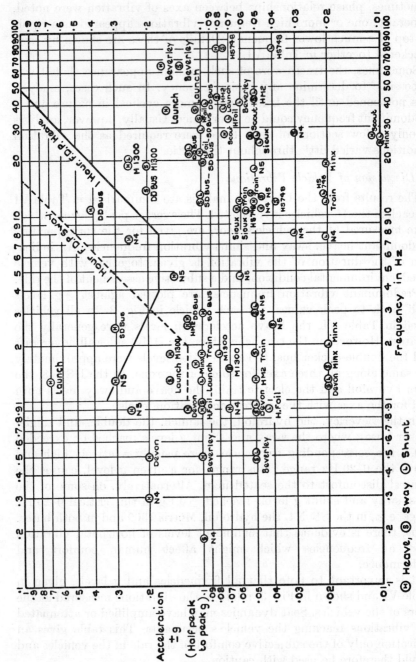

*Fig. 3* Predominant frequencies and acceleration levels measured in a range of vehicles. All data were obtained at the vehicle floor over a period of 1 min or longer.

Further measurements of the vibrations within existing types of transport require to be repeated with accelerometers small enough to be placed at the seat/man interface in order to determine the effective vibration input to the man. This would enable human performance and comfort to be related directly to the actual vibrations to which he is exposed.

## 4. *Concluding Remarks*

Three-axis continuous accelerometer records of the cabin floor vibrations from 15 different vehicles have been analysed. These records show that although heave vibration usually predominates, sway and shunt vibrations also exist at sufficient magnitudes to affect crew performance and passenger comfort. The vibration frequencies that have been recorded at the vehicles' floors range from 0.18 Hz to 80 Hz and cover almost the complete range of whole-body vibration frequencies which affect man. At the lower end of the range, large amplitude vibrations with frequencies of less than about 0.5 Hz can cause motion sickness. At higher frequencies, disturbing body resonances may occur that upset vision and consequently performance. A seated man's predominant resonant frequencies occur at approximately 5 Hz, 11 Hz and 20 Hz in heave and at 1.5–2 Hz in sway and shunt. These resonances may be modified in frequency and amplitude by the influence of a restraining harness and/or arm-rests, especially when low frequency sway is present.

Performance has been shown to be significantly reduced by vibrations existing concurrently in two axes, although the constituent vibrations would be acceptable if present along one axis alone.

Finally, since vibrations in all three axes have been shown to exist in current vehicles, vibration experiments and performance predictions should not be confined to single axis heave but should include both sway and shunt vibrations in combination with heave, to represent the conditions in a real vehicle.

## REFERENCES

Bolton, C. B. (1972). "Ventile Incompressible Cushions", Ergonomics Research Society, Industrial Spin-off from Military Ergonomics Conference Proceedings.

Hornby, R. C. and Wilson, R. (1967). "The Effects of Extended Practice on Performance in a Tracking Task", Aeronautical Research Council, Note 29887.

Huddleston, H. F. (1967). "Manual Tracking on a Visual Display apparently vibrating sinusoidally at 1–10 cycles per second", Report No. 399, Institute of Aviation Medicine, Farnborough.

International Organisation for Standardization. (1974). "Guide for Evaluation of Human Exposure to Whole-body Vibration". ISO 2631.

Lovesey, E. J. (1968). "The Influence of a Restraining Harness upon Human Comfort and Tracking Performance under Single and Multi-axis Heave and Sway vibration", unpublished Royal Aircraft Establishment Report, Farnborough.

Lovesey, E. J. (1971). "An Investigation into the Effects of Dual-axis Vibration, with Restraining Harness, Visual Feed-back and Control Force on a Manual Positioning Task", Farnborough Technical Report TR 71213, Royal Aircraft Establishment, Farnborough.

Lovesey, E. J. (1972). "An Investigation into the Effects of Dual-axis Vibration on Man". Ph.D. Thesis, Institute of Sound and Vibration Research, University of Southampton.

O'Hanlon, J. G. and Griffin, M. J. (1971). "Some Effects of the Vibration of Reading Material upon Visual Performance", Technical Report No. 49, Institute of Sound and Vibration Research, University of Southampton.

Shurmer, C. R. (1967). "A Review of the Effect of Low Frequency Vibration on Man and his Tracking Performance", Human Factors Study Note Series 4, No. 7, British Aircraft Corporation, Filton.

# 10. Vibration and Visual Acuity

*M. J. Griffin*

## I. Introduction
### A. MAN IN A MOVING WORLD

Man is aware of his environment by means of the information he receives from his senses. Classically these are the senses of touch, hearing, smell, taste and sight. Of these, sight is often considered to be the most necessary for his adequate performance in a system. A little consideration reveals that the process whereby the surrounding world of solid objects generates images in the eye and then perceptions of the size, colour, distance and position of objects is exceedingly complex. Indeed, the method of seeing is so wonderful that it may also seem improbable.

The characteristics of a perceived image of an object depend on the relative positions of the object and the observer's eye. Altering the position of either the object or the eye will normally affect the location, shape or size of the image of the object on the observer's retina. This normally results in the subject perceiving the relative motion and, sometimes, identifying it as being due to a movement of either himself or the object.

This motion may be a "signal" and contain information of value to the observer. Alternatively it may be of no such interest and is classified as "noise". In the latter case, while the motion may be either essential or incidental to the planned operation of the system, it becomes specially important if it prevents or impedes the input, output or information processing performance of the man in the system. It is common observation that various motions can have an adverse effect on man and it is also obvious that the ability to see is one faculty most often affected.

Motion implies both a physical displacement and a rate of change of displacement (velocity). It may also involve a rate of change of velocity (acceleration). The motion may either persist in some direction or oscillate about a mean position. It is the effects of oscillatory motions on vision which are the subject of this chapter.

## B. PURE AND APPLIED STUDIES

Human response is a highly variable factor—never can it be accurately specified by a single "magic number". Usually there are many uncontrolled variables which can have an effect. These make it necessary to state measures of both mean and variability in an adequate specification of the response. Attempts to classify the relevant variables have been previously published (e.g. Guignard, 1965; Griffin, 1972a) and these usually distinguish between variables characteristic of the man (intrinsic variables) and variables characteristic of the situation (extrinsic variables). The intrinsic variables are further subdivided as sources of between-subject variance (inter-subject variance) and within-subject variance (intra-subject variance). It is usual to find that there are a large number of intrinsic and extrinsic variables relevant to any human response to vibration experiment. The specification of the vibration conditions alone is therefore an inadequate description of the experimental variables.

In practice it is often difficult to measure, or even identify, some of the relevant variables. If results are to be applied in some particular context, either the experiment must be performed in this context (real or simulated) or, alternatively, the results must be extrapolated from a highly artificial experimental situation to the real-life environment. It will be shown later that many of the researchers experimenting with the effects of whole-body vibration on vision have selected, or been forced, to attempt to determine the effects of a few particular conditions that are experienced in a particular environment. In consequence there are only a few useful theoretical studies of the effect of whole-body vibration on vision. With the vibration of objects while the man remains stationary there are fewer variables of importance and there has been a greater concentration upon both systematically investigating the effect of variables and attempting to explain these effects.

## II. The Mechanism for Seeing

An understanding of the eye is essential for the critical appraisal of the information in the following sections. Some of the more relevant aspects are discussed here while a more complete account will be found in one of the many textbooks (e.g. Davson, 1962).

## A. THE EYE AND THE RETINA

The position of the eye is controlled by six muscles which serve to rotate it towards objects of interest. In the body of the eye, light is focused by the cornea and lens, passes through the pupil and then across the vitreous humour to produce a small inverted image on the surface of the retina.

The translation of light into electrical pulses (the language of the nervous system) is achieved by the light-sensitive rod and cone cells of the retina. These photoreceptors, some of which are only one micron across, form a complex interconnected mosaic from which signals are sent to inform the brain of the shape, colour and location of the objects whose images are falling on the retina. The psychology and physiology of the seeing process have some importance in the present context but the reader is referred elsewhere for the information (e.g. Davson, 1962; Gregory, 1966).

The motion of an observed object will tend to give rise to a similar, but reduced, motion of the object's image on the retina. If the motion is sufficiently large the image will then fall on a new set of photo-receptors. If the motion is of an oscillatory nature the image will constantly move back and forth across some confined area of the retina and a photoreceptor within this area may be expected to indicate alternately the presence and absence of the object. It may, however, produce a signal indicative of its average illumination so that the image has a "smeared" appearance. In these circumstances it is to be expected that it is the manner in which the photoreceptors and the brain cope with this constantly changing input that will determine the efficiency of the visual system. However, a "smear" will contain overlapping and confusion of detail that may be expected often to prove totally illegible. The moving object will be seen more clearly if its image can be stabilised on the retina so as to fall on some group of photoreceptors for as long as possible. This might be achieved if the eye rotates so as to follow the object. It will also be partly achieved at the nodal points of an oscillatory motion.

It is well established that the central portion of the retina (the fovea) contains cones in very close proximity to each other and this enables the detection of maximum visual detail. The ability to detect detail reduces as the image falls further away from the fovea. In daylight conditions the eyes are therefore oriented so that the image of a point of principal interest falls on the fovea. The ability to see detail in a moving object will be further reduced if it wanders outside the fovea.

## B. EYE MOVEMENTS

Fixation on a point in space is accompanied by two or three types of eye movement: drift, tremor and involuntary saccades. A drift is an irregular slow movement of the axis of an eye while the image remains within the fovea. The drift is accompanied by high frequency low amplitude oscillations of the axes of the eyes. During fixation on small targets the image may effectively wander over a central zone of the fovea about 6 minutes of arc in diameter. Maximum discrimination is achieved subjectively at all points within this zone but the position of the image within this area cannot be identified (Fender and Nye, 1961).

Eye drift appears to be uncorrelated in the two eyes and has a mean speed of approximately 5 minutes of angle per second and a maximum speed of 30 minutes of angle per second. It is generally agreed that the angular amplitude of eye tremor produces image displacements of the size of the retinal cones while the frequency of the movement is variously quoted from 20 Hz to 150 Hz. Saccades of both eyes coincide in time, amplitude and deviation. The small involuntary saccades that occur during fixation vary in amplitude from 2 minutes to 50 minutes of angle and in duration from 10 msec to 20 msec.

It is well known that if the image of an unchanging object becomes and remains, stationary, relative to the retina, it will effectively disappear (become an empty field) within 1–3 sec. Changes of illumination will aid vision under such conditions but a movement of the image is a necessary requirement for normal vision. Yarbus (1967) presents evidence to show that an image movement of about 20 minutes of arc per second is necessary for good vision and concludes that the drifts of maximum velocity, which occur several times a second, are the eye movements which prevent the formation of an empty field.

Yarbus (1967) has failed in an attempt to find an effect of tremor on vision. It is suggested that since the frequency of tremor is greater than the critical frequency of flicker fusion the result is not surprising. Ditchburn et al. (1959) have shown that low frequency oscillations (4–20 Hz and 0.05–1.10 minutes of angle) of an otherwise stationary image have a beneficial effect on visual discrimination. When the amplitude of oscillation exceeded 0.3 minutes of angle there was an increase in the fraction of time during which the object was observed. (The movements employed by Ditchburn et al. are not thought to be representative of normal eye tremor movements.) Krauskopf (1957) suggests that low frequency motion of the retinal image (1–5 Hz) will decrease contrast thresholds while high frequency (10–50 Hz) motions will increase them when normal retinal image motion is absent.

Since eye movements are essential for good vision it would appear quite possible that "normal" eye movements may not be sufficient for optimum vision. Some degree of vibration of an object relative to an observer could possibly improve the visibility of an object and, indeed, such improvements have been reported (e.g. Krauskopf, 1962).

However, the reported improvements are slight and unlikely to have any practical application in the present context.

## C. DYNAMIC VISUAL ACUITY

The visibility of moving targets has been studied by a number of authors (Ludvigh, 1953; Ludvigh and Miller, 1958; Miller, 1958). A few relevant aspects of these studies will be reviewed briefly since there is some similarity between low frequency oscillatory movements and the translational motions employed in studies of dynamic visual acuity. This similarity is inherent in the definition of dynamic visual acuity employed by Ludvigh and Miller who state that dynamic acuity is measured when the eyes are moving following the test object. Compulsive tracking of targets undergoing low frequency oscillation has been reported by several workers.

An article in the *Illustrated London News* (1 January 1938) attributed a velocity of 818 miles per hour to the deer botfly. This was questioned by Langmuir (1938) who showed that a simulated deer botfly was seen as a blur at 13 miles per hour and barely visible as a moving object at 26 miles per hour. He concluded that 25 miles per hour is a reasonable estimate of the speed of the flight of the deer botfly! It is thus demonstrated that acuity deteriorates as the relative angular velocity between the eye and the test object is increased. The manner of this deterioration with Landolt C targets has been shown by Miller (1958) to follow the semi-empirical equation:

$$Y = a + bx^3$$

where $Y$ is the size of the Landolt C at the threshold, $x$ is the angular velocity of the target and $a$ is the value of $Y$ under static conditions. This equation holds for both horizontal and vertical movement with angular velocities from 20 to 180 degrees per second and it is further shown that there is a high correlation between performance in the two directions. This implies that an individual's dynamic visual acuity (as described by the value of $b$) is dependent on the efficiency of his oculomotor pursuit mechanism rather than the strength of individual muscles. It has also been shown that increasing the level of illumination can improve the visibility of a moving target although the same increase will not improve acuity for the same type of target under static conditions. A study by Ludvigh and Miller (1958) has shown that there is little correlation between a subject's static acuity, $a$, and his dynamic acuity, $b$. In consequence of the wide range of dynamic acuity values it may be deduced that artificial means of magnification (which magnify both the size and the speed of the image of the target) may improve the dynamic acuity of some subjects and reduce the acuity of others. Imperfect eye pursuit movements, which result in continual motion of the image on the retina, would appear to be a more satisfactory explanation of loss of acuity than the fact that the target is partially viewed by the extrafoveal portions of the retina. In one of a series of studies of the perception of moving objects, Crawford (1960) has shown that for Landolt Cs which subtend 1 minute of arc, an error in the position of fixation of less than 1° and a velocity of fixation error less than 3° of arc per second do not individually interfere with perceptual ability. However, combined position and velocity errors of this magnitude had an appreciable effect on visibility.

## D. VISUAL ACUITY AND HUMAN PERFORMANCE

Good vision is largely the ability to see sharp images and judge the location of objects in space. This involves four categories of visual performance: (i) visual acuity, (ii) depth discrimination, (iii) form discrimination and (iv) movement discrimination. Visual acuity, the ability to see fine details, is naturally an important variable in depth, form and movement descrimination.

There are four distinct types of visual acuity: (i) minimum visible, (ii) minimum perceptible, (iii) minimum separable and (iv) minimum distinguishable. However, many practical tests of visual acuity are largely tests of luminance thresholds. Thus the ability to see a gap in a Landolt C is both a minimum separable acuity task and also a test of the luminance threshold for a small rectangular field bordered by a complex dark contour. In practice, values of visual acuity are dependent on many aspects of the visual display apart from the geometrical form of that display. Luminance and contrast, colour of illumination, exposure duration and location of the image on the retina are among the most common variables and their effects are reported in many reference works (e.g. Lythgoe, 1932; Westheimer, 1965).

Reductions in visual acuity are likely to be accompanied by decrements in human performance. The form and extent of the performance changes will be dependent on the nature of the reductions in acuity. In practice the visual acuity of a subject is often determined from his performance at some visual task and, in consequence, a relation between acuity and this particular performance is inherent in the definition of his acuity. However, the results obtained are highly characteristic of the selected performance indicator and it is difficult to use such results in predicting overall performance at the wide range of visual operations performed during, for example, flying or driving. Consequently, although it may be demonstrated that subnormal acuity occurs in certain situations, it is not to be assumed that there is necessarily any decrement in performance for those tasks which characterise the normal behaviour of any given operator in such a situation.

Studies by Burg (1968) and Burg and Coppin (1966) have found a significant relation between the rate of conviction for driving accidents and visual performance (including static and dynamic visual acuity). The large population investigated (17,500 subjects) included a number of subjects with extremely poor visual acuity. However, there was insufficient evidence to suggest visual criteria for the acceptance or rejection of driver license applicants. It has been found by Crossley (1969) that a group of trainee pilots requiring corrective lenses performed similarly to a matched group of pilots with normal vision during the first 16 weeks of flight training. Such studies establish their own criteria for acceptable performance according to the importance of success at the real task rather than by reference to arbitrarily selected psychological tasks. Therefore it is often highly desirable to evaluate experimental results in the context of real-life tasks and realistic performance criteria.

## III. Object Vibration
### A. INTRODUCTION

Various forms of vibrating object are seen in the wide range of modern transport systems as well as industrial and domestic situations. Studies of human ability to see such objects can yield information on the human visual system as well as indicating visual performance for the particular task. Thus the data obtained from studies of object vibration are of interest in other contexts including those cases where there is whole-body vibration with, or without, object vibration.

The published experimental investigations of the visibility of objects undergoing vibration are not very numerous and, chronologically, range from the reading and legibility experiments of Luckiesh and Moss (1938) Crook et al. (1947a b, 1948, 1949 and 1950) and Tinker (1948) to the tracking experiments of Huddleston (1970a, b) and the dual frequency experiments of Alexander (1972). The knowledge gained from such experiments will be reviewed in relation to the effects of individual physical variables (vibration frequency amplitude and direction, viewing distance etc.) on performance at various visual tasks.

### B. EFFECT OF VIBRATION FREQUENCY

Almost all experimenters agree that vibration frequency is an important source of variance.

## 1. *Pursuit Eye Movements*

Some experimenters (e.g. Drazin, 1962; Huddleston, 1970a, b; Alexander, 1972) have shown that, for a constant angular displacement of an object, the subject's performance (measured in terms of reading or tracking task errors) falls as vibration frequency is increased to some critical frequency. When the frequency is increased further, performance improves. There is evidence that this critical frequency appears to decrease with increasing angular displacement of the object and for displacements up to 4° double amplitude it is in the range 1–5 Hz. Drazin, Huddleston and Alexander employed very different visual tasks (dial reading, tracking performance and letter reading respectively) and little can be gained from comparisons of the different performance scores obtained by them.

The explanation of this frequency dependence is provided by the results of experiments measuring eye movements whilst viewing vibrating objects. Preliminary experiments in the range 1.4–3.4 Hz by Guignard and Irving (1962) involved the measurement of the frequency response of eye movements during vertical vibration of (a) the subject only and (b) the target only. In the first case it would be beneficial if the eye can "compensate" for the vibratory motion of the head while in the second case the eye would be required to "pursue" the motion of the object. The Guignard and Irving experiments led to the tentative conclusion that the frequency response of compensatory eye movements is higher than the frequency response of pursuit movements. Thus eye movements were found to be present in both situations but their efficiency can be increased when the motion is perceived by the subject via sensory modalities in addition to the visual perception of the moving target.

Drazin (1962) suggested that below about 3 Hz, pursuit eye movements are almost totally compulsive when the whole visual field is in motion. Limited recordings of the eye movements of one subject showed that as the frequency of vibration was reduced from 4 Hz to 3 Hz the times taken to inhibit these compulsive movements increased from 1 sec to 7.5 sec. At 2.5 Hz the subject could not inhibit the tracking after trying for 15 sec. Above 5 Hz Drazin suggested that this compulsion has less force and observers will have little difficulty in fixating on only the nodal points of the vibratory object. With reference to earlier work (Jones and Drazin, 1961; Trincker *et al.*, 1961) Drazin suggested that the increased dial reading errors found as frequency was raised to 3 Hz are a consequence of the limited frequency response of the eye. This produces progressive attenuation of pursuit movements at frequencies above 1 Hz.

Huddleston (1970a) measured the eye movements of six subjects performing a tracking task where the task and its surround were made to vibrate with 4° double amplitude at various frequencies. With 1 Hz, 2 Hz and 3 Hz vibration the eye attempted to follow the oscillations (in fact the subjects could not define any nodal images) but at 4 Hz the eye stayed near the centre of the oscillation. At 5 Hz the subjects attempted to view the upper nodal images but their gaze occasionally wandered elsewhere. At 6 Hz they appeared to have no difficulty in viewing the upper nodal image.

There is overwhelming evidence that the ability to see objects vibrating at low frequencies does depend on frequency. This was well illustrated by Huddleston (1969) who pooled the data obtained by various workers to obtain mean values of the amplitude and phase angle response of the eye. Figure 1 shows the mean phase angle response (for targets of 8.2° and 14.8° double amplitude) and mean amplitude response (for targets of 10° double amplitude) as calculated by Huddleston. For these vibration amplitudes it appears that pursuit tracking is unlikely to be effective above 1 Hz or 1.5 Hz. However, there is certainly insufficient data to be able to predict with any precision the relation between errors (however measured) and frequency.

## 2. Viewing Nodal Images

Object vibration experiments with frequencies greater than 10 Hz have been conducted by only a few authors (e.g. Crook, 1947, 1949; Dennis, 1965a; O'Hanlon and Griffin, 1971; Alexander, 1972; Griffin, 1973).

An extensive series of experiments on vibration and visual acuity were conducted by Crook et al. (1947a, b, 1948, 1949, 1950), but relatively little study was made of the effects of vibration frequency. Employing a number-reading task and frequencies of 9 Hz, 15 Hz and 30 Hz it was found that there were both increases in reading time and reading errors as the frequency was increased at constant vibration displacement.

Dennis (1965a) employed several frequencies above 10 Hz but, with different vibration levels at each frequency, the results do not lend themselves to establishing the effect of vibration frequency on visual acuity. The Landolt C reading experiments described by Alexander (1972) and O'Hanlon and Griffin (1971) are probably the most revealing concerning the importance of vibration frequency where nodal images are visible.

Employing vertical vibration of Landolt Cs (with the gap in the C orientated in a horizontal position—i.e. left or right) O'Hanlon and

Griffin recorded reading errors, reading time and a subjective rating of reading difficulty for a constant object double amplitude displacement of 2.5 mm and frequencies varying from 5 Hz to 30 Hz. This displacement corresponds to a double angle displacement of approximately

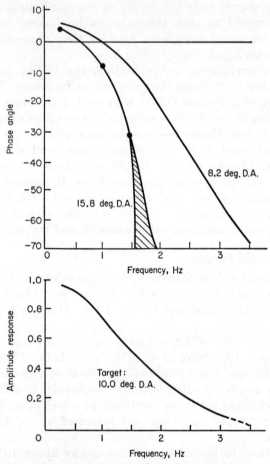

*Fig.* 1 Mean phase angle response and amplitude response of pursuit eye movements (from Huddleston, 1969). Curves indicate mean values obtained by various experimenters.

12 minutes subtended at the eyes of the eight subjects. It was found that mean reading errors, $E$, were directly proportional to the vibration frequency, $F$. In fact, for 24 targets:

$$E = 0.25F + 1.36$$

The reading time and difficulty rating also increased with increasing frequency. These results are shown in Fig. 2 and will be discussed again later.

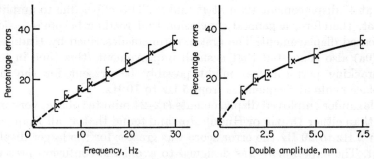

*Fig.* 2 The effects of vibration frequency and vibration amplitude on Landolt C reading errors (6/4 target size) (from O'Hanlon and Griffin, 1971).

With a similar reading task Alexander (1972) also found a linear frequency dependence from 5 Hz to 20 Hz. She employed object displacements of about 12 minutes and 24 minutes of arc and found that the relationship between errors and frequency is amplitude dependent.

The relation between vibration frequency and the threshold for visual perception of object vibration has been studied by Crook *et al.* (1949) and Griffin (1973). Employing numerical reading material and three subjects Crook found that "an increase in frequency from 18 Hz to 30 Hz caused a 127% increase in the threshold". Griffin found that the threshold for the detection of blur produced by a vibrating point source of light was independent of frequency from 5 Hz to 20 Hz. These two results might reflect a difference in the perception of higher frequencies (as proposed by O'Hanlon and Griffin, 1971) or, alternatively, the differences between the two tasks that were employed in the two very different experiments. For example, Griffin (1973) pointed out that the relation between blur and visual acuity is likely to be complex and highly dependent on the nature of the visual task.

## C. EFFECT OF VIBRATION AMPLITUDE

### 1. *Pursuit Eye Movements*

In their respective experiments Drazin (1962) employed three displacements and Huddleston (1970a) employed two different object displacements. Below about 4 Hz they both found that acuity decreased as the vibration amplitude increased. At higher frequencies (6 Hz and

8 Hz) Drazin found that the larger displacement amplitudes produced lower error scores than small displacements. This result was attributed to the confusion arising from the overlapping of the nodal images. It is shown that in this dial reading experiment the confusion would be less at 4° displacement than at 1° and 2°. This effect due to amplitude is not, therefore, a general conclusion that reading becomes easier at increased displacement! The first experiment described by Huddleston (1970a) also suggested that a small improvement (this time in terms of tracking performance) might possibly be present for the larger displacements at frequencies from 5 Hz to 10 Hz.

Alexander employed displacements (12–24 minutes of arc) very much less than either Drazin or Huddleston and found that at all frequencies from 2 Hz to 20 Hz the error score was greater for the larger displacement. The experiment was designed to avoid the confusion presented by the overlapping of images discussed by Drazin and therefore tends to confirm their importance—particularly in those conditions where the nodal images are employed. Twelve subjects participated in Alexander's experiment and she shows that, for frequencies below 5 Hz, as the vibration amplitude is increased the frequency of maximum error tends to decrease. However, errors were not exceptionally great in this range and she concludes that performance decrement in the pursuit range of viewing is not large until object displacements of the order of degrees, rather than minutes, of arc are encountered.

## 2. The Viewing of Nodal Images

Crook et al. (1947a, b, 1948, 1949, 1950) incorporated more than one vibration amplitude in several of their 14 experiments with object vibration. In Experiment 10, they employed a frequency of 17.5 Hz and five vibration amplitudes from 0.15 mm to 0.75 mm (with a viewing distance of 35 cm) but found no change in either reading errors or reading time due to alterations in the vibration amplitude. However, it was found in later experiments, especially Experiment 14, that performance was dependent on vibration amplitude when either of two other conditions (lighting and type size) was unfavourable. It was concluded that vibration double amplitudes of 0.5 mm are about the smallest that might impair performance when other conditions are optimal.

Employing their Landolt C reading task with a constant frequency of 16 Hz, O'Hanlon and Griffin (1971) found that reading errors, $E$, increased with vibration amplitude, $a$, such that

$$E = 9.8\sqrt{(a)} + 0.45 \quad \text{(if } a \text{ is in cm)}$$

This result (see Fig. 2) was obtained from six vibration levels (1.3–7.6 mm double amplitude) at a viewing distance of 1.01 m and with 24 Landolt Cs scaled down to the 6/4 size. With test objects 25% larger it was found that errors were much less and the above relation did not hold. Indeed, for this size of object, the errors were constant from 2.5 mm to 5 mm and decreased when the double amplitude was increased to 7.5 mm. In general the reading time and subjective rating of task difficulty increased as vibration amplitude was increased.

## D. EFFECT OF OBJECT ILLUMINATION

Crook *et al.* (1947a, b, 1948, 1949, 1950) employed more than one brightness level in several of their experiments. They eventually conclude that as brightness decreases from 15 ft Lamberts to 0.02 ft Lamberts the minimum vibration amplitude which impairs acuity reduces from 0.5 mm to 0.25 mm. There is thus evidence to show the presence of an interaction between vibration amplitude and object brightness. In view of this and other evidence (e.g. Morris, 1966; Rubenstein and Taub, 1967; Rubenstein and Kaplan, 1968) it is surprising that the importance of object illumination has not been studied more extensively.

## E. EFFECT OF OBJECT SIZE

O'Hanlon and Griffin (1971) report that:

> "A relatively small increase in test object size appreciably reduced reading errors—a 75% reduction in errors was produced by only a 25% increase in the size of the Landolt Cs. The same size increase resulted in up to 20% reduction in the time taken to complete the reading task."

Crook *et al.* (1947a, b, 1948, 1949, 1950) employed different type sizes in many of their experiments and also found that larger sizes were less affected by vibration. As might be expected, the effect of type size interacts with both brightness and vibration amplitude so that increased size is most beneficial when the combination of vibration amplitude and brightness is most unfavourable.

## F. EFFECT OF OBJECT VIEWING DISTANCE

Few experimenters have varied viewing distance so there is little experimental evidence of its effect. It seems reasonable to assume that an object vibrating with amplitude, $a$, and viewed from a distance, $d$, has a very similar retinal image to that of a similar object of twice the size seen at $2d$ and vibrating at an amplitude of $2a$. There are naturally limiting conditions for this assumption but, for example, an experiment described by Griffin (1973) suggests that the detection of blur caused by vibration is related to viewing distance as predicted by this theory.

For a constant size of object there will be increased reading difficulty as viewing distance is increased irrespective of whether the object is being vibrated. Employing frequencies above about 5 Hz it has been shown that, for constant levels of vibration, small increases in object size can result in a considerable improvement in reading ability; also, that increases in vibration amplitude are proportional to the square of the reading errors. (A doubling of errors is produced by a fourfold increase in vibration amplitude.) Thus, if a vibrating object is approached, there are corresponding increases in the sizes of the retinal images of both object displacement and object size. The limited experimental evidence suggests that the increase in object size will be more beneficial than the detrimental effect of the apparent increase in vibration amplitude. Reducing viewing distance may thus be beneficial when nodal images are being viewed.

In the absence of vibration, doubling the viewing distance would require the doubling of object size in order to maintain visual acuity. In the presence of vibration, doubling object size and viewing distance may be expected to improve acuity—unless the overlapping of nodal images causes significant confusion.

## G. EFFECT OF COMPLEX OBJECT MOTIONS

While there are understandable reasons for the selection of discrete single axis sinusoidal vibrations in most experiments, it remains a fact that such motions are the exception in real systems. In practice, motions often occur in more than one axis and consist of either a composite of several sinusoids or some form of random signal. In the available literature two experimental studies of such situations are reported.

Crook *et al.* (1947a, b, 1948, 1949, 1950) considered the dual axis situation with 23 Hz sinusoidal components in both the vertical and horizontal directions. By the selection of different phase relationships between these components they produced four different form patterns: one linear, two ellipses and one circle. In the first series of conditions the major axes of both ellipses, the diameter of the circle and the linear amplitude were all set to 0.8 mm (viewing distance 36 cm) and the minor axes of the ellipses were 0.25 mm and 0.53 mm respectively. The second series of conditions employed displacement amplitudes one-half those used in the first condition. Four subjects participated in the experiment and the effect of form pattern was not significant in terms of changes in reading time or errors.

This result is inconsistent with the predictions of a model of the method of seeing nodal images which is described in the next section.

This model would suggest that maximum difficulty would normally be experienced with the circular motion and the minimum difficulty experienced for the linear motion. Performance would be expected to be better for the first ellipse than the second. In fact, although the experimental effect due to form was not found to be significant, it is encouraging that the data for reading time and errors do approximate to this predicted ranking. Indeed, the authors concluded that "the circular form would be more unfavourable if secondary conditions were more severe".

The single axis multiple frequency situation was investigated in two experiments conducted by Alexander (1972). There would be considerable advantages in being able to predict performance under such complex vibration conditions from a knowledge of performance with single sinusoidal vibration. Thus Alexander compared performance for the combination of two frequencies with performance for each of the frequencies alone. Two such experiments were conducted: the first investigating the frequency effect of dual frequency vibration with components in the range 3–20 Hz; the second investigating the effect of varying component amplitudes in the 3 Hz plus 11 Hz and 20 Hz plus 11 Hz frequency combinations.

The experimental results are interesting but complex. It was found that when 2.5 mm double amplitude of 11 Hz vibration is added to the same displacement amplitude of 3, 4, 5, 6, 15 or 20 Hz vibration, the error score with the dual frequency is greater than that for the lower frequency component alone. However, the error score was less than, or the same order as, the error score found for the higher frequency alone! This trend was also followed by the measures of reading time.

The second experiment was conducted in two parts. The first investigated the effect of adding constant levels (2.5 mm double amplitude) of 11 Hz to various amplitudes of 3 Hz. The 11 Hz component had no significant effect on errors when the 3 Hz component was greater than 10.2 mm. At lower levels of 3 Hz, the 11 Hz component had an appreciable effect and below 2.5 mm of 3 Hz errors increased as the level of 3 Hz was decreased. However, the errors produced by 2.5 mm of the 11 Hz component alone were *greater* than the errors produced by this component added to any level of 3 Hz less than 10.2 mm! Indeed when 1.3 mm of 3 Hz were added to 2.5 mm of 11 Hz, errors were reduced by 25%. The second part of this experiment concerned 20 Hz and 11 Hz components added in various proportions keeping the total displacement constant at 5.1 mm. It was found that the task was most difficult when either component predominated (i.e. its level exceeded about 80% of the total displacement). Consequently, there was an optimum combination of the two components when they were of approximately equal magnitude.

Alexander had hoped to be able to predict performance from a knowledge of the waveform shape. She concludes that more knowledge of how subjects viewed particular waveforms (data such as might be obtained by monitoring eye movements) is necessary before any general rules can be offered. It was usually found that subjects were unable to state how they viewed the various dual frequency conditions.

There is evidence to show that both dual frequency and dual axis vibrations are important in determining the decrements in acuity caused by object vibration. The suggestion that dual axis vibrations present particularly difficult conditions must raise doubts about the applicability of current results to most real environments.

## H. CONCLUSIONS

There are a great number of variables that will interact with the effect of vibration on the ability to identify a vibrating object. The effects associated with vibrating frequency and amplitude, illumination, viewing distance, object size, dual axis and dual frequency vibration have been discussed. However, while the significance of these variables is poorly understood, there are other aspects of probable importance for which it does not seem possible to reach any useful conclusions. Questions concerning the nature of inter- and intra-subject variances, the effect of changing the form, colour or contrast of the object, the importance of the size of the vibrating visual field etc. must all be left unanswered.

On the relationship between vibration and visual acuity, it has been said that "there are in fact as many visual acuities as there are test objects". Visual acuity is determined by obtaining a measure of a subject's performance at a visual task. This performance may be measured in several ways: measures of speed, errors, omissions etc. There is, therefore, no single measure of acuity (either as regards the choice of test object or the measurement of performance). Laboratory and real-life visual tasks and measures of visual performance will differ to a considerable extent. Until the effects of all the relevant variables are known this must restrict (or possibly prohibit) the application of much of the experimental data to real situations.

The visual tasks have ranged through letters, numerals, dials, tracking tasks etc. Measures of performance may reasonably be expected to consist of both speed and accuracy. The need for both measures may be illustrated by the results of three experiments obtained over a period of 25 years. Luckiesh and Moss (1938) found that when their reading matter was vibrated the subjects found reading to be extremely fatiguing. However, the time taken to read two pages was unaffected by the vibration. They conclude that "these data clearly reveal the inadequacy of the criterion of speed of reading as a means of appraising ease of seeing". Tinker (1948) pointed out that:

> "All psychologists and workers in experimental education insist that there be a check on comprehension when measuring rate of reading. Rate of reading for them means how fast can a specific type of material be read with understanding."

Tinker produced a series of studies of the effect of several variables upon reading, including two on the effects of 5 Hz vibration (Tinker, 1948, 1953), and his argument to measure both accuracy and speed was later supported by an experiment conducted by Drazin (1962). He found that at about these frequencies the exposure time to the vibrating test object is an important factor.

In spite of the dearth of information there have been only two publications which have attempted to make general predictions on the basis of the experimental results. O'Hanlon and Griffin (1971) proposed a model of the viewing mechanism for the perception of nodal images. In brief, they propose that the ability of the eye to distinguish the presence of an element of visual detail is related to the time taken for the image of the detail to pass over some critical area (a few cones) on the surface of the retina. For a sinusoidal motion this time, $T$, is a maximum at the nodal image and is inversely proportional to the vibration frequency, $f$, and square root of the vibration amplitude, $a$. If this time is inversely related to reading errors, $E$, then:

$$E \propto f\sqrt{a}.$$

It will be recalled that the O'Hanlon and Griffin results took the form of errors being proportional to both frequency and the square root of the vibration amplitude. Alexander (1972) showed that the above equation also fitted her data.

While there is experimental backing for this relation it must remain of questionable value. The inverse relationship between the time, $T$, and reading errors (which is apparently similar to "Block's law") must break down outside a fairly narrow range of task difficulty. Further, it has been verified for only a few select conditions with a Landolt C reading task.

Griffin (1975b) claims that his data on the threshold of visual blur produced by object vibration can be used to predict "the minimum levels of vibration which would affect visual acuity". Limited evidence is presented in support of the hypothesis that when the image of a vibrating object cannot be distinguished from the image of an identical stationary object, visual acuity will not be affected. Thus the "threshold" of blur is chosen as the minimum level of vibration affecting visual acuity. Since the threshold of blur was shown to be largely dependent on the angle subtended by the vibration (approximately ± 1 minute of arc) the "acceptable" level of vibration will increase with increasing viewing distance. The application of the threshold level may be expected to be over-restrictive in all but the most critical conditions and so Griffin suggests that "displacements less than ± 1 minute of arc in any direction are unlikely to affect visual acuity while displacements greater than ± 2 minutes of arc may, depending on the difficulty of the task, affect reading ability". (This latter boundary is shown in Fig. 5 for a reading distance of 61 cm.)

## IV. Subject Vibration

### A. INTRODUCTION

The object vibration experiments reported by Crook *et al.* between 1947 and 1950 led to the identification of many relevant variables—but subsequent research was slow to progress beyond this level of discovery. Similarly, researchers into the effects of whole-body vibration on vision might have been expected to develop much from the work of Coermann (1947). However, the studies by both Crook *et al.* and Coermann have survived so that even after 20 years they are described as "largely dominant", "most extensive", etc.

If visual acuity is impaired when there is motion of the image of an object across the retina, we would expect that vibration of the head would be a critical factor in defining those situations in which body vibration impairs visual acuity. Head vibration occurs in most public transport systems (see Walsh, 1966; Griffin, 1972b) but applied studies of the effects of whole-body vibration on vision have usually been conducted in the context of military aircraft, tanks or spacecraft. (As in other areas of human factors research, such systems have held the monopoly of both the problems and the research effort.) Thus, of the 50 whole-body vibration and visual acuity experiments described in a recent analysis (Griffin, 1973), less than about 20% can be claimed as attempts at pure research and only about 10% have been conducted without some form of military support or objective. The predominance of military interest in research of this kind might be interpreted as an indication that only military personnel find themselves exposed to levels of vibration that affect visual acuity. However, such a conclusion is not possible while there remains inadequate information on the vibration to which people are exposed.

At least one author (Bryce, 1966) claims that as vibration levels are increased it is the visual effects which are usually the first to cause discomfort or disturbance for frequencies from 5 Hz to 19 Hz. With the general increase in human response to vibration research in the last decade (Griffin, 1972c), it is not surprising that there have been many recent experiments into the effects of vibration on visual acuity. More than half of the total number of relevant experiments have been performed in the United States. The remainder have been conducted in Great Britain with contributions from Japan, Germany, Canada etc.

The introduction to this chapter warned that the apparent distinction between pure and applied research was most evident in studies of the effects of whole-body vibration on vision. A primitive state of knowledge with regard to human response to vibration is the background to any experimentation in this area and this must seriously handicap all research. The principal problem is the poor understanding of the effects of the numerous variables relevant to both the real and the experimental situations. The following sections attempt to determine the importance of such variables by reference to the available research papers. Much of the literature has proved of no assistance in this attempt and will not be discussed. However, the majority of the available "research" literature on whole-body vibration and vision is included in the reference list at the end of the chapter.

## B. THE PRACTICAL DIFFERENCES BETWEEN WHOLE-BODY AND OBJECT VIBRATION

The visual effects caused by whole-body vibration differ from those produced by an identical vibration of an object for several reasons. The extent of any impairment in visual acuity is assumed to be dependent on the vibratory motions of the retinal image. For whole-body vibration these motions are due to movement of (or within) the eyeball. We therefore seek the answer to the pertinent question: how is the vibration input to the body related to the consequent eyeball motions?

In the following section the transmission of vibration to the body is briefly discussed. We might expect that for vibration from a seat, the displacement of the eye would become a smaller fraction of the displacement of the seat as the vibration frequency is increased. However, the system will have resonances and the retinal image motion will be affected by the resonances of both the eye and the various body parts between the seat and the eye. The "design" of the eye obviously incorporates the ability for its rotation in two angular axes (pitch and yaw) within the head. It also enables small movements in the other four axes. Consequently, we should not assume that a single axis of vibration at the seat will result in only this direction of motion at the eye. Finally, we will recall that low frequency vibrations of an object could be accompanied by a "pursuit" motion of the eye. In the case of whole-body vibration any such motion might reasonably be renamed a "compensatory" eye motion. However, the situations also differ in that whole-body vibration may be perceived other than by movements of images on the retina. This additional information could possibly result in a practical distinction between "compensatory" and "pursuit" eye movements.

## C. THE TRANSMISSION OF VIBRATION TO THE BODY

It is to be expected that the effects of whole-body vibration on visual acuity will be dependent on the nature and amount of head vibration. The head vibration is, in turn, normally dependent on the characteristics of the vibration at the various interfaces between the body and the environment. For practical purposes it has often been assumed that vertical vibration of the seat is the factor which determines head vibration although this is certainly a gross over-simplification for some environments. Based upon this simple conception, there have been a number of laboratory studies which attempt to relate the magnitude of vertical head motion to the magnitude of an applied motion of the seat. Many of these investigations have employed merely one or two subjects and demonstrated appreciable changes consequent upon alteration of body position and posture (e.g. Coermann, 1962; Edwards and Lange, 1964; Frovlov, 1970; Lange and Edwards, 1970). Other studies have found changes in the mechanical impedance of the body (impedance = force/velocity) due to changes in the level of acceleration of the environment (Vogt *et al.*, 1968), while Payne and Band (1971) have presented an elegant summary of the limited value of mechanical impedance measurements. In particular, it should be recognised that mechanical impedance is of dubious value if the mechanical response of the body is non-linear. Considering the small number of subjects employed in many of these experiments it is not surprising to find that some authors advocate linearity (e.g., Lange and Edwards, 1970; Lee and King, 1971) while others claim to have shown the response to be non-linear (e.g., Guignard and Irving, 1960; Edwards and Lange, 1964; Vogt *et al.*, 1968; Wittman and Phillips, 1969). Griffin (1975a) conducted an experiment with 12 seated subjects and six levels of vertical vibration at 12 frequencies from 7 Hz to 75 Hz. The principal finding was that body posture had a considerable effect on the vibration transmitted to the head. Figure 3 shows how the mean transmissibility of vertical vibration to the head changed as the subjects modified their posture so as to maximise and minimise the sensation of head vibration. Under these two posture conditions it was found that the fraction of vibration transmitted to the head was dependent on the vibration level. However, these non-linearities were relatively small and occurred predominantly at frequencies below 25 Hz. The standard deviations shown in Fig. 3 reflect fairly large intersubject differences. Further evidence of intersubject variability is provided by Guignard and Irving (1960), who suggest that there is greater damping at resonance with large subjects than with small subjects.

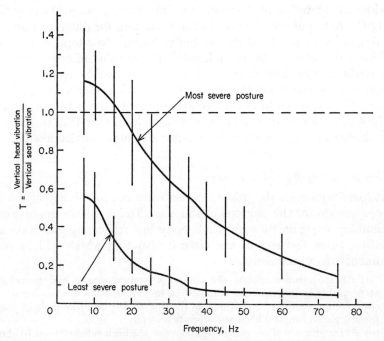

*Fig.* 3 The mean (and ± 1 standard deviation) of transmissibility, *T*, of 12 subjects at six levels of vertical vibration and in two postures (from Griffin, 1975a).

A number of authors have realised that the body and its various parts can undertake oscillation in six axes (three rotational and three translational). While the seat may only move vertically, the head may oscillate in any or all of the six possible axes. This is of interest since it is likely that the magnitude of lateral and pitch motions of the head, for example, are of some importance in determining the effect of head vibration on visual acuity.

## D. THE EFFECT OF VIBRATION FREQUENCY

It should now be apparent that the manner in which the effect of vibration on visual acuity varies with frequency will depend on the posture of the body and the position at which the vibration is measured. For particular postures and measurement positions the frequency effect will be partly due to the effective transmissibility of the vibration between the measurement position and the eye. It will also be a consequence of the relation between acuity and frequency of retinal image motion as was discussed in Section III.B.

In view of the large and important effects of posture, it is useful to consider the vibration of the head as an intermediate step. We may then study the dynamics of the eyes in the head and, for different postures, the dynamics of the head on the body. Failure to adopt such a subdivision will make it difficult to identify the location of any resonances and without this knowledge it becomes impossible to predict the importance of changing the dynamics of various parts of the body. Indeed, there is much to be said for attempting to assess the importance of vibration in an environment by measuring head vibration and relating it to similar measurements in laboratory and other environments.

### 1. *Compensatory Eye Movements*

At low frequencies the prime interest concerns the ability of the eye to compensate for the motions of the head. Drazin (1959) reports on a preliminary experiment with whole-body low frequency vibration and identifies three features of the aircraft situation which will be most detrimental to visual acuity:

"(i) At frequencies within the limits of compensatory eye movements attributable to labyrinthine stimulation, angular motion of the aircraft will elicit compensatory eye movements tending to displace the angle of regard from a visual target within the aircraft cockpit.

(ii) At frequencies of angular motion beyond the limit referred to at (i) above, the line of regard will be displaced relative to a visual target on the ground, thereby resulting in a loss of acuity.

(iii) In the case of translational motion of the head with respect to the aircraft, aircrew must make accurate pursuit movements of the head and eyes, so as to preserve fixation on a target within the cockpit. Such movements of the eye probably break down at some fairly low frequency—the exact frequency presumably depending upon amplitude—but even below this frequency they are not sufficiently accurate to prevent slight blurring of the retinal image."

Guignard and Irving (1962) conducted an experiment with 0.8° double amplitude of relative motion between object and observer for six frequencies in the range 1.4–3.4 Hz. Four subjects were exposed to the relative motion (achieved by (a) vibration of the target and (b) vibration of the object) and the results from two subjects lead the authors to conclude that the frequency response of compensatory eye movements during vibration of the man is higher than that of pursuit movements during vibration of the target. The mean for all four subjects shows that the turnover frequency is about 2 Hz for target vibration and about 3 Hz for vibration of the man. Additional evidence suggested that it is "labyrinthine impulses (presumably arising from otolithic stimulation, during linear vertical motion) which assist in ocular fixation".

Probably the most convincing distinction between compensatory and pursuit eye movements comes from a recent experiment by Benson (1972). He employed angular vibration in the yaw axis over the frequency range 0.5–10 Hz with a peak angular velocity of $\pm 20°$ per sec at all frequencies. The results of a number-reading task indicated that the pursuit reflex was insufficient at 0.5 Hz and apparently totally unable to aid vision above 2 Hz or 3 Hz. However, the vibration of the subject resulted in visual performance being maintained up to 6 Hz. A subject without semi-circular canal function performed similarly under the two conditions of object and subject vibration and thus gave confirmation of the presence of a vestibulo-ocular reflex in normal persons.

While other authors have devised methods of demonstrating the presence of such a reflex (e.g., Lee and King, 1971), the study by Benson is significant in that it appears to emphasise that angular head motion is the factor of importance in the compensatory reflex. Many previous experimenters have employed whole-body vertical vibration and, at best, measured vertical head motion. Such measurements can be misleading at low frequencies when there is an appreciable nodding motion of the head. In fact, the vibration level recorded will vary according to the position of the measurement transducer on the head. Further, the current information suggests that it is the angular head motions which should be related to some theoretical model of an efficient reflex system, while the translational motions may be considered to be relatively uncompensated. On this basis the overall effect of low frequency vertical whole-body vibration will be dependent on both vertical *and* angular head motion.

## 2. *The Viewing of Nodal Images*

For frequencies too high for the currently predicted compensatory eye movements to be beneficial, we are most concerned with the frequency response of the human body between the eye and the

11

vibration input. (The precise location of the boundary between high and low frequencies must await experimental clarification. Most would place it below 5 Hz or 10 Hz although it has been suggested (O'Briant and Ohlbaum, 1970) that some form of tracking might be possible up to about 20 Hz.) We should particularly consider the possibility that at some frequency the eyes may resonate within the head. The mechanical resonance of the living human eye appears to have been determined by only a few experimenters.

Thomas (1965) provided clear evidence of a mechanical resonance of the human eye of a subject and has shown that the resonance peak could be shifted to lower frequencies by increasing the effective mass of the eye. In the vertical plane Thomas demonstrated a resonance at about 30 Hz and suggested that, for vibration of the head, the eye/head velocity ratio is about 2 at this frequency.

Coermann (1947) was probably the first to attempt a systematic study of the effect of whole-body high frequency vibration on visual acuity. He measured vertical head vibration and studied the effect of frequencies from 15 Hz to 140 Hz on the ability of subjects to detect diverging black lines on a rotating drum. Incomplete results from five subjects strongly suggested some form of resonance "between the eye socket and the retina". Considerable differences between subjects were found and, while Coermann identifies three frequency ranges of maximum sensitivity (25–40 Hz; 60–90 Hz; 50–55 Hz) it is certainly not possible to generalise about "the resonant frequencies of the human eye". A somewhat similar experiment (Lange and Coermann, 1962) investigated the frequency range from 1 Hz to 20 Hz and concluded that decrements below 12 Hz were due to physiological stress while those above 12 Hz were due to image displacement on the retina. However no eye resonance was found below 20 Hz and, indeed, the authors state "the lowest resonant frequency of the eyeballs in the orbital cavity is above 20 cps for most human subjects".

Griffin (1975b) reports a whole-body vibration experiment in which 12 subjects underwent vertical sinusoidal vibration at frequencies between 7 Hz and 75 Hz. For each frequency the subjects were required to adopt postures that resulted in the maximum sensation of vibration and the head and then adjust the vibration level to produce just detectable blurring of a "point" source of light. Subjects were apparently able to follow these instructions without too much difficulty and the results are of some interest. It was hypothesised that, as in the object vibration situation described in Section III.H, subjects would adjust the vibration to a level that resulted in some critical displacement of the retinal image. If this was the case, the measurements of head motion at the "blur level" will indicate the effective transmissibility between head and retina. The results suggest that for all subjects this transmissibility is highly frequency dependent. However, the differences between subjects are considerable so that the *mean* response of the group of subjects does not clearly reflect the susceptibility of individuals to particular frequencies. To a first approximation it was found that from 15 Hz to 75 Hz constant vertical acceleration of the head gives rise to constant displacement of the retina. Expressed differently, this means that the effective transmissibility from head to retina is proportional to the square of the vibration frequency. Many previous studies have shown

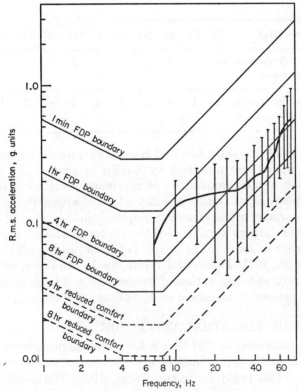

*Fig.* 4 The mean (and ±1 standard deviation) of vertical seat vibration of 10 subjects at blur level—see text (from Griffin, 1975b).

that human transmissibility from seat to head is roughly inversely proportional to frequency so it is not surprising to find that the mean experimental levels of seat vibration which produced blurring take a form which approaches a constant velocity curve (see Fig. 4). To aid comparison with other data this graph also shows some of the "fatigue decreased proficiency" (FDP) and "reduced comfort" contours derived by the International Standards Organisation (1970).

In relation to vertical head acceleration Griffin found that the frequency of maximum sensitivity varied from 25 Hz to 70 Hz and no more than two of the 12 subjects agreed on which frequency was "worst". Several subjects had more than one frequency of maximum sensitivity and both the local maxima and the absolute maxima are shown in Table I.

TABLE I: The location of frequencies of maximum sensitivity to vertical head vibration

| Frequency (Hz) | 15 | 20 | 25 | 30 | 35 | 40 | 45 | 50 | 55 | 60 | 65 | 70 |
|---|---|---|---|---|---|---|---|---|---|---|---|---|
| Number of subjects with absolute maxima | — | — | 2 | 1 | — | — | 2 | — | 2 | 1 | 2 | 2 |
| Number of subjects with local maxima | 1 | 1 | 6 | 2 | 2 | 2 | 3 | — | 3 | 1 | 3 | 4 |

The results obtained by Lee and King (1971) would appear to be in agreement with those obtained by Griffin in that, while individual subjects show several frequencies of maximum sensitivity, the overall effect is a head-to-eye transmissibility which is approximately proportional to the square of the vibration frequency in the range 12–70 Hz.

Many other authors have studied the effects of whole-body vibration at frequencies above 10 Hz (e.g., O'Briant and Ohlbaum, 1970; Ohlbaum et al., 1971; Mozell and White, 1958). However, all too often the excessively wide separation of frequencies and inadequate number of subjects prevent conclusions on the effect of frequency.

E. EFFECT OF VIBRATION AMPLITUDE

It is not surprising to find that a few experimenters have produced significant reductions in visual acuity by increases in vibration level (e.g., Loeb, 1954, 1955; Teare and Parks, 1963; Taub, 1964; Dennis, 1965a, b). However, with the majority of experiments having been conducted at one level for each frequency, there is little information upon which to base useful conclusions as to the relation between vibration amplitude and acuity. The supposition that man is a linear system would enable the necessary conclusions to be drawn from experiments on object vibration. However, there are also inadequate data upon which to base any such assumptions of linearity.

Discussion of vibration amplitude is thus primarily restricted to a consideration of a boundary between those levels that will, and those that will not, reduce visual acuity. Useful information on such a "threshold" is only provided by Griffin (1973). His data have been summarised in Fig. 4 and this figure might appear to answer the most fundamental question. However, the experiment revealed considerable inter- and intra-subject variances so that not only should care be exercised in making predictions from the mean value but it should also be recognised that this mean was obtained from only 10 subjects. Recognising these limitations, the graph implies that, when sitting on a hard seat vibrating in the vertical direction at the mean level given by the curve, about 50% of people (of similar type to the subjects used in the experiment) will not have impaired visual acuity, no matter what target they view or what sitting posture they adopt.

The graph demonstrates that some subjects are particularly sensitive to some frequencies and so data on the 50th percentile are possibly of little value for design purposes. However, the very limited data available show that if subjects in the above experiment were to adopt body postures which resulted in the least vibration of the head, the mean levels shown in the graph would have only very occasionally produced any visual blurring. Considering this and the extremely sensitive nature of the task it seems likely that, for most situations and most subjects, the mean levels of vibration shown in the graph will not reduce visual acuity. It may be noted that this conclusion does not appear to be contradicted by any other results available in the literature. Further progress beyond this point is obviously limited by our restricted knowledge of general response to vibration and, especially, the inadequacy of data on the magnitude of intersubject variability and the effects of changes in posture.

## F. EFFECT OF VIEWING DISTANCE

There would appear to be only five authors who have studied the effects of changing viewing distance. This is somewhat surprising since the application of simple mathematics shows that if, as many have assumed, visual acuity is impaired by head and eye displacements, reductions in viewing distance would be expected to be accompanied by corresponding reductions in acuity.

Dennis and Elwood (1958) employed several different viewing distances and found that subjects were able to detect Landolt C gap orientation more easily as viewing distance was decreased. This reduction was accompanied by a corresponding increase in the angular dimensions of the target. It is possible to conclude that, for Landolt Cs, the increase in apparent size more than offsets any increase in the magnitude of retinal image motion that may occur for nearer objects.

O'Briant and Ohlbaum (1970) and Ohlbaum *et al.* (1971) employed three viewing distances (40 cm, 1 m and 4 m) and would appear to conclude that angular displacement in the subject–target relationship is the critical factor. Thus, acuity is similar for all three distances at frequencies above about 15 Hz or 20 Hz where the vibration displacement is small. At lower frequencies, the high levels of vibration employed ($\pm 0.75$ g and $\pm 1.5$ g) caused displacements of several millimetres. Their results suggest that the resulting large angular displacements for near objects resulted in greater loss of acuity than smaller angular displacements for distant objects.

An experiment described by Griffin (1973) shows fairly conclusively that the lowest levels of whole-body vibration that cause visual blurring result in angular motions of the eye. For frequencies from 7 Hz to 60 Hz it was found that altering the viewing distance from 1·2 m to 6·1 m did not affect the blur threshold. (If the eye motion was translational the threshold would have increased by a factor of five.) This result does not conflict with the O'Briant and Ohlbaum findings because the two studies incorporated very different levels of vibration. It is reasonable to suppose that O'Briant and Ohlbaum produced large translational displacements of the heads of their subjects and this may have been the predominant motion at low frequencies. We would expect their findings to be the general situation at low frequencies where large displacements are not uncommon.

There is no experimental information available on the effect of changing viewing distance when pursuit or compensatory eye movements are important. The presence of at least some translational head motion implies that greater angular eye tracking movements will be required for those objects at near distances. The implications behind this conclusion offer an interesting line for future research.

## G. EFFECTS OF OBJECT SIZE AND OBJECT ILLUMINATION

The minimum size and illumination required to see an object during vibration have been used as measures of acuity (e.g., Schmitz and Simons, 1959; Rubenstein and Kaplan, 1968). Although the principal effects of these two variables could be studied with object vibration experiments, it seems possible that the size and illumination of a visual display could also affect the efficiency of compensatory and pursuit reflexes.

## H. EFFECTS OF COMPLEX VIBRATION AND OTHER FACTORS

Whole-body vibration studies are principally oriented towards seated subjects and whole-body vertical vibration. A number of visual acuity experiments have been conducted in connection with astronaut performance and, consequently, several authors have employed the semi-supine position (Faubert *et al.*, 1963; Taub, 1966; Rubenstein and Taub, 1967; Shoenberger, 1968). (Kinney *et al.* (1971) conducted an experiment with standing subjects.) Several experiments have been conducted with vibration in the $a_x$ direction (fore and aft relative to the man) (e.g., Dennis and Elwood, 1958; Hornick *et al.*, 1961; Faubert *et al.*, 1963; Taub, 1964, 1966; Clarke *et al.*, 1965; Shoenberger, 1968). Experiments with vibration in the $a_y$ direction (lateral relative to the man) have been made by Hornick *et al.* (1961), Taub (1964), Bryce (1966), Rubenstein and Kaplan (1968) and Shoenberger (1968). Two workers have used angular motion, Pradko (1964) and Benson (1972). Clarke *et al.* (1965) experimented with a combination of 11 Hz vibration and a constant acceleration of 3.85 g.

Most vibration experiments are conducted with distorted sinusoidal vibration. However, several authors have used other spectra. Dean *et al.* (1969) used a 2–20 Hz random spectra; Dean *et al.* (1964) used recorded helicopter vibration with peak levels at several frequencies from 4 Hz to 60 Hz; Faubert *et. al.* (1963) used various combinations of 11 Hz, 22 Hz and 140 Hz frequencies; while Hurt (1963) and Morris (1966) also employed low frequency random vibration.

Even with these experiments and the obvious hypothesis that vibration axis and spectra will be important variables in determining any reduction in visual acuity, there are no results which provide a suitable basis for discussion.

## I. GENERAL CONCLUSIONS

Our state of knowledge of human response to vibration is primitive. In consequence, few workers have been able to identify, control or monitor some of the most important variables in their experiments. While these experiments may have been "successful" in their particular context, the general applicability of the majority of the results is nil.

A few experiments have aided man's knowledge of how vibration affects vision and the work of Benson (1972), for example, will undoubtedly prove useful to subsequent researchers. On the other hand, it would be misleading not to comment that many experiments have been conducted without a clear definition of aims, without an understanding of the intricacies of vibration or vision, and without attempting to gather sufficient experimental data.

There are situations in which it would be useful to have a boundary between those vibration conditions that will, and those that will not, cause loss of visual acuity. Only the data provided by Griffin (1975b) come near to providing such information and, while his work has severe limitations (see Section IV.E), it appears to be the only general purpose guide. Figure 5 shows the relevant data for both object

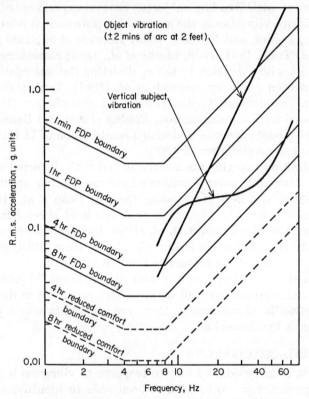

*Fig.* 5 Recommended vibration levels below which vibration is not normally expected to reduce visual acuity (from Griffin, 1973).

and vertical subject vibration (the object vibration data are shown for a 2 ft viewing distance).

Apart from the references already cited in this section, other useful references include Stevens (1946), Guignard (1959), Schmitz (1959), Drazin and Guignard (1960), Oshima (1962), Snyder (1962, 1965), Dennis (1963), Pradko (1965), Caiger (1966), Rushton (1967), Wells and Evans (1968) and Watanabe and Yoshida (1969).

## V. Object and Subject Vibration

### A. INTRODUCTION

Vibration is probably encountered most often by most people in the wide range of modern public transport systems (fixed-wing and rotary-wing aircraft, trains, cars, buses, lorries, motor cycles, hovercraft, hydrofoils etc.). Most of these vibrate both the man and the vehicle in which he travels. In consequence, the man vibrates and so does a large part of his visual field. Thus the object *and* subject vibration situation is that experienced reading a newspaper in a train, looking at instruments in a cockpit or a map in a car.

If the eyes were to remain fixed within the head, and the vibrations were of low frequency, the motions of the vehicle would be accompanied by similar motions of the man. The image of the interior of the vehicle would then maintain a fixed position on the retina of the eye. However, the vibrations are often not of low frequency and there are differences in both the amplitude phase and, possibly, direction of the subject and object motions. Further, we have seen that man appears to be equipped to compensate for some motions so, if the vehicle and the man were to move together at a low frequency, it would seem possible that this reflex could actually cause, rather than prevent, motion of the retinal image.

### B. EXPERIMENTAL INVESTIGATIONS

While several authors have vibrated both the subject and the object, the studies by Drazin (1959) and Lee and King (1971) are probably the most revealing. Over the frequency range 1–3 Hz and for three vibration amplitudes (2.84 cm, 5.71 cm and 11.43 cm) Drazin found that visual acuity is reduced progressively as either the amplitude or the frequency is increased. Assuming that the apparatus produced identical motions for both the subject and the objects, these results suggest that the mechanical response of the body greatly modified the vibration transmitted from seat to head. Alternatively, the compensatory eye reflex may have been destructive to normal vision. In either event it would appear that even at low frequencies the vibration of subject and object at the same level will not eliminate decrements in acuity. The experiment by Drazin would, of course, have been especially interesting if it had been complemented with separate results for object and subject vibration.

Adjusting the amplitude and phase of a vibrating object viewed by subjects moving at the same frequency was the task used by Lee and King (1971). When the vibrating object appeared stationary to the vibrating subject it was assumed that the amplitude of object vibration indicated the amount of eye movement. The authors are thus able to present information on "input to head" and "head to eye" transmissibility and phase angles. While the detailed results might well deserve more attention, the overall findings indicate that for a vibrating object to appear stationary to a vibrating subject the phase relation between the object and the subject's seat has to vary considerably for even small changes in frequency.

It would seem that simultaneous vibration of object and subject offers interesting possibilities for research. However, there is little evidence that visual acuity problems associated with vibration above 2 Hz can be alleviated by such an arrangement.

## VI. General Conclusions

*"All who attempt to read while riding on trains are aware of the frequently annoying vibration of the reading material. Subjectively it seems that the blurring caused by the vibration introduces a severe visual task which is apt to become fatiguing".*

More than 25 years after Tinker (1948) wrote these words we are little nearer to solving the problem. Indeed, one wonders whether we will see the passing of the train before we fully understand the problem of reading in trains!

The critical reader will have noticed the failure to discuss many aspects of the problem of vibration and vision (e.g., effects of infrasound, vibration of the eye lens etc.). In particular there has been little consideration of the effect of vibration on visual abilities other than visual acuity. Although a number of such studies have been conducted (e.g., visual search (Hawkins, 1972); peripheral visual acuity (Angelova, 1972)) it would seem that at present such research is of most value in stimulating further research rather than providing useful conclusions as to the effects of vibration.

A further omission might appear to be the question of whether object vibration is "better" or "worse" than subject vibration. Dennis (1965a) for example, demonstrates that the two situations give different results. By means of the approach given earlier in this chapter it is apparent that such a question is inadequately defined to enable the production of an unqualified answer—the difference between object and subject vibration will depend on the position at which the vibration is measured on the body of the subject. We may assume that identical retinal image motions will tend to produce identical acuity decrements. The relative sensitivity of the body will therefore depend on the transmissibility between the retinal image and the part of the body selected for making the vibration comparison. Since this transmissibility is likely to be highly frequency dependent it follows that the relative effects of object and subject vibration will also depend on the vibration frequency. Further consideration will also reveal that viewing distance can be a significant factor. Also, the subjective comments listed following the whole-body vibration experiment conducted by Griffin (1975b) demonstrate that the direction of eye motion may differ from the direction of the source of vibration excitation. The circular and elliptical retinal image motions observed during vertical vibration provided a clear qualitative distinction between object and subject vibration. Indeed, the question has re-emphasised the importance of identifying the relevant experimental variables but it has not, and cannot, provoke a useful practical answer.

This chapter has not provided an opportunity to discuss the effects of particular sources of vibration on vision. In fact there are exceedingly few studies that may be classed as rigorous attempts to establish the effect of "real" vibrations on visual acuity. Moreover, there are inadequate data on the vibrations encountered during everyday life to be able to make any general predictions as to how often human visual acuity is affected by vibration.

Reductions in visual acuity are probably the most quoted objective effects of vibration. However, with the exception of spacecraft, there remains little recorded evidence of environments in which this decrement has been established and is considered to be important. The extent to which this reflects the absence of a problem, rather than a failure to recognise or prove the presence of a problem, must remain a matter for speculation.

## REFERENCES

Alexander, C. (1972). "Performance Changes due to the Single and Dual Frequency Vibration of Reading Material", M.Sc. Thesis, University of Southampton, England.

Angelova, M. (1972). "The Effect of Vibration on Peripheral Vision", personal communication.

Benson, A. J. (1972). "Effect of Angular Oscillation in Yaw on Vision", U.K. Informal Group on the Human Response to Vibration Meeting, University of Sheffield.

Bryce, W. D. (1966). Report No. R. 286. National Gas Turbine Establishment, Pystock, Hants, England.

Burg, A. (1968). Highway Research Record Report No. 216, National Academy of Sciences, Washington, D.C., U.S.A.

Burg, A. and Coppin, R. S. (1966). Highway Research Record Report No. 122, National Academy of Sciences, Washington, D.C., U.S.A.

Caiger, B. (1966). "Some Problems in Control arising from Operational Experiences with Jet Transports", Stability and Control Specialists Meeting, AGARD, Cambridge, England.

Clarke, N. P., Taub, H., Scherer, H. F., Temple, W. E., Vykukal, H. B. and Matter, M. (1965). AMRL–TR–65–110, Wright–Patterson Air Force Base, Ohio, U.S.A.

Coermann, R. R. (1947). *Luftfahrtmedizen* 4 (2), 73–117 (also R.A.E. Library Translation 217 (1947)).

Coermann, R. R. (1962). *Human Factors* 4, 227–253.

Crawford, W. A. (1960). Air Ministry Flying Personnel Research Committee, Report FPRC Memo 150d, England.

Crook, M. N., Harker, G. S., Hoffman, A. C. and Kennedy, J. L. (1948). USAF Air Material Command: Memo-Report MCREXD–694–1Q.

Crook, M. N., Harker, G. S., Hoffman, A. C., Wulfeck, J. W. and Kennedy, J. L. (1949). USAF Air Material Command: Memo-Report MCREXD–694–1R.

Crook, M. N., Hoffman, A. C., Wessell, N. Y., Wulfeck, J. W. and Kennedy, J. L. (1947a). AML Memo Report, Serial No. TSEAA–694–1F.

Crook, M. N., Hoffman, A. C., Wessell, N. Y., Wulfeck, J. W. and Kennedy, J. L. (1947b). AML Memo Report, Serial No. TSEAA–694–1K.

Crook, M. N., Harker, G. S., Hoffman, A. C. and Kennedy, J. L. (1950). AF Technical Report No. 6246, U.S.A.

Crossley, J. K. (1969). "Pilot Performance and Refractive Error", AGARD Conf. Proc. No. 61, 26th Aerospace Medical Panel Meeting, Florence.

Davson, H. (1962). (ed.) "The Eye", Academic Press, London and New York.

Dean, R. D., Farrell, R. J. and Hitt, J. D. (1969). *Human Factors* 11 (3), 257–271.

Dean, R. D., McGlothen, C. L. and Monroe, C. L. (1964). Report No. D2. 90583, the Boeing Co., Seattle, Washington, U.S.A.

Dennis, J. P. and Elwood, M. A. (1958). Ministry of Supply: Directorate of Physiol. and Biol. Research, England, Report No. 78.

Dennis, J. P. (1963). *Occ. Psychol.* 37 (4), 277–282.

Dennis, J. P. (1965a). *J. App. Psychol.* 49 (4), 245–252.

Dennis, J. P. (1965b). *Ergonomics* 8, 193–205.

Ditchburn, R. W., Fender, D. H. and Mayne, S. (1959). *Journal of Physiol.* 145, 98–107.

Drazin, D. H. (1962). *Research* 15, 275–280.

Drazin, D. H. and Guignard, J. C. (1960). *In*: "Proceedings of the 5th European Congress of Aviation Medicine" (A. B. Barbour and H. E. Whittingham eds.), pp. 339–342. Pergamon Press, London.

Edwards, R. G. and Lange, K. O. (1964), AMRL–TR–64–91, Wright–Patterson Air Force Base, Ohio, U.S.A.

Faubert, D., Cooper, B. and Clark, C. C. (1963). Report ER 12838, Martin Co., Baltimore, Md., U.S.A.

Fender, D. H. and Nye, P. W. (1961), *Kybernetik* 1 (2), 81–88.

Frolov, K. V. (1970). *In*: "Dynamic Response of Biomechanical Systems" (N. Perrone ed.), American Society of Mechanical Engineers, pp. 146–150.

Gregory, R. L. (1966). *In*: "Eye and Brain: the Psychology of Seeing", World University Library, London.

Griffin, M. J. (1972a). Paper presented at the Int. Conference on Hand-Arm Vibration, Dundee, Scotland, July.

Griffin, M. J. (1972b). ISVR, Technical Report No. 58, University of Southampton, England.

Griffin, M. J. (1972c). "Human Response to Vibration Literature Collection of the University of Southampton". Paper presented to the U.K. Informal Group on Human Response to Vibration, Sheffield, England.

Griffin, M. J. (1973). "Whole-body Vibration and Human Vision", Ph.D. Thesis, University of Southampton, England.

Griffin, M. J. (1975a). *Aviat. Space Environ. Med.* **46**, 269–276.

Griffin, M. J. (1975b). *Aviat. Space Environ. Med.* **46**, 1033–1040.

Guignard, J. C. (1959). IAM Sci. Memo No. S. 21, R.A.F., I.A.M., Farnborough, Hants, England.

Guignard, J. C. (1965). *In*: "Textbook of Aviation Physiology" (J. A. Gillies ed.), pp. 812–894. Pergamon Press, London.

Guignard, J. C. and Irving, A. (1960). *Engineering* **190**, 364–367.

Guignard, J. C. and Irving, A. (1962). *Aerospace Medicine* **33**, 1230–1238.

Hawkins, N. M. (1972). "The Effect of Vibration on Visual Search", personal communication.

Hornick, R. J., Boettcher, C. A. and Simons, A. K. (1961). Final Report Ordnance Project No. TEI–1000, Bostrom Research Laboratories, Milwaukee, Wisc., U.S.A.

Huddleston, H. F. (1969). *Nature, Lond.* **222**, 572.

Huddleston, H. F. (1970a). *Journal of Applied Psychology* **54** (5) 401–408.

Huddleston, H. F. (1970b). AGARD, Conference Proceedings No. 55.

Hurt, G. J. (1963). NASA Technical Note D-1924.

International Organisation for Standardisation (1970). ISO/TC/108/WC7 (Secr. 19) 36.

Jones, G. M. and Drazin, D. H. (1961). Air Ministry FPRC Report, FPRC/1168, England.

Kinney, J. A. S., Luria, S. M. and Markowitz, H. (1971). *Human Factors* **13** (4), 369–378.

Krauskopf, J. (1957). *Journal of the Optical Society of America* **47** (8), 740–744.

Krauskopf, J. (1962). *Journal of the Optical Society of America* **52**, 1306.

Lange, K. O. and Coermann, R. R. (1962). *Human Factors* **4**, 291–300.

Lange, K. O. and Edwards, R. G. (1970). *Aerospace Medicine* **41** (5) 538–543.

Langmuir, I. (1938). *Science*, **87**, 233–234.

Lee, R. A. and King, A. I. (1971). *Journal of Applied Physiology* **30** (2), 281–286.

Loeb, M. (1954). Report No. 145 (Project 6–95–20–001), AMRL, Fort Knox, Ky., U.S.A.

Loeb, M. (1955). AMRL Report No. 165, Fort Knox, Ky., U.S.A.

Luckiesh, M. and Moss, F. K. (1938). *Industrial Medicine* **7** (10), 636–643.

Ludvigh, E. (1953). Project No. 001 075.01.03, Joint Report No. 3, U.S. Naval Air Station, Pensacola, Fla., U.S.A.

Ludvigh, E. and Miller, J. W. (1958). *Journal of the Optical Society of America* **48** (11), 799–803.

Lythgoe, R. J. (1932), Medical Research Council Special Report Series, No. 173, London.

Miller, J. W. (1958). *Journal of the Optical Society of America* **48** (11), 803–808.

Morris, D. F. (1966). Boeing Co. Document Report No. 7008.

Mozell, M. M. and White, D. C. (1958). *Journal of Aviation Medicine* **29** (10), 716–724.

O'Briant, C. R. and Ohlbaum, M. K. (1970). *Aerospace Medicine* **41** (1), 79–82.

O'Hanlon, J. G. and Griffin, M. J. (1971). ISVR Technical Report No. 49, University of Southampton, England.

Ohlbaum, M. K., O'Briant, C. R. and von Gierke, H. E. (1971). *Aerospace Medicine* **42** (1), 36–41.

Oshima, M. (1962). Proc. of IVth Int. Symp. on Space, Technology and Science, Agne Corporation, Tokyo.

Payne, P. R. and Band, E. G. U. (1971). Wyle Laboratories—Payne Division WP. No. 59101–6; AMRL–TR–70–35.

Pradko, F. (1964). Paper 4B presented at the 10th Annual Conference U.S. Army Human Factors R. and D., U.S. Army Tank Automotive Center, Warren, Michigan. Conf. Proc. (A.D. 478673), 154–168.

Pradko, F. (1965), *Shock and Vibration Bulletin* **34** (4), 173–190.

Rubenstein, L. and Kaplan, R. (1968). AMRL–TR–68–19, Wright–Patterson Air Force Base, Ohio, U.S.A.

Rubenstein, L. and Taub, H. A. (1967). AMRL–TR–66–181, Wright–Patterson Air Force Base, Ohio, U.S.A.

Rushton, W. A. H. (1967). *Nature*, Lond. **216**, 1173–1175.

Schmitz, M. A. (1959). Report No. 128, Bostrom Research Laboratories, Milwaukee, Wisc., U.S.A.

Schmitz, M. A. and Simons, A. K. (1959). ASME Paper No. 59–A–200, Bostrom Research Laboratories.

Shoenberger, R. W. (1968). AMRL–TR–67–205, Joint NASA/USAF Study, Wright–Patterson Air Force Base, Ohio, U.S.A.

Snyder, F. W. (1962). "Effects of Low Frequency Vertical Vibration on Human Performance", Paper presented at Aerospace Medical Association Meeting, Atlantic City, U.S.A.

Stevens, S. S. (1946). Summary Technical Report of Division 17 NDRC, **3**, Washington, D.C., U.S.A.

Taub, H. A. (1964). AMRL–TDR–64–70, Biophysics Laboratory, Wright–Patterson Air Force Base, Ohio, U.S.A.

Taub, H. A. (1966). AMRL–TR–66–57, Wright–Patterson Air Force Base, Ohio, U.S.A.

Teare, R. J. and Parks, D. L. (1963). Technical Report No. 4, Boeing Document, No. D3–3512–4. Wichita, Kansas, U.S.A.

Thomas, J. G. (1965). *Journal of the Optical Society of America* **55** (5), 534–537.

Tinker, M. A. (1948). *American Journal of Psychology* **61** (3), 386–390.

Tinker, M. A. (1953). *Journal of Education Research* **46**, 459–464.

Trincker, von D., Sieber, J. and Bartual, J. (1961). *Kybernetik* **1**, 21–28.

Vogt, H. L., Coermann, R. R. and Fust, H. D. (1968). *Aerospace Medicine* **39** (7), 675–679.

Walsh, E. G. (1966). *Bio-medical Engineering* August, **1**, 402–407.

Watanabe, A. and Yoshida, T. (1969). Proc. of the 8th ICMBE, Chicago, U.S.A.

Wells, A. M. and Evans, C. R. (1968). *Nature*, Lond. **217**, 1168–1169.

Westheimer, G. (1965). *Annual Review of Psychology* 359–380.

Wittman, T. J. and Phillips, N. S. (1969). *Journal of Biomechanics* **2**, 281–288.

Yarbus, A. L. (1967). *In*: "Eye Movements and Vision" (translated from the Russian by B. Haigh), Plenum Press, New York.

Young, L. R. (1965). *In*: "The Control of Eye Movements" (P. Bach-Y-Rita and C. C. Collins eds.), Pergamon Press, London.

# 11. Motion Sickness and Associated Phenomena

*J. T. Reason*

## I. Introduction

Notwithstanding the enormous technological advances in transport systems over the past half-century, the human nervous system still remains that of a self-propelled animal designed to move at foot-pace through an essentially two-dimensional environment under normal earth gravity. If we had been intended to move about in any way other than under our own power, we would have been equipped with an altogether different set of position and motion senses; for it is only under natural conditions of self-propelled locomotion that these senses—the eyes, the vestibular receptors and the non-vestibular proprioceptors—function in harmony to convey perfectly correlated position and motion information. That is, in biologically normal circumstances, they all tell the brain the same story regarding our orientation in space. But when we expose ourselves to an atypical force environment, as we do when we allow ourselves to be transported passively in any of the wide range of vehicles at our disposal, this delicate harmony is artificially disrupted to produce a mismatch between the signals communicated by these normally synergistic receptors. This state of affairs has been called "sensory conflict" (Lansberg, 1960) or "sensory rearrangement" (Held, 1961), and one of its more unpleasant consequences when the vestibular receptors are implicated (by the presence of a changing velocity component) is the disorder known as motion sickness whose principal characteristic is the nausea syndrome leading to vomiting.

Although it now enjoys widespread usage, the term "motion sickness" is not wholly accurate. For one thing, as we shall see later, its symptoms can be provoked not only by the presence of an unfamiliar motion but also by the absence of an accustomed one. For another, although we commonly refer to nausea and the subsequent vomiting as "feeling sick" and then "being sick", it is not a sickness in the strict sense of the word. Motion sickness is a truly functional disorder of the healthy individual which can occur in the absence of any pathogenic substance, structural damage, or the excess or deficiency of any physical substance. In fact, quite the reverse is true. Under extremely provocative conditions, it is the absence rather than the presence of symptoms that is indicative of true pathology since only those who lack an intact vestibular system are truly immune. Hill (1936) put the case well when he described motion sickness as a "normal response to an abnormal situation".

Despite these limitations, the term "motion sickness" has much to recommend it. In particular, it is now widely recognised as the general label for the family of maladies whose various members—seasickness, airsickness, carsickness, simulator sickness, swing sickness, space sickness and so on—are named for the circumstances that provoke them. Although at one time there was a tendency to regard these various forms of the disorder as separate entities, it is now apparent that a general label is more appropriate because regardless of their wide diversity of occurrence, they have important properties in common, both in regard to the nature of the symptom complex and to the essential characteristic of the provocative situation, namely some form of sensory rearrangement. The similarity between seasickness and other forms of motion sickness was first pointed out by Irwin in 1881: "a sickness identical in kind may be induced by various other motions than that of turbulent water". The accuracy of this statement has been amply borne out by the experience of recent years when the incidence of motion sickness has increased enormously as a function of the greater availability of many different forms of transport. Today, it is probably no exaggeration to claim that most people living in modern industrial societies have experienced this disorder in some degree at some time in their lives, most frequently in childhood—although there are many for whom it continues to be an all-too-common misfortune.

Although man's acquaintance with motion sickness probably dates back to the first dugout canoe, it is only within the last 30 years or so that anything like a consensus of scientific and medical opinion has emerged regarding its cause or treatment. With some notable exceptions, the earlier literature contained little more than a confused and often contradictory collection of clinical anecdotes, hunches, folklore and myths—many of which still persist in the minds of the travelling public. It is not within the scope of this chapter to evaluate the many different theories and preventive measures that have been aired in the literature, and nor would it be particularly helpful to do so. My purpose here is to sketch out some of the basic issues in the study of motion sickness. In particular, arguments are presented to support a "neural mismatch" theory of motion sickness, a view which satisfactorily embraces both the diverse occurrence of its symptoms and also the common pattern of adaptive effect and after-effect. Its central position in this chapter is felt to be justified because it succeeds in organising a large number of hitherto unrelated facts about motion sickness in a parsimonious and internally consistent fashion. But it is not offered as the final word on the subject; we are still a long way from reaching that point.

Before dealing with these basic issues, it would be helpful to outline the principal reactions associated with motion sickness, and to consider the various ways in which the disorder can develop under different stimulus conditions.

## II. The Nature of the Phenomenon

### A. CARDINAL SIGNS AND SYMPTOMS

The most commonly reported symptom of motion sickness is nausea. It is a profoundly unpleasant subjective experience relating to the epigastric region and usually heralding the approach of frank vomiting. Fully fledged nausea, the feeling of imminent vomiting, appears to be the termination of a fairly stereotyped sequence of events which begins with faint stomach awareness and progresses in severity through various degrees of queasiness until either vomiting intervenes or the provocative stimulus is removed. For many, the act of vomiting leads to a rapid recovery of well-being. But in some people the nausea persists after vomiting, leading to further bouts of vomiting and retching, and a continued decline in well-being. The persistence of nausea is not always the result of continued provocative stimulation. Once firmly established, the nausea syndrome quite often takes on a life of its own, waxing and waning independently of the circumstances which originally elicited it.

Vomiting or emesis is defined as the forceful expulsion of the gastro-intestinal contents through the mouth. It is usually preceded by a build-up of nausea, but it can occur in the absence of any premonitory symptom. It should also be stressed that vomiting is not the inevitable consequence of nausea. In experimentally induced motion sickness, the strength and duration of the provocative stimulus can be adjusted so that vomiting does not occur (Kennedy and Graybiel, 1965). Similarly, there are a number of relatively susceptible individuals who apparently find it difficult to vomit, and thus remain at the point of acute nausea for lengthy periods. It seems likely that these people suffer considerably more than those who can vomit readily. It should not necessarily be assumed, therefore, that the act of vomiting automatically signifies a more severe case of motion sickness than one in which only the nausea syndrome is present.

Along with vomiting, the two most frequently reported signs of motion sickness are the presence of pallor and cold sweating. In a fair-complexioned person, pallor is evident as a whitish-greenish tinge in the skin of the face which is usually first detected in the region of the nose and mouth. Cold sweating, on the other hand, may be defined as that sweating which occurs in the absence of an adequate thermal stimulus. It appears to serve no useful purpose, and the mechanism is probably part of a primitive response pattern.

## B. ASSOCIATED REACTIONS

While pallor, cold sweating, nausea and vomiting constitute the most reliable and consistent features of the motion sickness syndrome, other reactions are frequently reported and observed in conjunction with them. They generally show a much greater variability both between provocative situations and between individuals than do the "big four" reactions described in the preceding section.

Objective reactions include increased salivation, sighing, yawning and hyperventilation. Gastric signs such as belching and flatulence are commonly associated with the development of nausea. Several investigators have noted a diminution in urinary output during motion sickness. Taylor and his co-workers (1957) made an extensive study of this phenomenon and found a highly significant positive correlation between measures of antidiuresis and the severity of the motion sickness reactions in experimentally induced sickness. They concluded that the onset of motion sickness is associated with the release of a circulating antidiuretic hormone.

Of particular interest are the associated "head" reactions. These include headache, usually of the frontal variety, and complaints of a tightness around the forehead, a constriction of the throat or, under certain stimulus conditions, a "buzzing in the head". Other more idiosyncratic reactions are social indifference, mental confusion, a feeling of coldness in the face and extremities, anxiety, depression, weakness, anorexia and an overall increase in bodily warmth.

Drowsiness or somnolence in situations which provoke sickness has been reported by several investigators (Field, 1942; Tyler and Bard, 1949; Schwab, 1954; Graybiel et al., 1960; Clark and Graybiel, 1961; Wood et al., 1965). The fact that it is not an integral part of the motion sickness syndrome is suggested by its presence in subjects who are otherwise unaffected by the provocative vestibular stimulus, and by its persistence after other ill-effects have vanished as the result of adaptation to continuing exposure. In a recent study (Reason and Graybiel, 1971), involving a 3-day exposure to gradually increasing cross-coupled angular accelerations, persistent and overwhelming drowsiness together with abnormally long hours of sleep were the most dramatic effects observed in the three experimental subjects. Although it can be argued that drowsiness is a consequence of physical confinement and forced inactivity, there are good grounds for believing that prolonged, repetitive vestibular stimulation is the primary cause. It seems as if the experimental devices and vehicles which swing, rock, roll, pitch and spin adult subjects have an effect very similar to that induced in infants when their cradles or prams are rhythmically rocked or shaken. Graybiel *et al.* (1960) suggest that the diencephalic sleep centre is affected by repeated vestibular stimuli. In a later publication, Graybiel (1969) put forward the view that this drowsiness is evoked by labyrinthine signals passing via the vestibular nuclei to the ascending reticular formation and thence to the lateral hypothalamic area. Whatever the neural pathways involved, however, it is evident that repetitive vestibular stimulation has a powerful soporific effect, and one which is likely to constitute a serious, although as yet largely neglected, problem in long-haul transport systems. From the available evidence, it seems reasonable to conclude that drowsiness and motion sickness are parallel but distinct phenomena that can be induced simultaneously by the same vestibular stimulation, although drowsiness can exist in the absence of motion sickness, and vice versa.

## C. VARIETIES OF RESPONSE

In the past, many clinicians found it convenient to distinguish two types of motion sickness: that in which "head reactions" were the primary complaint, and that in which "gut reactions" (primarily the nausea syndrome leading to vomiting) were most prominent. It used to be thought that the apparent predominance of either the "head" or the "gut" symptoms reflected constitutional differences between people (Danvers, 1892; Hill, 1936; Holtermann, 1956). But in the light of more recent research (Komendantov and Kopanev, 1963; Reason and Graybiel, 1970a), it seems more likely that head and gut reactions represent different stages in the temporal development of a single symptom complex. The particular reactions observed at any one time appear to depend upon the complex interaction of three factors: the severity of the provocative stimulus, the basic susceptibility of the individual and the length of time for which he is exposed.

As a rough approximation, it can be suggested that when the provocative conditions are mild and the exposure of long duration, relatively susceptible individuals will first present "head" symptoms which may be superseded later by "gut" symptoms. But, under the same conditions, relatively resistant individuals may show only mild "head" symptoms or remain symptom-free. On the other hand, when the exposure to the provocative stimulus is both sudden and severe, the susceptibles tend to develop "gut" reactions—the nausea syndrome— almost immediately. Head symptoms may be present, but they tend to be overshadowed by the gastric reactions. In the case of more resistant subjects, however, the latency of the gastric reactions is much longer and may be preceded by a phase in which head reactions predominate. In highly resistant people, of course, these "head" symptoms may be the only manifestation.

While the specific form of the head symptom is highly variable and idiosyncratic, there is sufficient commonality among the forms and latencies of the gut reactions to permit a fairly reliable description of the stages in their development. This is given in the next section.

## D. SEQUENCE OF EVENTS LEADING TO VOMITING

The very first reactions to a motion stimulus tend to be reflex phenomena that are not strictly a part of the motion sickness syndrome. These include nystagmus eye-movements and vertigo due to the vestibular stimulation, and also autonomic responses mediated by the ascending reticular formation that are triggered by any novel and arousing stimulus. These initial reactions can occur irrespective of whether the subject subsequently develops motion sickness.

The first signs of sickness proper are likely to be a faint pallor in the region of the mouth, and the beginnings of a cold sweat on the thermal sweat areas (as distinct from the arousal sweat areas—see McClure et al., 1971). Along with this comes faint stomach awareness, something which is not yet queasiness, just the unfamiliar sensation of being able to "feel" the stomach. If the provocative stimulus is removed at this stage, recovery occurs in a matter of seconds (Reason and Graybiel, 1970a). This state has been described by Graybiel et al. (1968) as the Malaise II level of severity, and is sufficiently well defined in most individuals to be used as an end-point in experimentally induced motion sickness.

Compared with what lies ahead, the development of gut reactions up to this point is relatively slow. From here on, should the provocative stimulus continue, well-being deteriorates very rapidly and this phase of development has been termed the "avalanche phenomenon". Once the "avalanche" has begun, acute nausea is almost inevitable. Moderate queasiness quickly replaces stomach awareness and this, in turn, is rapidly superseded by fully fledged nausea, or what Graybiel has defined as the Malaise III level of severity. Should this state persist then acute vomiting frequently intervenes; but not, as mentioned earlier, in all cases. The "avalanche" is also signified by an increase in the intensity of the pallor and cold sweating already established, as well as by the presence of increased salivation, feelings of bodily warmth, constriction of the throat, tightness of the head and often severe depression. If the stimulus is removed at the Malaise III level, recovery can still occur fairly rapidly for most people; but there are some in whom the symptoms persist for many hours after the stimulus has been removed. If, however, the nauseogenic stimulus is not removed at the Malaise III level, vomiting usually occurs within seconds.

## III. The Role of the Vestibular System

One incontrovertible fact about motion sickness is that an intact vestibular system is necessary for the production of symptoms. The essential part played by the vestibular receptors in the aetiology of this disorder was established at the end of the nineteenth century through the pioneering work of Irwin, de Champeaux, William James, Reynolds, Pollack, Minor and others. More recent studies by Sjöberg (1931), Brown et al. (1941), Graybiel (1965) and Johnson et al. (1951) have provided additional confirmation of these early observations.

The evidence is of two kinds. First, there are those studies demonstrating the immunity of labyrinthine-defective (L-D) subjects to provocative situations in which normal subjects succumb very rapidly to motion sickness. From these, perhaps the most convincing evidence has been provided by Graybiel and his colleagues who, over a period of 10 years, have systematically evaluated the reactions of L-D individuals to a wide variety of provocative circumstances and found no indication of motion sickness in any of them. The second kind of evidence has been derived from surgical interference studies with animals. In these, animals of demonstrated susceptibility were subjected to bilateral destruction of the labyrinthine receptors and then re-exposed to the provocative stimulus whereupon they were found to be unaffected.

Although the involvement of the vestibular system had been indicated by observations made some 50 years earlier, it was not until the Second World War that theories of motion sickness attempted to specify the role played by the vestibular receptors. But once convinced of the vital role played by this sensory system, most investigators focused their attention exclusively on vestibular activity and phrased their explanations solely in these terms. In other words, they tended to ignore the fact that the vestibular system was but one part, albeit for sickness an essential part, of the basic orientation system which also included vision and the non-vestibular proprioceptors. As a result, the years between 1945 and 1960 were dominated by the view that motion sickness was caused by an excessive stimulation of the vestibular system induced by the non-physiological accelerations imposed on the head through vehicular motion.

Having adopted this limited "sense-bound" approach, it was inevitable that one of the main concerns of these theorists should be to determine which of the two vestibular receptors, the semi-circular canals or the otoliths, was primarily responsible for the disorder. This led to a rather sterile series of investigations in which efforts were made to establish whether sickness resulted mainly from angular accelerations stimulating the semi-circular canals, or from the linear accelerative components of vehicle motion registered by the otoliths. The outcome of this work was that the otoliths were thought to be the receptors primarily involved.

## IV. The Otolith Overstimulation Theory

In recent years, the theory that motion sickness is principally due to the unnatural or excessive stimulation of the otoliths by imposed linear accelerations has been most vigorously championed by Dutch investigators (van Egmond et al., 1954; Jongkees, 1967). It has been stated in its most emphatic form by de Wit (1953): "Seasickness is caused by the overstimulation of the otolith system. The part played by the other [sense] organs in the determination of the position of the body is only secondary." These views accorded closely with the consensus of theoretical opinion during and immediately after the Second World War as can be judged from the principal reviews of that period (McNally and Stuart, 1942; Tyler and Bard, 1949; Chinn and Smith, 1953).

The case for the primacy of otolithic overstimulation rested mainly on three pieces of evidence:

(1) Early investigators (Mach, 1875; Dodge, 1923) placed the threshold for the detection of angular accelerations in the region of $2°/sec^2$, and early analyses of ship motions (Quix, 1923; Sjöberg, 1931) suggested that the maximum angular accelerations imposed on passengers exceed that value by only a very small amount, if at all. On this basis it was argued that the angular motions produced by the rolling of a ship are insufficient to create an adequate stimulus for the semi-circular canals. By contrast, the linear accelerations associated with

pitching and scending were found to be many times greater than the estimated threshold for linear motion which Mach found to be in the region of 0.012 g. Thus it was assumed that the otoliths alone were responsible for the production of seasickness.

There are many reasons why this is an unsatisfactory argument. In the first place, the threshold values obtained by Mach and Dodge considerably underestimate the true sensitivity of the canals as shown by more recent threshold studies using improved methodology (Clark and Stewart, 1968). Second, the above case for otolithic overstimulation is predicated on what Lowenstein (1970) has termed "the mistaken orthodoxy" that the canals only respond to angular accelerations and the otoliths only to linear accelerations. Many recent studies have shown that while this functional distinction may hold for naturally occurring movements, it breaks down in the unusual force environments created by vehicles and laboratory devices (Benson and Bodin, 1965, 1966a, b; Melvill Jones and Milsum, 1966; Benson et al., 1967; Correia and Guedry, 1967; Lowenstein, 1970). Thus it is no longer particularly meaningful to infer the primacy of either the otoliths or the canals on the basis of whether the eliciting motion consists mainly of either linear or angular accelerations. Third, there is a methodological criticism of the studies upon which these arguments were based. Apart from the many technical problems involved in estimating the forces that a vehicle exerts upon its passengers (see Morales, 1949), these investigators have largely ignored the fact that the head is capable of independent motion so that the measurements of vehicle motion do not necessarily bear any relation to the actual accelerative stimulus delivered to the vestibular system. Just as the failure to control for these independent head motions by providing adequate head restraint has cast doubts on the findings of many studies concerned with making quantitative estimates of the effective provocative stimulus, so it also invalidates the case produced by the supporters of the otolithic over-stimulation theory.

(2) Shipboard observers have failed to observe nystagmus during seasickness and, from this, have argued that the canals are not involved (Oriel, 1927; Chinn and Smith, 1953). Therefore, it was maintained, only the otoliths were implicated.

Even taking it at its face value, this argument is extremely dubious, and does not stand up to the most casual scrutiny. In the first place, failure to detect nystagmus in motion sick individuals without the aid of sophisticated recording apparatus does not necessarily mean that it was not present either at the time or during the preceding exposure period. But this is really immaterial since this whole argument is based on the erroneous assumption that nystagmus eye-movements are only elicited by adequate canal stimulation. It has now been established that well-defined compensatory nystagmus can be evoked by the continually changing stimulus to the otoliths engendered by constant-velocity rotation about Earth-horizontal or off-vertical axes (Benson and Bodin, 1965; Correia and Guedry, 1967). Not only does this mode of stimulation produce nystagmus, but it is also extremely effective in producing sickness, so that the two frequently coexist. Thus the apparent absence of nystagmus in seasickness can provide absolutely no support for the otolith overstimulation viewpoint.

(3) Finally, there is the well-established observation that adopting the supine position, or simply tilting the head back while in the sitting position, affords considerable protection against sickness. The overstimulation theorists have attributed this to the fact that otoliths are less responsive to vertically acting linear accelerations in this position of the head. This follows the general theory of Quix (1923) that the otoliths are maximally sensitive in the head-upright position, and minimally sensitive in the inverted position—the so-called "blind-spot". Quix also believed that this blind-spot extended to the supine position as well.

While the prophylactic effects of the supine position can indeed be explained in terms of the otolith overstimulation theory, it is by no means the only possible explanation. An equally plausible alternative is that the supine position inevitably brings with it a considerable degree of head restraint, thus limiting the independent head motions that Johnson and his co-workers (1951) have found to be positively correlated with individual susceptibility. We will take up this point later.

We have just examined the three major props of the otolith theory and have found them to be lacking in substance. Thus, the case for the otolith overstimulation point of view, even on its own terms, is an extremely weak one. But the case against this theory becomes overwhelming when one considers the number of important motion sickness phenomena that escape explanation by this theory. Some of these phenomena are listed below—since they will be considered again at later points in this chapter, only a brief mention will be made of them here.

## 1. *Visually induced Sickness*

The appearance of symptoms in situations where the disturbing motion is perceived visually and where there is no direct vestibular stimulus, but only one that is implied through past experiences with the visual input. An obvious example is "Cinerama sickness" where symptoms are readily produced by watching (from a stationary seat) a motion picture shot from a moving vehicle, say, a roller-coaster car.

## 2. *Coriolis Sickness*

The fact that head movements executed out of the plane of rotation on a spinning platform can rapidly produce symptoms (the Coriolis vestibular reaction induced by cross-coupled angular accelerations). Here the otolithic response is in most important respects identical to that which occurs during a natural head-tilt in a stationary environment. Thus there can be no question of there being an excessive otolithic input.

## 3. *Space Sickness*

Motion sickness is readily induced by head tilts executed in conditions of zero-gravity in which there is no effective otolithic input—so-called "space sickness".

## 4. *Mal de Débarquement*

The occurrence of *mal de débarquement*, or the sickness which appears at the *cessation* of a provocative stimulus, provided that the exposure has been of sufficient duration and quality to allow the acquisition of some degree of adaptation. These after-effects are seen most clearly after repeated head movements aboard a rotating platform where they are induced, following rotation, by executing the same head motions that precipitated symptoms during the rotational period. This phenomenon cannot be explained by the otolith theory since it occurs during the course of self-induced natural head motions.

Clearly, an adequate theory of motion sickness must address itself not only to the essential role played by the intact vestibular system, but also to accounting for these hitherto unexplained phenomena. Furthermore, it must also explain why motion sickness can occur in such a wide variety of differing circumstances, and why the phenomenon of adaptation appears to be common to all of them. It is believed that the most satisfactory explanation of motion sickness at this time is provided by the "sensory conflict" theory, considered in detail below.

## V. The Sensory Conflict Theory

The notion that motion sickness could have its origins in the discrepant information signalled by normally synergistic position and motion senses was first put forward by Irwin in 1881. In addition to labyrinthine factors, he argued that seasickness is promoted by the "discord between the immediate or true visual impressions and a certain visual habit or visual sense of the fitness and order of things". Similar ideas were later advanced by Claremont (1931) and Brooks (1939), but it was not until the 1960's that the theory gained widespread support (Groen, 1960; Lansberg, 1960; Guedry, 1965; Gillingham, 1966; Reason, 1969, 1970). The theory as it is elaborated below also owes a considerable debt to ideas generated outside the field of motion sickness, principally by von Holst (1954), Sokolov (1960) and Held (1961).

The sensory conflict or "sensory rearrangement" theory is most conveniently presented in the form of answers to two related questions. First, what is the essential qualitative nature of the stimulus that provokes motion sickness? Second, what are the mechanisms underlying the acquisition of "protective adaptation", and also its sequel, *mal de débarquement*? Implicit in this theory, as we shall see later, is the notion that motion sickness is best understood as being a maladaptation phenomenon.

## A. THE ESSENTIAL NATURE OF THE PROVOCATIVE STIMULUS

One of the problems facing the theorist is the wide diversity of circumstances that cause motion sickness. This is reflected by the many names that have been used to designate this disorder—seasickness, train sickness, carsickness, airsickness, swing sickness, simulator sickness and, most recently, space sickness. What do they all have in common?

The basic premise of the sensory conflict theory is that all situations which provoke motion sickness are characterised by a condition of sensory rearrangement in which the motion signals transmitted by the eyes, the vestibular system and the non-vestibular proprioceptors are at variance not only with one another, but also—and this is the crucial factor—with what is expected on the basis of previous transactions with the environment. In other words, the important nauseogenic conflict exists between what is presently being signalled by the spatial senses and what is expected on the basis of past experience.

The second premise is that irrespective of what other spatial senses are party to these conflicts, the vestibular system must be implicated either directly or indirectly in order that sickness shall ensue. This proviso also tells us something about the nature of the effective motion signal. For example, it dictates that the motion input must involve a changing rather than a constant velocity component, since the vestibular receptors only respond to alterations in linear and angular velocity, that is, to accelerations and decelerations. This holds true even when no direct vestibular stimulus is present as in the case of

"Cinerama sickness" induced by a visual input previously associated with vestibular stimulation. If the visual stimulus were one which, under actual conditions, would be associated with constant velocity motion on the part of the observer, then no sickness would occur. To be effective, the visual stimulus has to be one which implies an accelerative stimulus being delivered to the vestibular system, as, for example, in the case of a moving picture shot from the passenger's position on a roller-coaster car.

Although there may well be others, we can specify two main types of sensory rearrangement present in situations which produce sickness:

*visual–inertial rearrangement* (where the term "inertial" includes both the vestibular and the nonvestibular proprioceptors)—this constitutes an intermodality conflict;

*canal–otolith rearrangement*—this constitutes an intra-labyrinthine or intra-modality conflict.

Under natural conditions of self-propelled locomotion, both pairs of receptors work in close harmony to provide us with correlated information about our position in space. But in unusual force environments, or under conditions of passive motion, this harmonious relationship can be disrupted to produce three basic types of sensory conflict. If A and B represent portions of normally correlated receptor systems—visual–inertial or canal–otolith systems—then these three conflicts can be represented as follows:

*Type* 1: when A and B *simultaneously* signal contradictory or uncorrelated information.
*Type* 2: when A signals in the absence of an *expected* B signal.
*Type* 3: when B signals in the absence of an *expected* A signal.

From these two kinds of sensory rearrangement and three conflict types, we can derive six basic conflict situations in which motion sickness might reasonably be expected to occur. The characteristics of each of these situations are enumerated below, together with examples drawn from both the laboratory and vehicular transport in which motion sickness has been experienced.

### 1. *Type* 1 *Visual–inertial Conflict*

This is the situation in which both the eyes and the inertial receptors are simultaneously signalling motion, but of an unrelated or incompatible kind—incompatible, that is, with expectations based on previous experience. Examples include watching the motion of the waves from the side of a pitching, scending and rolling ship, observing the passing landscape from the side or rear windows of a moving vehicle which is changing either direction or speed, and making head motions while wearing an optical device that distorts visual input. The latter is a feature of studies investigating adaptation to optical devices which either invert or reverse the visual field, or simply displace it. Stratton (1897), Ewert (1930), Kohler (1955) and Smith and Smith (1962) have all observed or experienced dizziness, nausea and other prodromal symptoms when moving the head either actively or passively during the initial period of distortion and immediately following the restoration of normal vision.

### 2. *Type 2 Visual–inertial Conflict*

These are the situations mentioned earlier in which motion sickness is provoked by seen motion in the absence of the normally related cues from the inertial receptors. One example is "Cinerama sickness", mentioned earlier, where a stationary observer views a motion picture shot from a vehicle that is changing either speed or direction, or both (Benfari, 1964). In a recent study, Parker (1971) observed that subjects were readily made motion sick by watching a film taken from a car driving down a mountain road. However, when the same film was run backwards, no ill-effects were observed. This is in accordance with the sensory conflict theory which argues that visually induced sickness arises from the absence of vestibular signals in the presence of visual motion information which, in the actual vehicle, would be accompanied by corroborating inputs from the semi-circular canals and otoliths. When the sickness-inducing film was run backwards, the visual motion did not elicit stored expectations of vestibular concomitants since the seen combination of real (visual) and implied (vestibular) stimulation would not, in all probability, have been encountered in actual vehicle motion.

Another example of this kind of conflict is simulator sickness. It is now well established that motion sickness can be produced by the operation of a fixed-base vehicle simulator incorporating an appropriately moving visual display (Miller and Goodson, 1960; Barrett and Thornton, 1968; Sinacori, 1968; Reason and Diaz, 1971). The argument that simulator sickness is due to the unfulfilled expectations of a vestibular input created by the seen motion is supported by the additional finding (Miller and Goodson, 1960; Reason and Diaz, 1971) that experienced vehicle operators are considerably more susceptible to this disorder than trainees, or those with little or no previous experience of the real vehicle motion. This is presumably because the expectations of the former are more firmly entrenched than those of the latter, and hence conflict more drastically with the "rearranged" sensory inputs encountered in the simulator.

## 3. *Type 3 Visual–inertial Conflict*

This is defined by the presence of an inertial input—from the vestibular system primarily—in the absence of an expected correlated visual signal. Perhaps the most familiar example is the case of the car passenger who attempts to read a map while being driven along a winding, bumpy road. His inertial receptors signal the motion of the vehicle while his eyes, being fixed on the map which is stationary with respect to him, inform him that he is not moving relative to his immediate environment. However, the same kind of conflict is present in all modes of passive transport where the passenger lacks a clear view of the world outside the vehicle. Thus it contributes to occurrences of symptoms in the sea-traveller or aircraft passenger seated in an enclosed cabin while his vestibular system is subjected to changing patterns of linear and angular accelerations. His vision is restricted to the interior of the craft which is stationary with respect to him. It is well known that navigators and other aircrew with limited or no external reference suffer a much higher incidence of airsickness than do pilots actually flying an aircraft. But it has also been noted that pilots make unusually susceptible passengers in aircraft. One explanation is that, deprived of the external visual reference associated with control of the aeroplane, pilots are subjected to a more acute sensory conflict since they have learned to integrate the visual and inertial inputs characteristic of flight.

This type of sensory conflict has also been studied under more controlled conditions. Manning and Stewart (1949) investigated the effects of visual reference upon the incidence of swing sickness, and found that when subjects could only see the interior of the small compartment in which they were swung they were considerably more disturbed by sickness than when they were allowed a full view of their surroundings. More recently, Reason and Diaz (1970) required subjects to make 90° head movements in a rotating device under three conditions of visual reference: with full view of the exterior, with eyes closed, and with vision restricted to the illuminated interior of the device. In the latter condition of internal visual reference, subjects experienced significantly more sickness and acquired protective adaptation more slowly than in either of the other two conditions, even though the provocative vestibular stimulus was identical.

### 4. *Type* 1 *Canal–otolith Conflict*

This is a situation in which the two normally synergistic vestibular receptors, the canals and the otoliths, simultaneously signal contradictory position and motion information. The best example is the Coriolis vestibular reaction which occurs when a subject, seated on a platform rotating at constant angular velocity, moves his head about some axis other than the axis of platform rotation (Fig. 1). During and immediately following the head motion, the subject experiences a sensation of apparent rotation about an axis which is orthogonal to both head tilt and platform axes, while the otoliths continue to signal the head tilt more or less correctly. Semi-circular canals, previously unstimulated by the platform rotation, are brought into the plane of this rotation by the head motion, causing an accelerative cross-coupled stimulus to be delivered to the cupula–endolymph systems of these canals. When the head motion is of short duration, the strength of the cross-coupled stimulus is determined by the angular velocity of the platform and the angle through which the head is moved. A good description of the mechanics of the Coriolis reaction is given by Guedry and Montague (1961).

The Coriolis reaction thus represents a clear case of a type 1 canal–otolith conflict in which an unusual force environment causes the canals and otoliths to send conflicting messages concerning the position of the head. As Guedry (1969) has pointed out, this situation could only be replicated by having the skull split in two and the halves travel in different directions. Small wonder, therefore, that it is an especially potent stimulus to motion sickness. Provided he possesses an intact vestibular system, anyone can be made motion sick, given sufficient quantity and duration of cross-coupled stimulation. As a consequence of these effects, the Coriolis reaction is foreseen as a major hazard in projected spacecraft that rotate to provide artificial gravity and has been the subject of considerable research interest in recent years. Some of this work will be discussed at a later point.

### 5. *Type* 2 *Canal–otolith Conflict*

This is characterised by the presence of a canal signal in the absence of an expected corroborating signal from the otoliths. The effects of this are seen most dramatically in space flight. In zero-gravity flight, an angular motion of the head will evoke a normal response from the semi-circular canals since they are largely gravity-independent, but in the absence of a gravito-inertial vector there will be no related signal from the otoliths. The nature of the otolithic activity in these circumstances is not yet clearly understood, but it will certainly differ from

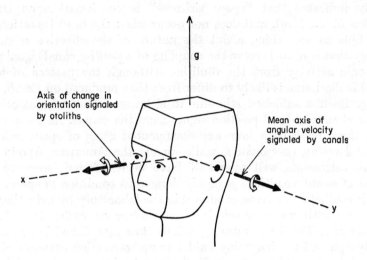

Head tilt on rotating table

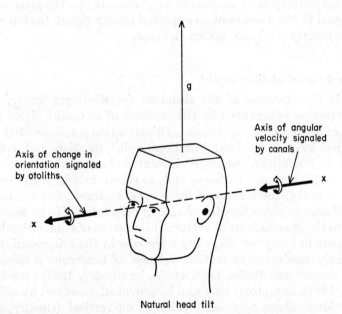

Natural head tilt

*Fig.* 1 Natural head tilt compared with that made on a rotating platform.

that obtained under 1 g conditions and hence will conflict with Earth-based expectations. Evidence from cosmonauts and astronauts clearly indicates that "space sickness" is contingent upon tilting motions of the head, and does not occur when the head is stationary. This tells us something about the nature of the effective stimulus, namely that it must involve the coupling of a *positive* canal signal with the tonic activity from the otoliths. Although the pattern of tonic otolithic discharge is likely to differ from that produced on Earth, it is not by itself a sufficient stimulus to sickness; it must be associated with a change-of-head-position signal from the canals. At the present time, there have been four well-documented cases of space sickness among Russian cosmonauts, while among the American Apollo and Skylab astronauts well over half have been affected, some to the extent of acute vomiting—a highly dangerous condition in space.

This conflict can also be produced in the laboratory by irrigating the outer ear with water which is either hotter or colder than blood temperature. The temperature gradient thus established between the endolymph and the irrigating fluid sets up convection currents within the endolymph which cause a displacement of the cupula, and hence deliver illusory signals of apparent bodily rotation in the absence of corresponding otolithic signals. Here we have a situation analogous to that accompanying head motions in weightless flight—the presence of a canal signal in the absence of an expected otolith signal. Such a caloric stimulus readily produces motion sickness.

## 6. *Type 3 Canal–otolith Conflict*

This is the converse of the situation described previously. Here, motion sickness is provoked by the presence of an otolith signal in the absence of an expected canal signal. This situation can be created in the laboratory by two devices: "barbecue-spit" rotation and counter-rotation. In the former, the subject is rotated about an Earth-horizontal axis like a chicken on a barbecue spit, as shown in Fig. 2. At constant angular velocity, there is no effective canal stimulus, but the otoliths are continuously signalling the changing orientation of the head with respect to the gravito-inertial vector. This pattern of stimulation has no counterpart in everyday life, except perhaps in the fairground, and is particularly conducive to motion sickness as numerous studies have shown (Benson and Bodin, 1965, 1966a, b; Guedry, 1965; Correia and Guedry, 1967). Symptoms may also be provoked, however, by spinning an individual about any axis which is off-vertical (Guedry, 1969; McClure *et al.*, 1971).

A counter-rotating device consists of a secondary turntable mounted on a centrifuge of short radius, where the secondary turntable rotates at the same rate as the main centrifuge, but in the opposite direction. As a result, an individual seated on the secondary turntable remains facing in the same direction since the counter-rotation of this turntable

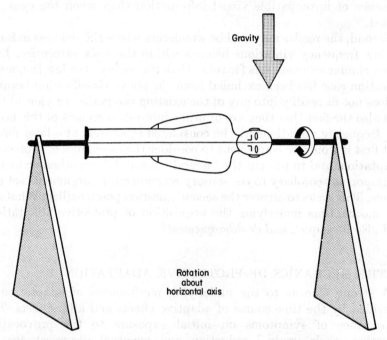

*Fig.* 2 Schematic of a "barbecue-spit" rotation system.

cancels out the rotation of the primary drive axis. The subject is not exposed to an effective canal stimulus, but receives continuous otolith and gravireceptor stimulation due to the resultant force vector whose direction is changing constantly with respect to his head through 360°. Using such a device, Graybiel and Johnson (1963) found a relatively high incidence of sickness, although susceptible subjects were generally better able to withstand this type of rearranged stimulus than the cross-coupled accelerations described earlier.

Two general points need to be made about this scheme for classifying nauseogenic conflict situations. First, canal–otolith conflicts are usually complicated by the presence of visual information which may increase or reduce the sick-making properties of the total stimulus depending

12

on the particular situation. A pure canal–otolith conflict can only occur when vision is occluded. In transport situations, for example, canal–otolith conflicts are often exacerbated by being part of a wider visual–inertial conflict. Evidence has already been cited (see Reason and Diaz, 1971) to show that a type 1 canal–otolith conflict in the form of cross-coupled accelerations is considerably more nauseogenic in the presence of incompatible visual information than when the eyes are closed.

Second, the reader may well be wondering where the sickness induced by low frequency vibrations belongs within these six categories. Like many similar schemes, it is far tidier than the reality. The low frequency vibration case has been excluded from the above classification because it does not fit readily into any of the existing categories. In view of this and also the fact that they are of prime interest to readers of this book, low frequency vibrations will be considered separately at a later point. But first it would be convenient to consider the mechanics of protective adaptation, and to present the "neural mismatch" hypothesis which is an important corollary to the sensory rearrangement arguments set out above. This seeks to answer the second question posed earlier: What are the mechanisms underlying the acquisition of protective adaptation, and also its sequel, *mal de débarquement*?

## B. THE MECHANICS OF PROTECTIVE ADAPTATION

A strong clue as to the underlying mechanisms of adaptation is provided by the time-course of adaptive effects and after-effects. The appearance of symptoms on initial exposure to the provocative situation, their gradual reduction and eventual disappearance on continued exposure, and their reappearance on returning to the previously typical environment are sufficiently uniform over a wide range of eliciting conditions to suggest that they are mediated by common central mechanisms (Guedry, 1965; Reason, 1969, 1970).

To explain the occurrence of these different phases in the adaptation cycle, I have borrowed concepts from von Holst (1954), Groen (1960), Lansberg (1960), Sokolov (1960) and others and expressed them in the form of a simple model, termed the "neural mismatch hypothesis". This postulates the existence of two neural components illustrated in Fig. 3. First, a neural storage unit that retains the informational characteristics of previous inputs from the position and motion senses—for example, their intensity, direction, temporal spacing and so on; and, second, a comparator unit that matches up the most recent contents of the neural store (stimulus traces) with the informational characteristics of the prevailing sensory inputs from the spatial senses, particularly the eyes and the vestibular receptors.

The processes underlying the sequence of events observed in the adaptation cycle are shown in Fig. 4. Along the ordinate I have expressed the amount of discrepancy between the sensory inputs and the

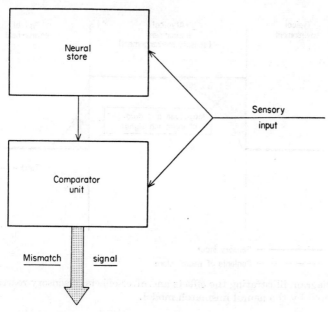

*Fig.* 3 Basic components of the neural mismatch model.

contents of the store in spatial terms. The abscissa shows the time-scale. The bold unbroken line indicates changes in the sensory input, while the dotted line shows the corresponding changes in the contents of the neural store.

In the typical environment, the influx from the spatial receptors and the contents of the store are perfectly compatible as the result of long experience with the natural conditions of self-propelled locomotion. But during the initial stages of exposure to the atypical or rearranged environment (a convenient example would be making head movements aboard a rotating device), the contents of the neural store are markedly different from the signals arriving from the spatial senses. The store information remains appropriate to the typical conditions experienced earlier, while the prevailing sensory inputs are radically altered due to the changed force environment. This discrepancy is detected by the comparator unit, which, in response, generates a mismatch signal reflecting both the extent and the direction of the discrepancy. The mismatch signal is directed along reflex pathways to the neuronal and neurohumoral mechanisms responsible for the production of symptoms. It is assumed that the severity of the symptoms is in direct relation to the strength of the mismatch signal.

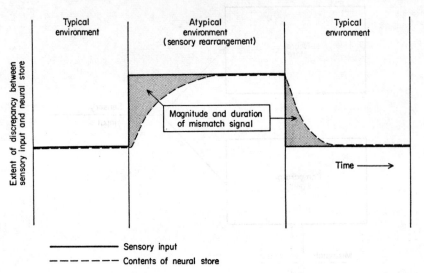

*Fig.* 4 Diagram illustrating the effects and after-effects of sensory rearrangement as predicted by the neural mismatch model.

With continued exposure, the contents of the neural store are gradually updated by incorporating elements of information about the rearranged sensory inputs, so that eventually they are compatible with the characteristics of the provocative environment. When this occurs, the mismatch signal is no longer generated, and symptoms disappear. At this point, the individual is said to be adapted to his rearranged environment.

On returning to the previously typical environment, the recent contents of the store, having adjusted to the rearranged conditions, are again at variance with the incoming sensory information. This causes the reinstatement of the mismatch signal and with it the reappearance of symptoms and other reactions characteristic of the initial exposure phase. Where these latter have a sign, they are in the opposite direction to those experienced during the initial rearrangement phase. But on remaining in the typical environment, the contents of the store are rapidly readjusted to be compatible with the existing sensory input. This part of the adaptation cycle is likely to occur much more rapidly than the initial adaptation to the rearranged conditions since the informational characteristics of the typical environment will be over-learned. That is, the appropriate stimulus traces are well consolidated and easily retrievable from the store for matching within the comparator. Similarly, when the subject again encounters the same conditions of rearrangement, adaptation is likely to proceed far more rapidly than on the first occasion owing to the presence of stored stimulus traces from the previous exposure. If the individual continues to move in and out of this environment, the time will come when both transitions will be free from symptoms, as in the case of the experienced sailor who is evidently able to retrieve the appropriate stimulus traces from store before a mismatch signal of sufficient strength to trigger motion sickness can be generated. This is the rationale for the "adaptation schedules" discussed in a later section.

These arguments do not explain why motion sickness should occur at all, nor why it takes the particular form that it does. These questions are not answered by any theory at the present. The principal strength of the sensory conflict theory and its corollary, the neural mismatch hypothesis, is that motion sickness is regarded not as an isolated vestibular phenomenon but as a part of a wide range of effects that can be elicited by sensory rearrangement.

## VI. Quantitative Studies of Oscillatory Stimulation

### A. VERTICAL OSCILLATION

Adequate studies of the relationship between motion sickness incidence and the stimulus parameters of vertical oscillation are sparse, and even the best of them—the Wesleyan University Studies under the direction of Wendt—had serious methodological flaws such as the failure to control for independent head motions and a high ambient temperature. But this problem is partly offset by the fact that the few studies performed in this area have come up with relatively consistent findings, at least with regard to the relationship between sickness and the frequency of oscillation. This relationship is most simply presented by considering in some detail the results of the Wesleyan University (and later University of Rochester) vertical oscillator studies (Alexander et al., 1947).

Using a modified elevator, Wendt and his co-workers compared the sickness rates produced by 16 different waveforms in which four aspects of the waves were either controlled or varied in a counterbalanced design: rate of work done, energy per wave, time per wave and acceleration level. The principal dependent variable was the Sickness Index computed by giving a score of 1 for profuse sweating or unequivocal nausea, and a score of 2 for vomiting. The index was then given by the following formula:

$$\frac{\text{Total score for the group} \times 100}{\text{Total number of subjects}}$$

The motion of the elevator was not a regular sinusoid, but consisted of symmetrical acceleration pulses of $\pm 0.2 - \pm 0.65$ with durations of 0.38–2.08 sec.

Readers requiring a clear summary of this work (with diagrams of the waveforms unavailable in the original papers) should follow the advice of Wendt himself and consult the excellent review by Baker (1966). Those needing more detailed procedural information should consult the original papers, of which the final paper contains a summary of the principal conclusions by the investigators themselves (Alexander *et al.*, 1945a, b, c, d, 1947). Also of interest is a recent publication by Wendt (1968), in which he evaluates the results of the whole project. For our present purposes, however, we will restrict our attention to a reworking of the Wesleyan data by Benson (1973) which reveals a high negative correlation between the incidence of sickness and frequency of oscillation that was not made evident by previous analyses.

Disregarding the different peak accelerations at each stimulus condition, and using the raw data as presented by Baker (1966), Benson obtained a clear negative correlation between the incidence of sickness and the frequency of oscillation over the range of frequencies investigated: 0.22–0.59 Hz. This is shown in Fig. 5(a). In an attempt to improve this correlation, several ways of normalising the sickness index for a unit stimulus were tried. The highest coefficient was obtained using the integral of the modulus of the acceleration waveform per unit time—see Fig. 5(b). Benson comments on this relationship as follows:

"Unfortunately, no experimental observations were made at frequencies lower than 0.22, so it is not possible to conclude with any certainty that oscillation at 0.27 Hz represents the optimum frequency for the induction of motion sickness as was inferred by Alexander *et al.* (1947). Obviously an inflection must occur, for the sickness index is nil at zero frequency. Current work by McCauley and Hanlon (personal communication), who are studying the effects of vertical sinusoidal oscillation at frequencies below 1 Hz on human subjects, suggests that the inflection lies between 0.2–0.3 Hz, but confirmation of this finding must await completion of a long series of experimental trials."

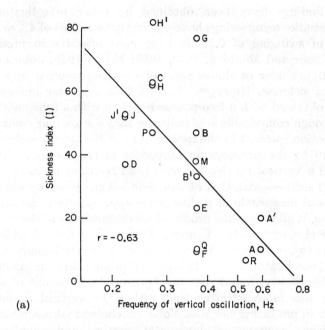

(a)

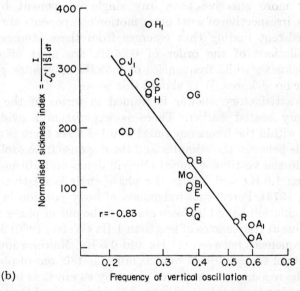

(b)

*Fig.* 5(a) and (b) Benson's reworking of the Wendt data from the Wesleyan University studies. Letters refer to particular waveforms used (see Alexander *et al.*, 1947).

Similar findings have been obtained by other investigators. A number of studies using swings have shown that a radius of 4.5 m and a frequency of swinging of 0.25 Hz were most effective in producing sickness (Fraser and Manning, 1943, 1950; Noble, 1945; Johnson and Taylor, 1961). Faster or slower rates of swinging resulted in a lower incidence of sickness. However, the fact that a greater incidence of sickness is obtained with a two-pole swing than with a four-pole swing moving through comparable arcs indicates that the angular component of swing motion (present in the former but not the latter) makes some contribution to the nauseogenic properties of the motion. Manning (1943) used a vertical accelerator with head restraint to compare the incidence of sickness with that obtained on a 3 m, 90° swing where the frequency and magnitude of g change are approximately the same on both devices. While the swing produced a 50% incidence of sickness, the vertical accelerator produced none. The main point of difference between the two devices was the absence of a tangential component on the vertical accelerator. Noble (1945) and Cipriani (1942), using dogs of known susceptibility, found that the horizontal component of a two-pole swing was more effective than either the vertical or angular components in producing sickness. Noble concluded that a combination of the various components—horizontal, vertical and angular—was considerably more effective than any single component by itself. Nevertheless, irrespective of what other motion components are present, the one consistent finding that emerges from these studies is that vertical oscillations of the order of 0.25 Hz are most effective in producing sickness, while frequencies of 0.55 Hz or greater generally elicit little or no sickness. Why should this be so?

The most satisfactory answer is framed in terms of the sensory conflict theory stated earlier. There is experimental evidence to suggest that within the frequency range of 0.1–1.0 Hz there is a change of phase angle between the stimulus and the response from otolithically driven cells in the vestibular nuclei (Melvill Jones and Milsum, 1966), while between 1.0 Hz and 2.0 Hz the phase angle is relatively stable (see Benson, 1973). Perceptual judgments of body position in vertical sinusoidal oscillation have also been shown to be out of phase with the actual stimulus at frequencies of less than 1 Hz (Walsh, 1960; Malcolm, 1971). At frequencies between 0.1 Hz and 0.5 Hz, Malcolm found that the judgments of some subjects were as much as 180° out of phase, and 48% of all the responses were out of phase by as much as 90°.

Because we do not yet fully understand the dynamics of the transduction of linear accelerations by the otolith organs and other gravi-receptors, it is not yet possible to specify the exact nature of the sensory conflicts involved in low frequency vibration. Our present state of knowledge is best summarised by quoting again from Benson (1973):

> "Undoubtedly, during vertical oscillation in the frequency range where motion sickness occurs, there is confusion and uncertainty in the perception of motion. The nature of the sensory mismatch or conflict is difficult to identify. It may perhaps be dependent on the dynamics of the otolith organ in the frequency domain where its function changes from a 'static' receptor, signalling head position relative to gravity, to that of a 'dynamic' receptor responding to brief movements of the head. In addition, the absence of compatible signals from the vertical canals which are normally synergistic with those from the saccular and utricular maculae as the head is rotated in a sagittal or coronal plane, no doubt also contributes to the sensory mismatch during vertical oscillation."

Restated in terms of the classificatory schema outlined earlier, this could mean that we are dealing here with either a Type 1 or a Type 3 canal–otolith conflict, depending upon whether the head is free to move. But if the eyes are open, then wider visual–inertial conflicts are going to be involved, the nature of which will depend on the degree of external visual reference. In addition, conflicts are also likely to exist between the otoliths and other mechanoreceptors, which, as yet, have no place in the existing schema.

## B. ANGULAR OSCILLATION

Most of the evidence with regard to the nauseogenic properties of angular oscillation has emerged as incidental findings; few if any studies have specifically examined the relationship between sickness incidence and stimulus characteristics in this particular mode. Niven and Hixson (1961), in a series of experiments using the Human Disorientation Device in Pensacola, failed to observe any sickness in subjects exposed to moderate stimuli over a wide frequency range (0.02–0.2 Hz, constant peak acceleration $\pm 40°/\text{sec}^2$). Nor was sickness found in a more recent study by Benson and Sternfeld (1973) over a stimulus range of 0.01–5 Hz, with a constant peak velocity of $\pm 30°/\text{sec}$.

In an investigation primarily concerned with assessing dynamic visual acuity, Benson and Guedry (1971) exposed subjects for 20 min to a sinusoidal angular oscillation where the peak velocity was 160°/sec and the periodic time 25 sec (0.04 Hz). The subjects were either upright so that the stimulus was about the yaw (z) axis of the head, or with their heads positioned so that the stimulus acted about an axis through their ears—the pitch or y axis. In the former situation, where the oscillatory motion acted primarily on the horizontal canals, only 1 of 10 subjects experienced any symptoms of motion sickness. Of particular interest, however, was that when the subjects adopted the latter position so that the vertical canals were stimulated, 6 subjects were nauseated in less than 10 min and only 2 completed the 20 min schedule. And even when the exposure period was reduced to $7\frac{1}{2}$ min, 5 of the 11 subjects became sick.

Benson (1973) attributed the higher incidence of sickness during angular oscillation in pitch to the greater sensory conflict existing between canal signals and other motion cues when the subject lay on his side on the turntable. He postulated three factors that may contribute to this more intense conflict:

> "One factor is that the vertical canals, stimulated by angular motion in pitch, exhibit a greater phase advance than the lateral canals to angular oscillation at low frequency (Melvill Jones et al., 1964; Benson and Guedry, 1971). In addition there are greater changes in the force environment with larger force gradients in the z axis of the body when motion occurs about the y axis than when rotation is about the z axis. It must also be remembered that during natural angular motion in pitch, the head changes its orientation to the gravitational force, so that when the vertical semi-circular canals signal a pitching movement of the head there will be a concomitant and compatible signal from the otolithic maculae. When the rotation axis is vertical and the head so orientated that the vertical canals are stimulated, there is no changing stimulus to the otolith organs, provided the head is close to the axis of rotation."

The last point is particularly important since it underlines the basic argument of the sensory conflict theory, namely that motion sickness arises from a discrepancy between what is currently being signalled by the spatial senses and what we have come to expect from previous transactions with the natural environment.

In the next section, we will review some of the correlates of motion sickness susceptibility, and in particular we shall consider how the sensory conflict theory can help us to pinpoint some of the more important sources of individual variation in this respect.

## VII. Factors Influencing Susceptibility

Among those possessing an intact vestibular system, there are wide individual differences in motion sickness susceptibility, and the extent to which any one person is prone appears to be a relatively stable and enduring characteristic among his or her contemporaries. Within broad limits, the degree of individual proneness is predictable from one provocative situation to another (Hemingway, 1946; Birren and Fisher, 1947; Birren, 1949; Graybiel, 1964; Reason, 1967). The one notable exception to this general intra-personal consistency is individual susceptibility to sickness in zero-gravity conditions which appears to show little or no relationship with Earth-bound assessment of susceptibility (Graybiel, 1971). Some of the more important factors known to influence motion sickness proneness are considered below.

## A. AGE

There is overwhelming evidence to show that motion sickness susceptibility fluctuates markedly with age (Tyler and Bard, 1949; Chinn and Smith, 1953; Money, 1970). Sickness rarely occurs before 2 years of age, probably since for a large part of that time infants are moved passively anyway, but it then increases with age until it reaches a peak somewhere between 10 and 13 years. Certainly there is a highly significant decline in susceptibility between the ages of 12 and 21 (Reason, 1967). This decline continues through young adulthood to middle age and beyond. Chinn et al. (1950) surveyed 5000 subjects on transatlantic troopship crossings and found a 31% incidence of seasickness between the ages of 17 and 19 years, which fell to 13.2% between the ages of 30 and 39 years. A similar decline with age has been found on civil aircraft (Lederer and Kidera, 1954). A recent survey by the present writer found that motion sickness was an extremely rare occurrence beyond the age of 50, and this could not be attributed simply to a reduced exposure on the part of older people.

One explanation for the decline in susceptibility beyond puberty could be that the information traces consolidated during previous exposures to an increasingly wide variety of provocative situations do not fade with time but remain in some readily accessible form; perhaps in a long-term storage unit. The possibility of such a long-term store is strongly indicated by the results of a recent investigation in which it was found that the protective adaptation acquired during a series of graded exposures to cross-coupled angular accelerations was still largely intact when the subjects were tested some 6 months later (Reason and Diaz, 1972). It is not unreasonable that the process of adaptation should follow a long-term pattern of retention similar to that observed in other types of learning.

The increased resistance associated with advancing years may also be augmented by a diminution in the strength of the mismatch signal responsible (within the terms of the sensory conflict theory) for triggering motion sickness reactions. This may be due either to some reduction in the activity of the sensory transducing mechanisms (see the subsequent section dealing with "receptivity"), or because the older person no longer experiences the same degree of sensory incongruity.

## B. SEX

There is no doubt that women are more susceptible than men. This was frequently noted by ship's physicians during the nineteenth century and has subsequently been confirmed by numerous investigations covering a wide range of provocative circumstances (Lederer and Kidera, 1954; Kaplan, 1964; Reason, 1967; Reason and Diaz, 1971).

The basis for this sex difference is not fully understood. One possibility is that it may be associated with the female endocrine system. Schwab (1954) observed that women appear to be more susceptible during the time of menstruation, and there is considerable anecdotal evidence to indicate that pregnancy increases the likelihood of motion sickness.

## C. RECEPTIVITY AND ADAPTABILITY

Within a fairly homogeneous group of healthy young men, there is evidence that a considerable part of the residual variation in motion sickness susceptibility (after age and sex factors have been eliminated) may be accounted for by two primarily perceptual factors: *receptivity* and *adaptability*.

### 1. *Receptivity*

The term "receptivity" refers to the idiosyncratic way the central nervous system transduces or codes stimulus energy. Three separate studies (see Reason, 1968) have indicated that individuals reporting an extensive history of motion sickness tend to be more "receptive" to a given level of stimulus energy, irrespective of modality. That is, they transduce this input more effectively so that the subjective experience it evokes is more intense than that produced within less "receptive" individuals by the same objective level of stimulus energy. These characteristic differences in subjective experience reveal themselves both in reactions to vehicle motion and also in a number of laboratory procedures including the spiral after-effect, kinaesthetic figural after-effects (Petrie, 1966) and the slope of psycho-physical magnitude functions.

Why should "receptives" be more susceptible to motion sickness than "non-receptives"? To answer this, we need to refer back to the neural mismatch hypothesis discussed earlier. It is suggested that the connection between motion sickness susceptibility and receptivity lies in the magnitude of the initial discrepancy between the prevailing sensory influx and the contents of the neural store. Receptives, because of their greater awareness of the intensity of the conflicting sensory cues, will suffer more intense symptoms than non-receptives since at any given level of sensory rearrangement, they will produce a greater mismatch signal. In a rotating environment, for example, an objective angular velocity of 5 rev/min may elicit in a receptive individual a neural response equivalent to that produced by, say, 7 or 8 rev/min in a less receptive person. This argument is similar in many respects to that advanced by Barrett and Thornton (1968) to account for the significant relationship they found between susceptibility and "field dependence". In brief, therefore, it seems that receptives receive sufficient incongruity in the total stimulus flux to trigger the nausea syndrome at relatively low intensities; while non-receptives require greater physical energy levels to evoke the same condition.

This hypothesised relationship between intensity coding and motion sickness susceptibility has also received support from work carried out in other laboratories. Komendantov and Kopanev (1963) cite several Russian studies which indicate that susceptibility is related to Pavlov's (and later Teplov's) "strong" and "weak" nervous system typology. A high degree of proneness is found to be characteristic of "weak" nervous systems. The similarity between this and the receptivity dimension can be seen from Teplov's description (see Gray, 1964) of the "strength" typology—"... the strong nervous system acts as if it damped down stimulation, while the weak nervous system acts as if it amplified it". On this basis, and from their respective relationships with susceptibility, it is reasonable to suggest some degree of identification between "receptives" and "weak" nervous system individuals.

A similar identification can be made, at least in part, between Eysenck's introverts (Eysenck, 1955) and the receptive end of the above continuum. According to Eysenck's cortical inhibition theory of extraversion–introversion, introverts will react to a given level of stimulation with a more intense neural response than extraverts owing to both their lower potential for reactive inhibition and their greater neural excitability. Although never firmly established, there are indications in the motion sickness literature that introverts are more prone than extraverts. Perhaps the most solid evidence was obtained by Kottenhoff and Lindahl (1960). They found negative correlations between extraversion (as measured by the Maudsley Personality Inventory) (see Eysenck, 1959) and susceptibility as gauged from experimental exposure to a combination of bodily rotation and optical inversion of the visual field, and from a personal history questionnaire.

In a recent study, Parker (1971) found that highly susceptible subjects showed significantly greater amounts of volar sweating while viewing a visually disorienting film (the scene taken from a car driving down mountain roads). He interpreted these findings as supporting the "receptivity" hypothesis, arguing that if the highly prone subjects were more receptive to the disturbing visual stimuli, "then there would be more central nervous system work expended in processing the incoming information and this increased use of energy could be reflected as increased volar sweating".

## 2. Adaptability

Here, the term "adaptability" refers to that rate at which an individual typically adjusts to conditions of sensory rearrangement in which inputs from one or more of the spatial senses are artificially distorted to render them incompatible with information being signalled by functionally related senses. Numerous studies, particularly the long-term investigations carried out in the Pensacola Slow Rotation Room (Graybiel, 1964; Reason and Graybiel, 1972), have shown that normal individuals differ widely and consistently in the rates at which they adjust to a rearranged force environment. Clearly, the typical rate at which an individual adapts to a nauseogenic situation will have a close bearing on his overall susceptibility to motion sickness.

Recently, a technique called the Coriolis Adaptation Test (Reason and Graybiel, 1970) has been developed to assess differences in adaptability as they appear in a rotating environment. A number of studies involving this test have shown that individuals who require a large amount of exposure to neutralise their Coriolis vestibular reactions (i.e. who are "slow" adapters) suffer a greater decline in well-being and present more severe symptoms over a given period of stimulation than do those who adjust rapidly. Furthermore, these "slow adapters" also report a significantly more extensive history of motion sickness on a wide range of vehicles than do the "fast adapters" (Reason and Graybiel, 1972). Slow adapters also tend to be more introverted than fast adapters—a fact which may contribute to the previously mentioned relationship between introverts and susceptibility.

Within the terms of the neural mismatch theory, defective adaptation can result from one or a combination of several factors. It could reflect the inability of the neural store to accommodate traces of the re-arranged sensory influx. In other words, the contents of the store could resist change and thus perpetuate the mismatch signal. This could be analogous to a failure to "learn" the informational characteristics of the atypical environment. Alternatively, there could be a breakdown or inefficiency in the mechanisms responsible for retrieving the appropriate stimulus traces from the store for comparison with the prevailing sensory inputs. Or there could be something akin to "forgetting" occurring within the store. That is, traces laid down in the store lack the necessary degree of permanence; either they fail to be consolidated or they are erased through interactions with newer stored material. Any of these failings, either singly or in combination, could contribute to unusually slow rates of adaptation, or to the absence of adaptation as noted by Hemingway (1945) and Tyler and Bard (1949).

## 3. *The Relative Contributions of Receptivity and Adaptability*

To what extent are these two factors related within the individual, and what are their relative contributions to motion sickness susceptibility? In a recent study designed to find answers to these questions, receptivity and adaptability measures were administered to a large sample of healthy young men together with questionnaire and exposure indices of susceptibility (Reason and Graybiel, 1972). The results indicated that no systematic relationship existed between receptivity and adaptability. In other words, these two perceptual factors constituted orthogonal dimensions of interpersonal variation where an individual's position along one was largely independent of his position along the other.

From this finding, it was possible to classify four susceptibility types on the bases of the neural mismatch theory. Each is distinguished by the degree of symptomatology on first exposure to the provocative stimulus, and by the subsequent persistence of these symptoms with further exposure. Figure 6 shows how these four types relate to the neural mismatch notions expressed previously in Fig. 4. The predicted characteristics of each type can be summarised as follows:

(i) *High receptivity–slow adapter* (*HR–SA*): the most susceptible type—the high receptivity will (theoretically) ensure that reactions are initially severe, and the slow rate of adaptation guarantees that they will persist for a relatively long time.

(ii) *High receptivity–fast adapter* (*HR–FA*): it is expected that this type will suffer initially severe reactions, but that these will diminish rapidly due to the fast rate of adaptation.

(iii) *Low receptivity–slow adapter* (*LR–SA*): this individual is likely to suffer mild symptoms for a relatively long time.

(iv) *Low receptivity–fast adapter* (*LR–FA*): the least susceptible type—suffers (if at all) mild symptoms for a relatively short time.

To test these predictions, the subjects were retrospectively split into four subgroups corresponding to these types and a comparison was made of several indices of motion sickness susceptibility. According to the predictions, the HR–SA should have been the most susceptible and

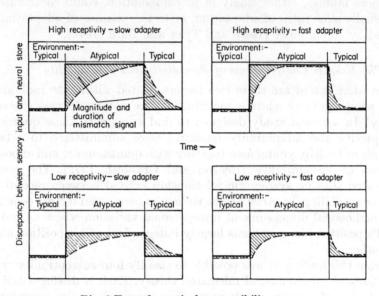

*Fig.* 6 Four theoretical susceptibility types.

this indeed turned out to be the case; but the HR–FA group rather than the LR–FA group was the least susceptible—contrary to prediction. Further examination of the data revealed that adaptability rather than receptivity was the primary factor influencing both general susceptibility and perrotational discomfort. However, the receptivity predictions were supported for the slow adapters. This suggested that receptivity factors contribute to susceptibility among the slow adapters but not among the fast adapters in whom the rapid rate of adjustment appears to suppress their influence. A positive and significant correlation was found between receptivity and susceptibility within the slow adapter group; but within the fast group, the correlation coefficient was zero. From this analysis, it was concluded that adaptability is the most potent factor contributing to individual variation in motion sickness susceptibility. But among relatively slow adapters, receptivity also plays a part in determining individual proneness.

## 4. *The Long-term Retention of Adaptation*

So far in this discussion, we have concentrated upon differences in the rates at which individuals adapt to what is effectively their first prolonged exposure to a rearranged force environment. But this is only one possible dimension of variation. There is another source of individual differences which may or may not be related to these "initial-exposure" measures of adaptability, and that is the extent to which subjects *retain* this adaptation on subsequent exposures to the same stimulus.

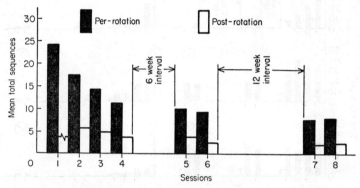

*Fig.* 7 Retention of protective adaptation—group data.

This issue has been examined in a recent study (Reason and Diaz, 1972) in which eight young men were exposed to eight rotational sessions over a total period of 24 weeks. The direction of rotation was alternated for each subject in a balanced design. The first four sessions occurred at 1-week intervals, then there was an interval of 6 weeks followed by two more sessions at 1-week intervals. Then came a gap of 12 weeks followed by the two final sessions, again separated by an interval of 1 week. The principal measure was the number of head movements required on each block to attain a predetermined adaptation criterion, characterised primarily by the absence of illusory sensations of motion during head movements. Figure 7 summarises the group data, while Fig. 8 shows individual patterns of initial adaptability and subsequent retention of adaptation.

From Fig. 7 it is clear that the mean number of head movements required to achieve the same operationally defined level of adaptation at 5 rev/min showed a steady decline over the first four sessions, indicating a gradual build-up of adaptational savings from one session to the next. Furthermore, this adaptation was retained intact after both the first interval of 6 weeks and the second of 12 weeks. Also of

13

interest is the fact that adaptation acquired in one direction appeared to transfer to the opposite direction, as well as to subsequent sessions in the direction of rotation.

Turning now to the individual patterns of initial adaptability and retention, it can be seen from Fig. 8 that no systematic relationship existed between the initial rate of adaptation (the number of head

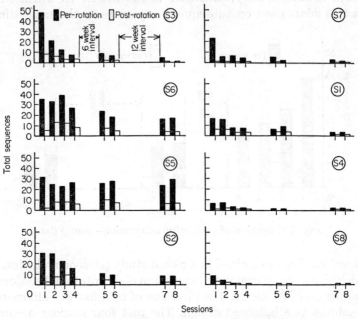

*Fig.* 8 Retention of protective adaptation—individual data.

movements to criterion on Session 1) and the subsequent degree of retention. These findings indicate that it is not sufficient to base predictions of susceptibility on a single adaptation test. We need to know not only this initial rate of adaptation, but also the extent to which this protection is retained with the passing of time.

## 5. *Practical Implications for Screening*

Evidence has been cited to show that both receptivity and adaptability contribute to variation in motion sickness susceptibility. But, although these factors appear to be independent of one another within the individual, they do not have equal influence upon susceptibility. Adaptability is clearly the most potent factor, yet receptivity plays some part in determining susceptibility among slow adapters only.

However, a measure of adaptability acquired on a single test does not give any prediction of the subsequent retention of protective adaptation; two or more tests are required to assess this important dimension of retentiveness. These findings have been integrated into a procedure for screening out high-risk individuals when age and sex factors are held constant. The logic of this procedure is shown schematically below (Fig. 9).

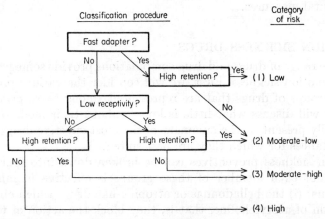

*Fig.* 9 Suggested screening procedure for identifying high risk individuals.

This scheme is of course extremely tentative. In the first place, the moderate categories of risk cover a wide range, and the *a priori* grounds for indicating that certain individuals will fall into, say, the moderate–low category rather than the moderate–high category are not strong. But these are relatively minor limitations since the primary aim of the procedure is to eliminate, or at least "tag", the high-risk individuals. A more serious problem is the degree to which we can generalise from findings obtained in a specific kind of environment; namely, a rotating device. Can we assume, for example, that adaptability and retentiveness measures obtained under these laboratory conditions will be predictive of reactions in flight or on hovercraft. There are two pieces of evidence to suggest that these assumptions are partially justified. First, there are the positive and significant correlations between adaptability and motion sickness questionnaire scores reflecting proneness to a wide variety of provocative circumstances. Second, a number of investigators (Lansberg, 1960; Ambler and Guedry, 1971) have shown that reactions to brief but severe exposures to cross-coupled angular stimuli are of value in predicting the incidence of sickness in flying training.

## VIII. The Prevention of Motion Sickness

The motion sickness literature abounds with suggested methods for preventing motion sickness, many of them absurd and few of them effective. No attempt will be made to review these methods here; instead, we shall concentrate on three types of preventive measure which have shown themselves to be of both practical and theoretical interest: (a) drugs, (b) adaptation schedules and (c) postural or behavioural measures.

### A. MOTION SICKNESS DRUGS

A wide range of drugs and drug combinations provide some protection against motion sickness. First, we will consider the various pharmacological groups of drugs that are represented among these preventives, then we will discuss what little is known about their mode of action, and finally present a brief summary of the most effective drugs and the circumstances for which they are best suited.

Motion sickness preventives can be broken down into four groups, though not each member of these groups is effective in minimising symptoms: (i) the belladonnas or atropine-like drugs which antagonise the action of acetylcholine, that is, they block the action of the parasympathetic nervous system; (ii) antihistamines which, in addition to antagonising histamine, also have an atropine-like effect; (iii) phenothiazines which have a tranquillising effect and are sympathetic blocking agents; and (iv) various combinations of these and other drugs including barbiturates and amphetamine.

As far as the present writer can judge, the first recorded use of anticholinergic drugs as a motion sickness preventive was in 1869 when an anonymous correspondent to the *Lancet* recommended a combination of chloroform and tincture of belladonna against seasickness. Although their prophylactic effects have been known for a long time (see Oriel, 1927), the belladonnas did not come into widespread use until during the Second World War when extensive trials by mainly British investigators indicated that one member of this class, 1-hyoscine hydrobromide (trade name, Scopolamine), was the single most effective preventive available (Glaser and McCance, 1959). Subsequent research has clearly confirmed the efficacy of hyoscine (Wood *et al.*, 1965; Brand and Perry, 1966; Wood, 1968). When taken by mouth in doses of 0.6–1.0 mg 1 hour before the expected exposure, hyoscine provides relatively quick-acting though short-term protection against motion sickness. But at these dosages it does produce some marked side-effects, particularly drowsiness, a dry mouth and some blurring of vision. Synthetic belladonnas, such as procyclidine (Kemadrin) and cycrimine hydrochloride (Pagitane), produce fewer side-effects but also confer less protection (Renzi and Milch, 1958).

In 1949, Gay and Carliner treated a case of hives with the antihistamine, dimenhydrinate (Dramamine). The patient was a pregnant woman who had, incidentally, been a lifelong sufferer from severe carsickness. But whilst taking the drug, she found herself to be completely free of any motion sickness symptoms. Other American investigators took up this serendipitous observation and subjected a wide range of antihistamines to extensive field trials both at sea and in the air (Chinn and Smith, 1953, 1955). As the result of this and later work, a number of antihistaminic drugs were found to give satisfactory protection. Among the most effective were cyclizine (Marezine), meclizine (Bonamine), diphenylhydramine (Benadryl) and buclizine (Bucladin). Side-effects were generally less pronounced than with the belladonnas, but drowsiness and some dizziness were reported.

So far, only a few phenothiazines have been found effective. Of these, the two best appear to be trifluoperazine (Stelazine) and promethazine (Phenergan). Another phenothiazine, chlorpromazine (Thorazine), was found to be completely ineffective in man, but was a powerful preventive against swing sickness in dogs (Chinn and Smith, 1955). In a recent study (Wood, 1968), it was found that certain phenothiazines, particularly tiethylperazine (Torecan) in 10 and 30 mg doses, actually increased susceptibility to the sickness induced by cross-coupled accelerations. Another drug, meprobromate, which also reduces sympathetic activity, had a similar effect. Typical side-effects of the phenothiazines are drowsiness, hypertension and mental depression.

Various drug combinations have also been used with some success. For example, antihistamines such as Benadryl or Dramamine are frequently used with Scopolamine and a barbiturate or vitamins $B_1$ and $B_6$. In general, however, these combinations have not yet shown themselves to be more effective than a full-strength dose of their most effective component (Wood et al., 1965). The one notable exception was a combination of hyoscine and d-amphetamine (Wood, 1968) which proved more effective than any other preparation in delaying the onset of symptoms in the Pensacola Slow Rotation Room. This combination has since been used by the Apollo astronauts, but legal limitations on amphetamine are likely to restrict its general use.

How do these preventives achieve their effect? The first thing that needs to be clearly stated is that no drug has yet been found which is completely effective in preventing sickness; these drugs only serve to increase the amount of exposure an individual can stand before he experiences symptoms. It is evident that none of these drugs increases resistance through its specific pharmacological action. As Brand and Perry (1966, p. 920) put it: "It seems very improbable that the effect is due to the ability to antagonise—at least at peripheral sites—the actions of either acetylcholine or of histamine." However, most of these drugs have a cortical depressant effect, and there is some evidence that hyoscine, for example, modifies the sensory transduction process in the direction of rendering individuals temporarily less receptive to the intensity of stimulation (Benson and Reason, 1965; Croucher and Hindmarch, 1973). A great deal more research is required before we can be certain of the precise mode of action of these drugs; but for now, the important thing is that in Wood's (1968) words: "The proper drug at the proper time will greatly increase an individual's chance of avoiding motion sickness."

What is the proper drug and in what circumstances is it most appropriate? To some extent the answer to this question depends on which side of the Atlantic you are. British investigators strongly favour l-hyoscine hydrobromide, while Americans tend to recommend antihistamines such as cyclizine. However, there is evidence (Brand and Perry, 1966; Wood, 1968) to indicate that both classes of drug are appropriate but in different circumstances. Where the traveller seeks protection against a short but relatively severe exposure such as a Channel crossing in a ship or hovercraft, then hyoscine given orally in doses of 0.3–0.6 mg 1 hour before departure is recommended. But for longer journeys in which the motion is likely to be milder, the anti-histamines are most satisfactory because they are longer acting and have less severe side-effects. Cyclizine 50 mg, Dramamine 100 mg, Benadryl 50 mg and Meclozine 50 mg will provide useful protection against long-duration motion where repeated medication is needed. Cyclizine, Dramamine and Benadryl act in about 2 hours and should be repeated after 4–6 hours. Meclozine takes about 3–4 hours to act and exerts an effect for between 12 and 24 hours (Brand and Perry, 1967).

## B. ADAPTATION SCHEDULES

Perhaps the only certain way of avoiding motion sickness in a particular nauseogenic situation is through the acquisition of sufficient protective adaptation. This, as Hill (1936) pointed out, is "Nature's own cure". To acquire a satisfactory degree of protective adaptation, we need to interact actively with the provocative stimulus. As in gaining other forms of immunity, we have to expose ourselves to the sick-making agency in order to increase our natural resistance to it. Research at

Pensacola and in our own laboratory at Leicester indicates that adequate and lasting protection against specific nauseogenic environments, like the rotating room, can be conferred *without loss of well-being* by exposing individuals to gradually increasing levels of cross-coupled stimulation (Reason, 1970, 1973). The result is that during subsequent exposures to this particular situation, the rate of adaptation is greatly speeded up and, with it, the risk of motion sickness either removed or considerably diminished.

The rationale for these procedures, termed "adaptation schedules", is provided by the neural mismatch hypothesis. The subsequently accelerated rate of adaptation is presumed to be a function of the presence within the neural storage unit of appropriate pre-formed stimulus traces. If these pre-formed traces are well established, then it appears that they can be retrieved for comparison with the prevailing sensory inputs before a mismatch signal of sufficient strength to generate symptoms can be activated. Once consolidated, these pre-formed traces remain effective for long periods of time, probably being retained in some form of long-term storage (Reason and Diaz, 1972).

While the theoretical justification for these procedures is relatively clear-cut, their practical application is more difficult. The major problem is that protective adaptation tends to be highly specific (Guedry, 1965). Although there is some evidence that well-consolidated adaptation does generalise in a limited way to altered provocative circumstances (Reason and Graybiel, 1972), the more universal finding is that protection acquired through adapting to one kind of motion stimulus does not transfer to qualitatively different stimuli. Thus, sailors who have adjusted satisfactorily to the characteristic motion of a small vessel such as a frigate or destroyer can become seasick when exposed to the considerably more sedate motion of a larger vessel such as an aircraft carrier. Consequently, the application of adaptation schedules is presently restricted to situations where we understand the primary sick-making characteristics of a particular situation, and where we can effectively simulate them in the laboratory. And even where we can fulfil these conditions, the procedures are both time-consuming and expensive so, for the present at least, we must restrict ourselves to highly selected populations such as astronauts and pilots for whom the penalties of inflight sickness can be high.

To date, work in this area has largely been directed towards the prevention of motion sickness aboard projected spacecraft that rotate to provide artificial gravity (Reason, 1973). However, it is our firm belief that the general principles underlying the design of this particular schedule can also be applied to the prevention of sickness in other circumstances, particularly among aircrew in conventional aircraft during training.

The schedule presently recommended for the prevention of sickness in a rotating environment is summarised diagrammatically in Fig. 10. The principal aim underlying this research was to devise a schedule that would produce the maximum amount of protective adaptation with the least cost in either time or discomfort. The basic units of the

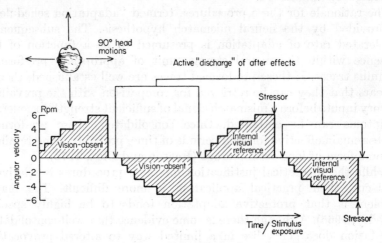

*Fig.* 10 A suggested pre-flight adaptation schedule.

schedule consist of sequences of eight 90° head movements executed in four quadrants: front, back, left and right. The initial speed of rotation is 1 rev/min and proceeds through a series of 1 rev/min steps up to a terminal velocity which can be adjusted to operational circumstances. It can be seen that there are four blocks of these controlled head movements, two in the clockwise direction and two in the counter-clockwise direction. The actual number of these blocks and their duration can be adjusted to suit both the basic susceptibility of the individual and the nature of the subsequent real exposure. However, it is important that the blocks should alternate in direction to confer "all-round" protection.

Other features of the schedule reflect specific research findings. It has been found, for example, that adaptation proceeds more quickly if the number of head movements executed at each velocity step is graded to the absolute speed of rotation, giving proportionately more head movements to the higher steps (Reason and Graybiel, 1970b). It has also been shown that it takes less exposure with a smaller risk of symptoms to attain a predetermined level of adaptation if the eyes are kept closed during the first half of the schedule (Reason and Diaz, 1971). Discordant visual information exacerbates the nauseogenic properties of the cross-coupled stimulus and if this is initially absent it can be introduced at a later point without marked ill-effects. But if the discordant visual information is present from the outset, then progress can be slow and the risk of symptoms high. Another study (Reason and Graybiel, 1969) revealed that protective adaptation acquired in one direction of rotation transfers more readily to the opposite direction if the subject is allowed to "discharge" his after-effects during an inter-mediate period at zero velocity.

Finally, periods of "stressor activity" can be slotted into the latter stages of the schedule to assess the degree of generalised protection attained. These stressor tests can be tailored to suit the particular circumstances for which protection is required, but essentially they should consist of exposing subjects to more extensive head movements in all directions. If these tests indicate that insufficient protection has been acquired, then further blocks can be added to the schedule until this criterion is satisfied.

## C. POSTURAL AND BEHAVIOURAL MEASURES

There is now a great deal of evidence (see Money, 1970) to show that, where the situation permits, adopting the supine position markedly reduces the risk of motion sickness. On swings, the incidence of sickness in the supine position was found to be one-fifth of that in the sitting position (Manning and Stewart, 1949) and similar advantageous effects of this position have been observed on both ships and trains. As mentioned earlier, part of this effect may be due to the fact that lying in the supine position necessarily restricts independent motions of the head which are known to be positively correlated with motion sickness susceptibility (Johnson et al., 1951). Certainly, the provision of some form of mechanical head restraint is helpful in reducing the likelihood of sickness, particularly on aircraft during moderate turbulence (Johnson and Mayne, 1953). In a rotating environment or in weightless space flight, the nauseogenic stimulus is only applied when the head is tilted, so that fixing the head will guarantee immunity against sick-ness—unfortunately, this simple expedient will also ensure that the astronaut will be unable to perform most of his operational duties. In a car with high-backed seats, passengers can gain a considerable amount of protection from simply holding their head against the support and moving it as little as possible. Even voluntary head restraint is likely to help. Where head movements are essential, they should be carried out slowly and preferably when the car is not involved in a turning manoeuvre. This advice, of course, only applies to passengers; drivers are in any case relatively immune.

Because we can exert a considerable influence upon our susceptibility through our own voluntary actions, the traveller is, to a large extent, the master of his own state of well-being. If he follows a few simple rules predicated upon the sensory conflict theory, he can greatly reduce the likelihood of becoming motion sick on almost any mode of transport.

The cardinal rule is to behave in a way that will minimise as far as possible the degree of mismatch between the various available sources of motion and position information. As we have seen, intra-labyrinthine conflicts can be reduced by adopting the supine position or keeping the head still. Similarly, visual–inertial conflicts can be alleviated by controlling the direction of gaze, or, where this proves impossible, by closing the eyes. In a car, for example, it is important to maintain a forward-looking direction (just as the driver does) and to avoid side-ways or backwards glances that present the brain with uncorrelated visual information. Aboard ship, it is helpful to fixate the horizon or some visible landfall; almost all other directions of looking will provide visual information that is discordant with the prevailing inertial inputs. Where it is impossible to avoid visual–inertial conflicts—below decks, for example, or in a totally enclosed vehicle—it is often helpful to the passenger if the eyes are closed. This, at least, is a "natural" way of removing incompatible motion information.

Finally, there are a number of anecdotal and research observations to indicate that mental activity involving some engaging task reduces susceptibility (Tyler and Bard, 1949; Guedry, 1964). By contrast, asking subjects to concentrate upon the imposed motion and to describe their symptoms tends to increase susceptibility (Correia and Guedry, 1967). Why concurrent mental activity should promote resistance is not understood, but it is possible that it involves some pre-empting of the cortical pathways implicated in the production of symptoms. The moral for the traveller: keep your mind on other things than the state of your stomach and engage yourself in some form of mental activity—where this does not, like reading a book in a moving vehicle, aggravate that which is already hard to bear.

## IX. Conclusion

One of the most important consequences of the sensory conflict theory and its corollary, the neural mismatch hypothesis, is the kind of research strategy they dictate when we attempt to specify the nauseo-genic properties of a particular transport situation. Many previous workers, operating within an "overstimulation" framework, restricted their attention to the purely vestibular components of the provocative stimulus. They sought relationships between symptomatology and the physical properties of the motion stimulus, and from these they hoped to establish which of the vestibular receptors was primarily involved. But to seek limited quantitative relationships of this kind is to run the risk of missing the essential character of the provocative stimulus, that is, that *all* the spatial receptors are implicated in one way or another— even though it is only the involvement of the vestibular system that actually triggers the motion sickness reactions. The sensory conflict theory directs us, in the first instance, to make a qualitative analysis of the sick-making situation as a whole. In other words, we need to establish at the outset which sources of motion information are available to the passenger, and in what manner and to what extent they conflict with one another. This theory also tells us that we cannot hope to understand the degree to which a person is susceptible to a particular situation without first establishing his previous "exposure-history". Finally, the sensory conflict viewpoint instructs us that motion sickness is not an isolated phenomenon, but just one of the many consequences of sensory rearrangement.

Motion sickness is a self-inflicted condition. Nobody *has* to suffer; if we had remained as self-propelled animals, it would have been largely unknown. As it is, motion sickness is one of the penalties we pay for our enormous capacity to modify our natural environment and increase our powers of locomotion. Since we are increasing these powers at a positively accelerating rate, the problem of motion sickness and allied disorders will get worse rather than better. Aside from taking the unlikely step of turning back the technological clock, the only lasting solution will stem from a better appreciation of our built-in limitations with regard to passive motion and a more complete understanding and exploitation of our very considerable powers of adaptation.

## REFERENCES

Alexander, S. J., Cotzin, M., Hill, C. J., Ricciuti, E. A. and Wendt, G. R. (1945a).
    *J. Psychol.* **19**, 49–62.
Alexander, S. J., Cotzin, M., Hill, C. J., Ricciuti, E. A. and Wendt, G. R. (1945b).
    *J. Psychol.* **19**, 63–68.
Alexander, S. J., Cotzin, M., Hill, C. J., Ricciuti, E. A. and Wendt, G. R. (1945c).
    *J. Psychol.* **20**, 3–8.
Alexander, S. J., Cotzin, M., Hill, C. J., Ricciuti, E. A. and Wendt, G. R. (1945d).
    *J. Psychol.* **20**, 9–18.

Alexander, S. J., Cotzin, M. and Klee, G. R. (1947). *J. exp. Psychol.* **37**, 440–448.

Ambler, R. K. and Guedry, F. E. (1971). *Aerospace Med.* **42**, 186–189.

Baker, C. H. (1966). Motion and human performance: a review of the literature. *Human Factors Research Inc. Tech. Rept.* 770–771.

Barrett, G. V. and Thornton, C. L. (1968). *J. appl. Psychol.* **52**, 304–308.

Benfari, R. C. (1964). *Perceptual and Motor Skills* **18**, 633–639.

Benson, A. J. (1973). "Physical Characteristics of Stimuli which induce Motion Sickness", unpublished Medical Research Council (London) Committee Paper.

Benson, A. J. and Bodin, M. (1965). The effects of the direction of a linear acceleration vector on postrotational vestibular responses in man. *AGARD Conference Proceedings Series No. 2*, 9–22.

Benson, A. J. and Bodin, M. A. (1966a). *Aerospace Medicine* **37**, 144–154.

Benson, A. J. and Bodin, M. A. (1966b). *Aerospace Medicine* **37**, 889–897.

Benson, A. J. and Guedry, F. E. (1971). *Aerospace Medicine* **42**, 593–601.

Benson, A. J. and Reason, J. T. (1965). "The effects of hyoscine upon the perception of motion after-effects", unpublished report.

Benson, A. J. and Sternfeld, M. L. (1973). Influence of Linear acceleration on the Response of the Vestibulo-ocular Reflex to Angular oscillation", unpublished report.

Benson, A. J., Guedry, F. E. and Jones, G. M. (1967). *J. Physiol. (Lond.)* **191**, 26–27.

Birren, J. E. (1949). Motion sickness: its psychophysiological aspects. *In*: "Human Factors in Undersea Warfare", National Research Council, Washington, D.C.

Birren, J. E. and Fisher, M. B. (1947). *J. appl. Psychol.* **31**, 288–297.

Brand, J. J. and Perry, W. L. M. (1966). *Pharmacological Review* **18**, 895–924.

Brand, J. J. and Perry, W. L. M. (1967). The use of drugs in the prevention of motion sickness in the Services. *Medical Research Council: Royal Naval Personnel Research Committee Report No.* 08/1101, S.S. 178.

Brooks, M. (1939). *Med. Rec.* N.Y. **150**, 23–26.

Brown, G. L., McArdle, L. B. and Magladery, J. W. (1941). Interim report on clinical investigations into airsickness. *Flying Personnel Research Committee Report*, 410.

Chinn, H. I. and Smith, P. K. (1953). *Pharmacol. Rev.* **7**, 33–82.

Chinn, H. I. and Smith, P. K. (1955). *Internat. Rec. Med.* **168**, 13–22.

Chinn, H. I., Noell, W. and Smith, P. K. (1950). Prophylaxis of motion sickness. *Arch. internal Med.* **86**, 810–822 (also in *Sch. Av. Med. Proj. Report*, No. 21–32–014 Report No. 4).

Cipriani, A. (1942). An analysis of the forces encountered on the simple swing used in the study of motion sickness. *Proc. Conf. Motion Sickness*, Nat. Res. Council, Canada, *Rept. No.* C744, *App.* 1.

Claremont, C. A. (1931). *Psyche* **11**, 86–90.

Clark, B. and Graybiel, A. (1961). *Aerospace Medicine* **32**, 93–106.

Clark, B. and Stewart, J. D. (1968). *Percept. Psychophys.* **3**, 253–256.

Correia, M. J. and Guedry, F. E. (1967). *Acta Otolaryngol.* **62**, 297–308.

Croucher, T. and Hindmarch, I. (1973). *Psychopharmacologica* (Berl.) **32**, 215–222.

Danvers, H. (1892). *Lancet* i, 1295–1296.

Dodge, R. (1923). *J. exp. Psychol.* **6**, 1, 107.

Ewert, P. H. (1930). *Genet. Psychol. Monogr.* **7**, 177–363.

Eysenck, H. J. (1955). *J. abn. soc. Psychol.* **51**, 94–106.

Eysenck, H. J. (1959). "Manual of the Maudsley Personality Inventory", University of London Press, London.

Field, W. S. (1942). Induced motion sickness in naval ratings. *Proc. Conf. Motion Sickness*, Nat. Res. Council, Canada, *Rept. No.* C738, *App. D.*

Fraser, A. M. and Manning, G. W. (1943). The effect of variation in the radius (frequency of maximal change in g) and the arc (quantity of maximal change in g) of the swing on the incidence of swing sickness. *Report to Assoc. Comm. on Av. Med. Res.* N.C.R., Canada.

Fraser, A. M. and Manning, G. W. (1950). *J. Appl. Psychol.* **2**, 580–584.

Gay, L. N. and Carliner, P. (1949). "The Prevention and Treatment of Motion Sickness. I: Seasickness", Johns Hopkins University and Hospital Allergy Clinic Report.

Gillingham, K. K. (1966). "A Primer of Vestibular Function, Spatial Disorientation and Motion Sickness", Review 4–66, U.S.A.F. School of Aerospace Medicine, Aerospace Medical Division (A.F.S.C.), Brooks Air Force Base, Texas.

Glaser, E. M. and McCance, R. A. (1959). *Lancet* **1**, 853–856.

Gray, J. A. (1964). "Pavlov's Typology", Pergamon Press, Oxford.

Graybiel, A. (1964). Vestibular sickness and some of its implications for space flight. Chapter XI. *In*: "Neurological Aspects of Auditory and Vestibular Disorders" (W. S. Fields and R. R. Alford eds), Charles C. Thomas, Springfield, Illinois.

Graybiel, A. (1965). "Functional Disturbances of Vestibular Origin of Significance in Space Flight". *In*: 2nd International Symposium on Basic Environmental Problems of Man in Space, Paris, France.

Graybiel, A. (1969). *Aerospace Med.* **40**, 351–367.

Graybiel, A. (1971). Personal communication.

Graybiel, A. and Johnson, W. H. (1963). *Annals of Otology, Rhinology and Laryngology*, **72**, 357.

Graybiel, A., Clark, B. and Zarriello, J. J. (1960). *A.M.A. Arch. Neurol.* **3**, 55–73.

Graybiel, A., Wood, C. D., Miller, E. F. and Cramer, D. B. (1968). *Aerospace Med.* **39**, 453–455.

Groen, J. J. (1960). *Acta Oto-laryngol., Suppl.* **163**, 59–66.

Guedry, F. E. (1964). *Acta Oto-laryngol.* **58**, 377–389.

Guedry, F. E. (1965). Psychophysiological studies of vestibular function. *In*: "Contributions to Sensory Physiology" (W. D. Neff ed.), Academic Press, London and New York.

Guedry, F. E. (1969). Conflicting sensory orientation cues as a factor in motion sickness. *Fourth Symposium on the Role of the Vestibular Organs in Space Exploration*, *NASA SP*-187, Naval Aerospace Medical Institute, National Aeronautics and Space Administration, Pensacola, Fla., U.S.A.

Guedry, F. E. and Montague, E. K. (1961). *Aerospace Med.* **32**, 387–500.

Held, R. (1961). *J. nerv. ment. Dis.* **132**, 26–32.

Hemingway, A. (1945). Incidence of airsickness in cadets during their first ten flights. *A.A.F. School of Aviation Medicine, Project* 170, *Report No.* 5, Randolph Field, Texas, U.S.A.

Hemingway, A. (1946). *J. Aviation Med.* **17**, 80–85.

Hill, J. (1936). *Br. Med. Journal*, Oct.–Dec., 802–807.

Holtermann, H. (1956). *Münchenen Medizinische Wochenschrift* (München) **98**, 229–231.

Irwin, J. A. (1881). *Lancet*, ii, 907–909.

Johnson, W. H. (1961). *Annals of Otology, Rhinology and Laryngology*, **70**, 777.

Johnson, W. H. and Mayne, J. W. (1953). *J. Aviation Med.* **24**, 400–411.

Johnson, W. H. and Taylor, N. B. G. (1961). *Aerospace Med.* **32**, 205–208.

Johnson, W. H., Stubbs, R. A., Kelk, G. F. and Franks, W. R. (1951). *J. Aviat. Med.* **22**, 365–374.

Jongkees, L. B. W. (1967). On the otoliths: their function and the way to test them. *In: Third Symposium on the Role of the Vestibular Organs in Space Exploration*, NASA SP–152, 307–331, Naval Aerospace Medical Institute, Pensacola, Fla., U.S.A.

Kaplan, I. (1964). *Ind. Med. Surg.* **33**, 648–651.

Kennedy, R. S. and Graybiel, A. (1965). The dial test: a standardised procedure for the experimental production of canal sickness symptomatology in a rotating environment. *Naval School of Aviation Medicine, NSAM*–928, Pensacola, Fla., U.S.A.

Kohler, I. (1955). *Acta Psychologica* **11**, 176.

Komendantov, G. L. and Kopanev, V. I. (1963). Motion sickness as a problem of space medicine (English translation). *In: U.S. Joint Pub. Resch. Serv.*, Washington D.C., No. 18,395, **2**, 84–99.

Kottenhoff, H. and Lindahl, L. E. (1960). *Acta Psychologica* **17**, 89–112.

Lansberg, M. P. (1960). "A Primer of Space Medicine", Elsevier, Amsterdam.

Lederer, L. G. and Kidera, G. J. (1954). *Internat. rec. Med.* **167**, 661–668.

Lowenstein, O. (1970). Paper given to Brain Research Association, Birmingham, England.

McClure, J. A., Fregly, A. R., Molina, E. and Graybiel, A. (1971). Response from arousal and thermal sweat areas during motion sickness. *Naval Aerospace Medical Research Laboratory Report NAMRL*–1142.

McNally, W. J. and Stuart, E. A. (1942). *War Medicine* **2**, 683–771.

Mach, E. (1875). "Grundlinien der Lehre von den Bewegungsempfindungen", Leipzig.

Malcolm, R. (1971). Human responses to vestibular Stimulation and some Implications to the Flight Environment, Ph.D. Thesis, McGill University, Montreal.

Manning, G. W. (1943). Acclimatisation to swing sickness. *Report to Assoc. Comm. on Av. Med. Res.*, N.R.C., Canada.

Manning, G. W. and Stewart, W. G. (1949). *J. appl. Physiol.* **1**, 619–628.

Melvill Jones, G. and Milsum, J. H. (1966). Patterns of vestibular neuronal response to rotation of the linear acceleration vector. *Proceedings of the 37th Annual Scientific Meeting, Aerospace Med. Assocn.*

Melvill Jones, G., Barry, W. and Kowalsky, N. (1964). *Aerospace Med.* **35**, 984–989.

Miller, J. W. and Goodson, J. E. (1960). *Aerospace Med.* **31**, 204–212.

Money, K. E. (1970). *Physiol. Rev.* **50**, 1–39.

Morales, M. F. (1949). Motion sickness: physical considerations regarding its etiology. *In*: "Human Factors in Undersea Warfare", 399–414, National Research Council, Washington, D.C.

Niven, J. I. and Hixson, W. C. (1961). Frequency response of the human semicircular canals. I. Steady-state ocular nystagmus response to high-level sinusoidal angular rotations. *U.S. Naval School of Aviation Medicine, Report No.* 58, Pensacola, Fla., U.S.A.

Noble, R. L. (1945). *Canad. J. Res., Sect. E* **23**, 212–225.

Oriel, G. H. (1927). *Lancet* ii, 811–813.

Parker, D. M. (1971). *J. gen. Psychol.* **85**, 87–92.

Petrie, A. (1966). "Individuality in Pain and Suffering". University of Chicago Press, Chicago.

Quix, F. H. (1923). *Monograph. Oto-rhino-laryngol. Intern.* **8**, 828–987.

Reason, J. T. (1967). "Relationships between Motion Sickness Susceptibility, Motion After-effects, and Receptivity", Ph.D. Thesis, University of Leicester.

Reason, J. T. (1968). *Br. J. Psychol.* **59**, 385–393.

Reason, J. T. (1969). *Int. J. Man–Machine Studies* **1**, 21–38.

Reason, J. T. (1970). Motion sickness: a special case of sensory rearrangement. *Adv. Sci.*

Reason, J. T. (1973). Adaptation studies on motion sickness. *Proceedings of Xth World Congress of Otorhinlaryngology, Excerpta Medica*, No. 276.

Reason, J. T. and Diaz, E. (1970). The effects of visual reference on adaptation to Coriolis accelerations. *Flying Personnel Research Committee Report No.* 1303.

Reason, J. T. and Diaz, E. (1971). Simulator sickness in passive observers. *Flying Personnel Research Committee Report No.* 1310.

Reason, J. T. and Diaz, E. (1972). "Long-term Retention of Protective Adaptation to Motion Sickness", unpublished report.

Reason, J. T. and Graybiel, A. (1969). Adaptation to Coriolis accelerations: its transfer to the opposite direction of rotation as a function of intervening activity at zero velocity. *Naval Aerospace Medical Institute Report No.* 1085, Pensacola, Fla., U.S.A.

Reason, J. T. and Graybiel, A. (1970a). *Aerospace Med.* **41**, 166–171.

Reason, J. T. and Graybiel, A. (1970b). *Aerospace Med.* **41**, 73–79.

Reason, J. T. and Graybiel, A. (1971). "The Effectiveness of a 3-day Adaptation Schedule designed to prevent Motion Sickness in a slowly Rotating Device", unpublished report.

Reason, J. T. and Graybiel, A. (1972). Factors contributing to motion sickness susceptibility: adaptability and receptivity. *AGARD Conference Proceedings No.* 109.

Renzi, A. A. and Milch, L. J. (1958). *J. aviat. Med.* **29**, 587–589.

Schwab, R. S. (1954). *Intern. Record Med.* **167**, 631–637.

Sjöberg, A. A. (1931). *Acta Otolaryngol. Suppl.* **14**, 1–136.

Smith, K. U. and Smith, W. M. (1962). "Perception and Motion", W. B. Saunders, Philadelphia and London.

Sokolov, E. N. (1960). Neuronal models and the orienting reflex. *In*: "The Central Nervous System and Behaviour" (M. A. Brazier ed.), J. Macy, New York.

Stratton, G. M. (1897). *Psychol. Rev.* **41**, 341, 463.

Taylor, N. B. G., Hunter, J. and Johnson, W. H. (1957). *Canad. J. Biochem. and Physiol.* **35**, 1017–1027.

Tyler, D. B. and Bard, P. (1949). *Physiol. Rev.* **29**, 311–369.

van Egmond, A. A., Groen, J. J. and de Wit, G. (1954). *Internat. Rec. Med.* **167**, 651–660.

von Holst, E. (1954). *Br. J. Anim. Behav.* **2**, 89.

Walsh, E. G. (1960). *J. Physiol.* **155**, 53–54P.

Wendt, G. R. (1968). Experiences with research on motion sickness. *Fourth Symposium on the Role of the Vestibular Organs in Space Exploration, NASA SP–187,* Naval Aerospace Medical Institute, National Aeronautics and Space Administration, Pensacola, Fla., U.S.A.

Wood, C. D. (1968). Use of drugs in the prevention of motion sickness. *Fourth Symposium on the Role of the Vestibular Organs in Space Exploration, NASA SP–187,* Naval Aerospace Medical Institute, National Aeronautics and Space Administration, Pensacola, Fla., U.S.A.

Wood, C. D., Kennedy, R. S. and Graybiel, A. (1965). *Aerospace Med.* **36**, 1–4.

# Appendix: International Standards in the Vibration Field

*D. M. Cowley*

## Human Exposure to Vibration

International Standards are issued by two main bodies, the International Organisation for Standardisation (ISO) and the International Electrotechnical Commission (IEC). The relevant technical committees which might include the subject of human response to vibration within their terms of reference were initially ISO/TC43 "Acoustics" which first met in 1953, and IEC/TC29 "Electro-acoustics". The ISO and IEC agreed to set up a joint steering committee to avoid any possible conflict between the two bodies. Further discussion led ultimately to the setting up of a Working Group ISO/TC108/WG7 "Human Exposure to Vibration".

This Group held its first meeting in 1964 under the Chairmanship of Dr. von Gierke of the U.S.A. Experts from France, Germany, the Netherlands, Sweden and the U.S.A. attended and agreed on the following Scope:

"To propose criteria for various degrees of acceptability of vibration and shock environments to man. Levels for industrial situations and for operators as well as passengers of transportation vehicles will be specified with the goal of ensuring safety and preformance capability (including comfort) of man. The acceptability of ground transmitted shock and vibration environments in residential houses will be included. Instruments and measurement procedures connected with shock and vibration work involving human subjects shall also fall under this scope. The effect of the whole mechanical spectrum up to ultrasonic frequencies shall be included provided that such mechanical energy is transmitted to the human body by structures or liquid. Vibrations of parts of the human body excited by airborne sound waves, particularly infrasonic noise, shall also be included in the scope. However, excluded from the scope are effects of such vibrations on the human ear."

The Group decided that first priority should be given to a document defining acceptable limits of vibration exposure for industrial situations, transport vehicles and residential premises. A German proposal was taken as a starting point for discussion. Entitled "Classification of the influence of mechanical vibration on man" it was substantially the same as the VDI publication "Assessing the Effects of Vibrations on Human Beings" which was largely based on the work of Dieckman on K values and was believed to be the only known document of its kind in practical use at the time. However, the scope of this proposal was rather limited—for example, it dealt in principle with instantaneous perception of vibration, took no account of the effects of duration of exposure and did not attempt to make recommendations concerning possible tolerances. The Group accordingly decided that more information, to be obtained from research and experience, and any specifications existing in this field, should be collected and circulated to all members before the next meeting was held. It was hoped to obtain enough information by this means to enable the Group to give really useful guidance on the evaluation of vibration effects on man. Initially, however, it was the scarcity of consistent quantitative data concerning man's perception of vibration and his reactions to it that made it difficult to reach agreement on an objective basis on essential matters such as time dependency, choice of corner frequencies for plotting acceleration/frequency weighting curves and weighting for direction (i.e. vertical or horizontal).

Meetings were held in 1965, 1966 and 1967 during which time experts from several more countries including Czechoslovakia, Japan and the U.K. joined the Group and several draft proposals were reviewed and revised. Partly no doubt for the reasons given above, members of the Group found themselves undecided as to the main purpose of the document they were aiming to produce: were they to try to specify rigid limits for human exposure to vibration or merely to provide guidelines? They finally decided that limits should be stated but that it should be made clear that they were recommendations and should not be applied too rigidly, and that a warning should be given against extrapolation. Although some compromises were inevitable, on matters such as corner frequencies, for example, it was agreed that there was a real need for some general guidance and that the Group should produce as good a document as it could on the basis of the information available. Notable points on which it was felt that little guidance could be given for the present were frequencies below 1 Hz and possible differences between time-dependent and time-independent effects on performance of tasks. (It is also of interest to note that, as their discussions proceeded, members of the Group came to feel that its title did not satisfactorily reflect its interests and it was eventually changed to the much more general "Human exposure to mechanical vibration and shock".)

After the 1967 meeting, a First Draft Proposal embodying the Group's decisions to date was prepared and later circulated to all members of the main Committee ISO/TC 108. In order to make clear what the Group's aims had been, as described above, the Foreword to that document contained the following statements:

> "In view of the complex factors determining the human response to vibrations, and in view of the paucity of consistent quantitative data concerning man's perception of vibration and his reactions to it, the present recommendation has been prepared first to facilitate the evaluation and comparison of data gained from continuing research in this field and, second, to give provisional guidance as to acceptable human exposure to vibration. The limits proposed in this Guide seem to be a fair compromise between the available data and should satisfy the need for recommendations that are simple and suitable for general application. The limits are defined explicitly in numerical terms to avoid ambiguity and to encourage precise measurement in practice. However, when using these criteria and limits, it is important to bear in mind the restrictions placed upon their application.
>
> Because of the wide variety of possible conditions and effects of human exposure to vibration, and because of the existing shortage of firm data, more detailed guidance is hardly warranted at the present time. Nevertheless, it is hoped that the Guide will not only prove useful in the assessment of existing or predicted vibration environments but will also stimulate the reporting and critical evaluation of new findings about the effects of vibration on man.

Comments received on this proposal were considered by the Working Group at a meeting in 1969 and some revisions were made. The resultant document was reviewed at a further meeting of the Working Group in 1970 and accepted by the Technical Committee, subject to a few minor modifications, for submission to the ISO Central Secretariat for circulation as a Draft ISO Recommendation.* The

---

* In 1971, the ISO Council agreed to issue ISO Standards (rather than ISO Recommendations) and Technical Reports, as described above.

proposal was approved by the required majority of members (the U.S.S.R. disapproved and the U.K. considered that it should be issued as a Technical Report rather than an International Standard) and was published as International Standard ISO 2631 in 1974 with the title "Guide for the Evaluation of Human Exposure to Whole-body Vibration".

The Standard recognises three basic types of human exposure to vibrations which may be briefly described as vibrations transmitted simultaneously to the whole-body surface or substantial parts of it, vibrations transmitted to the body as a whole through the supporting surface, and vibrations applied to particular parts of the body such as the head or limbs. However, it states that the recommendations apply chiefly to the case where vibration is applied through the principal supporting surface to the body of a standing or seated man, although they may also be used provisionally—and subject to due regard for all the circumstances—for the reclining or recumbent man.

Limits of exposure are specified for vibration transmitted from solid surfaces to the human body in the frequency range 1–80 Hz and are applicable within a given range to periodic vibrations and to random vibrations with a distributed frequency spectrum. The frequency range, its subdivisions and corner frequencies are selected in accordance with ISO/R 266 "Preferred Frequencies for Acoustical Measurements" and with national standards of several countries.

The extrapolation of any part of the standard to frequencies outside the range 1–80 Hz was explicitly forbidden. It was recognised that much more investigation was needed in the range below 1 Hz where the symptoms associated with vibration are different in character from the effects of higher frequency vibrations and often depend on individual factors which are not simply related to the intensity, frequency or duration of the motion concerned. At the other end of the scale, it was considered that the effects of vibrations at frequencies above about 80 Hz are dependent on so many possible variables that no generally valid recommendations can as yet be formulated.

Stated to be applicable only to situations involving people in normal health (i.e. persons considered fit to carry out normal living routines, including travel, and to undergo the stress of a typical working day or shift), the limits of exposure are set in accordance with three generally recognisable criteria which can be broadly described as preserving working efficiency, safety or health and comfort. For the purposes of the Standard, the limits are designated "Fatigue, decreased proficiency boundary", "Exposure limit" and "Reduced comfort boundary" respectively. They are specified in terms of vibration frequency, acceleration magnitude, exposure time and direction of vibration relative to the torso, defined in accordance with the recognised anatomical axes of the human body.

The Standard includes sections dealing with the characterisation of vibration exposure and a vibration evaluation guide. The former covers direction of vibration, location of measurement, intensity of vibration, measuring equipment, random or broadband analysis and exposure time and these points are qualified or explained as necessary. Limits are specified for vibration at the point of entry into the human body in the anatomically longitudinal direction and in the transverse plane. Linear vibrations are measured in the appropriate directions of an orthogonal co-ordinate system originating at the location of the heart.

It is acknowledged that there are circumstances in which angular or rotational vibrations may be more disturbing and users of the standard are urged to measure and report on angular vibrations in roll, pitch and yaw wherever practicable in order to add to the so-far rather scanty information on human response to such excitation.

Whatever type of transducer or pick-up is used for measurement, the primary quantity used to describe the intensity of vibration is acceleration expressed in metres per second squared (m/s²). The magnitude of a vibration should be expressed as a root-mean-square (rms) value.

The section containing the evaluation guide defines and explains the limits of exposure recommended for the Fatigue, decreased proficiency boundary, exposure limit and reduced comfort boundary. Figure 1 shows the longitudinal $(a_z)$ acceleration limits as a function of frequency and exposure time for the Fatigue, decreased proficiency boundary. The Standard includes another graph showing the way in which human tolerance decreases for various frequencies of vertical vibration with an increase in exposure time and there are two comparable graphs for the horizontal $(a_x, a_y)$ vibration exposure limits; there are also tables giving numerical values for the Fatigue, decreased proficiency limits for vibration acceleration in the vertical and horizontal directions.

It will be noted that Fig. 1 gives weighting factors of $+6$ dB and $-10$ dB for the exposure limit and reduced comfort boundary respectively. This is based on the assumption that human beings may be able to tolerate higher levels of vibration on occasion without impairing their health or risking their safety than they might be expected to do when carrying out tasks demanding varying degrees of skill and concentration. On the other hand, conditions which may be tolerated by people at work may very well be unacceptable to them under other conditions, for example, passengers travelling in transport vehicles, whether by air, land or sea, and people occupying residential, office or hospital premises. The limits set in ISO 2631 are generally in accordance with experimental observation and experience, but users are warned that a simple hierarchical relationship between the vibration intensities likely to impair health, working efficiency or comfort might not exist in all circumstances.

As has been shown, the recommended limits are related to exposure time. A normal daily working time of 8 hours is assumed and it is stated that, if the daily exposure to vibration is less than 8 hours, the tolerable acceleration level increases with decreasing exposure time.

The limits given in the graphs and tables apply when the exposure is continuous for a given period and numerical values are tabulated for 1 min, 16 min, 25 min, 1 hour, 2.5 hours, 4 hours and 8 hours. It is noted that where interrupted daily exposure or division of exposure into several intervals occurs, the effects of vibration might be mitigated by some degree of recovery which, if it occurred, would allow the tolerable total exposure level given in the Standard to be extended. In the absence of quantitative data on the recovery effect, this is not allowed for in the Standard. Directions are given for dealing with exposure to vibration interrupted by pauses during the working day but with the intensity of vibration remaining the same and the cases where the vibration level varies appreciably with time or the total daily exposure is composed of several individual times at different levels. Where exposure to vibration, whether continuous or intermittent, goes on for more than 24 hours, the limits specified are taken to apply to each 24-hour period or any part of it, so that, in computing an equivalent total exposure time, the period of integration for total exposure is 24 hours.

These are the main features of ISO 2631 which, as already stated, was published in spite of its acknowledged deficiencies because it was felt that it did at least

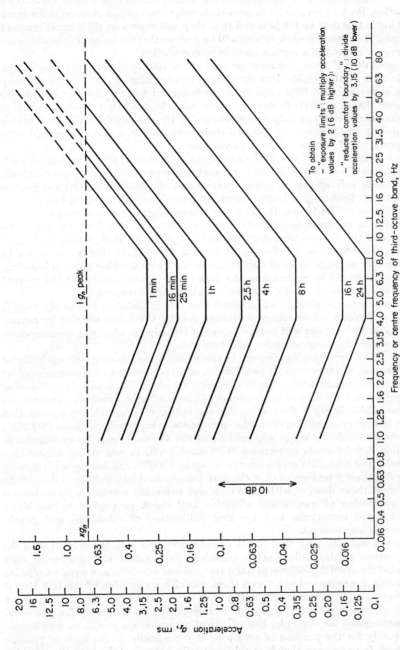

*Fig.* 1 Longitudinal ($a_z$) acceleration limits as a function of frequency and exposure time: "fatigue, decreased proficiency boundary".

provide some much-needed guidance in the field of human exposure to whole-body vibration. It also provides a common basis for procedure and evaluation for those working in this field and it is hoped that they will report on their experiences of applying it so that the next version will be more authoritative on points which are at present subject to a certain amount of speculation.

A good deal of space has been devoted to the history of ISO 2631 because the production of this Guide was the main preoccupation of the Working Group since it was set up in 1964 until the Draft Standard was circulated to all the ISO Member Bodies in 1971. It should also be borne in mind that during this period the document was not only under discussion by the members of the Working Group but was referred by them to their national Committees concerned with the problems of human exposure to vibration.

The composition of the BSI Committee is probably fairly typical of such committees; it includes doctors, researchers, representatives of aeronautical, automobile, railway and shipping interests and of agricultural, civil and general engineering. Government bodies represented include the Ministry of Defence, the Department of Trade and the Forestry Commission. Proposals and comments by national committees—including any reservations they had on particular features of the Guide—were duly transmitted to the Working Group and many were taken into account before the Guide was finalised, so that it should not be seen simply as the product of a small group of experts working away in isolation. Rather, it should be regarded as the best compromise available at the present time between the views of numerous experts in many countries.

It cannot be too strongly emphasised that it is intended to be exactly what it says—a "Guide", whose recommendations may be taken into account by anyone concerned with exposure of human beings to vibration in whatever circumstances but applied with common sense and discretion.

One ISO Committee making use of the Guide is that dealing with agricultural tractors and machinery in its preparation of a standard for the measurement of vibration on tractors and other self-propelled vehicles which is aimed at promoting the safety and comfort of the operator. Concerned with absolute measurement on the vehicle in three directions, this committee recommends instrumentation using frequency-weighting networks appropriate to limits selected from ISO 2631.

Before considering other applications of the Guide, it may be of interest to mention developments concerning the Group itself. It was stated earlier that several of the original Working Groups set up by ISO/TC 108, having subsequently extended their programmes of work, were transformed into Sub-Committees; the first were those dealing with balancing and balancing machines, measurement and evaluation of mechanical vibration and shock as applied to machines, vehicles and structures, and use and calibration of vibration- and shock-measuring instruments.

Even during the time that the Working Group was mainly occupied with the preparation of the Guide, other questions were raised and discussed; they included the special problems of hand transmitted vibration and matters relating to human exposure to impact and there was also recognition of the fact that it was necessary to envisage continuing work on the Guide, partly with the object of supplementing it with further recommendations on weighting for particular circumstances—for example, the effects of vibration on people in buildings—and partly for the purpose of reviewing it periodically in the light of possible feedback from users so that it could eventually be revised. In 1972 the Working

Group was elevated into a Sub-Committee with five Working Groups of its own to deal with the following matters: standardisation of terminology in human vibration and shock work; supplements and amendments to ISO 2631; hand-transmitted vibration; human impact testing and evaluation; and biodynamic modelling.

Programmes for the new Working Groups were reviewed at the first meeting of the new Sub-Committee held in September 1972. With regard to terminology, it was recalled that work on an International Standard for general vibration and shock terminology was virtually complete, but the Chairman of the Group concerned stressed that it would deal only with terms required in this particular field and these were intended to supplement the general terminology.

As far as the second Working Group was concerned, it was felt that the most important point not yet resolved by the Guide was the relationship between random and sinusoidal vibrations. Other matters to be considered would include the question of whether the frequency shape should be changed, especially for frequencies below 1 Hz, and the effects of vibration on people in buildings and in ships. It may be mentioned in passing that the BSI Committee agreed with the Group's view on its first priority but also thought that the question of time dependency needed a good deal more study as far as decreased proficiency was concerned. With regard to a correction table for vibration as related to buildings, the Group agreed that, for special conditions, values combining curves proposed by German and U.K. experts should be adopted and Japanese experts would make proposals for suitable instrument cut-offs. A Yugoslavian expert would prepare a document for ship vibration analogous to that for buildings.

A question on which work has been in progress for some time is the evaluation of human exposure to whole-body vibration below 1 Hz. Although ISO 2631 refers to the "special problems in the frequency range below 1 Hz associated with symptoms such as motion sickness", it makes no recommendations concerning lower frequencies and, in fact, as already mentioned, forbids extrapolation to cover them. It is in just this frequency range that much of the vibration en-countered in many forms of transport occurs and its effects range from mild discomfort to acute distress, but little guidance was available to help designers of various types of vehicles to overcome this problem.

This may have been partly due to the complexity of the problem, since the discomfort or distress experienced in this frequency region might well depend on factors other than the motion itself, e.g. vision, odours, age, sex etc. It may also have been due in part to the lack of useful data from laboratory and field studies clearly linking human reaction with motion input.

With the aid of critical surveys and analysis of such laboratory and field studies as were available, some proposed recommendations were formulated and these were intended not only to give some design guidance but also to stimulate research in this neglected area.

The recommendations cover vibration transmitted to the body in the frequency range 0.10–1.0 Hz and apply especially to discrete frequency and narrow band vibration. The suggested limits relate to two criteria, namely to minimise the severe discomfort associated with motion sickness and allied symptoms and to preserve comfort. They are confined to $a_z$ (longitudinal) linear motion and to vertical vibration only. Limits are given as a function of frequency and exposure times for periods of 30 min, 2 hours and, tentatively, 8 hours and the acceleration/time relationship follows a "constant energy" law ($a^2 t = $ constant). The limit given for frequencies between 0.6 Hz and 1.0 Hz is said to be largely an extrapolation due to lack of data, but there is some evidence to suggest that motion sickness rarely occurs in that frequency range. Designers concerned to minimise motion sickness are therefore recommended to try to eliminate vibration or at least reduce it wherever possible in the 0.1–0.3 Hz region in particular.

The severe discomfort boundary applies to what might be termed "infrequent travellers"—i.e. the general public. Frequent exposure often increases tolerance and both civil and military vehicle operators will normally be less susceptible to the effects of vibration than the general travelling public. For such people the boundary could probably be raised or, if retained, applied to a greater proportion of that particular population.

Other factors that have to be taken into account are sex and age. It appears that women are more prone to motion sickness than men (so that, in order to give equivalent cover, the limits would have to be lowered by about 20%) and young children are in general more sensitive to vibration than elderly people, and it is difficult to find a realistic means of adjusting the limits to provide for this age effect.

As with most problems concerning human exposure to vibration, much study, both in the field and in the laboratory, is still needed and it is hoped that any recommendations that may be published will stimulate further research in this field.

Another Sub-Committee of ISO/TC 108 that will need to take account of the Guide's provisions—and certainly of any recommendations on low frequency vibration—is SC2, which is concerned with mechanical vibration and shock as it concerns machines, vehicles and structures. Work has been in progress for some time on vibration in ships and it is considered that vibration limits for ships or any vehicle or structure should allow not only for what they can stand but also for what the occupants can tolerate. Note that this principle is being applied in the case of tractors and other self-propelled vehicles as reported above.

The question of hand-transmitted vibration is one of great concern to a number of countries. "Reynaud's phenomenon" or "Vibration-induced White Finger (VWF)" is a condition which afflicts many people in industries where vibrating tools such as chain saws, pneumatic drills, portable grinders etc. are used. Considerable research has been carried out in several countries and proposals for vibration limits have been put forward by Czechoslovakia, Japan, Sweden and the U.K. Because of the difficulty of reaching firm decisions on matters such as the best way of measuring the frequency spectrum, possible correlation between the energy absorbed and vibration damage and the frequency bands of most interest from the energy absorbing point of view, it was agreed that any proposals on this subject would probably be issued in the form of an ISO Technical Report. It may be mentioned in passing that the BSI has already published the U.K. proposals in the nationally equivalent form of a Draft for Development which invites users to report on their experiences of applying its recommendations.

Very little has been said here about the work on human exposure to impact since it is really outside the scope of this appendix, but it may be of interest to mention that work is in hand on human impact testing and evaluation, including such features as characterisation of human exposure to shock and biodynamic modelling. The latter may well be relevant to the hand–arm vibration group as a Japanese expert has raised the question of hand–arm impedance and the possibility of producing a model for evaluating this factor.

The work of ISO/TC 108/SC 4 with which we have been mainly concerned in this appendix must be seen as continuous since further information on the effects of vibration on man will always be required, as long as he is subjected to new environmental conditions, and instruments and equipment are developed to investigate their effects.

There are other Sub-Committees and Working Groups under the general umbrella of ISO/TC 108 that are or may be concerned with the activities of the Sub-Committee dealing with human exposure to vibration. SC2, referred to above, is an obvious candidate since its work necessarily overlaps with that of SC4. The Sub-Committee dealing with vibration and shock measuring instruments will also be concerned when SC4 has decided what is wanted with regard to instrumentation.

The Working Group on vibration isolators and dampers may also have an interest eventually since the question of hand tool isolation may be raised at a future date.

Another group whose work is related to that of SC4 is one concerned with "Generalized Terrain-dynamic Inputs to Vehicles". It is obviously difficult to assess the effects of vibration on people in vehicles unless the input is standardised in some way and the group is endeavouring to establish a method of defining the surface in terms of one spectral density but no conclusions have yet been reached.

It is hardly possible at the time of writing to predict what conclusions may ultimately be reached in the field of International Standards on human exposure to vibration. ISO 2631 offers the best guide so far available to those concerned with the effects of vibration on human beings but it is acknowledged to be subject to further modifications. Questions of the relationship between random and sinusoidal vibrations, low frequency vibrations etc. are still very much under discussion. Continuing increases in the stresses imposed on human beings may well make it impossible ever to write "Finis" to deliberations in this field, but it can at least be said that adequate machinery exists to ensure that they result in some fruitful recommendations.

# INDEX

## A

Abnormal individuals, 19, 35
Acceleration limits, 353
Accelerative cross-coupled stimulus, 314
Acceptable levels, 73, 144
Accidents (driving), 35, 142, 269
Acoustic filter, 39
Active anti-vibration seat, 242
Adaptability, 330, 334
Adaptation, 318, 339
Adaptation schedules, 338, 339
Aerodynamic infrasound, 7, 19, 21, 31
Aero-engines, 10
Age, 327
Air bag, 129, 130
Air compressor, 81
Air-conditioning, 37, 42, 66, 81
Aircraft vibration, 258, 260
Air transport, 10
Alcohol, 112
Alleviation of vibration, 242
Alpha rhythm, 115
Amplitude response (eye), 271, 272
Analysis of infrasound, 6
Anechoic room noise, 15
Angular acceleration, 152
Angular oscillation, 325
Angular oscillation effects, 201, 291
Annoyance, 65 ff.
Annoyance and loudness, 61 ff., 65 ff.
Annoyance and speed, 69
Annoyance in transportation, 68
Antidiuresis, 302
Artificial gravity, 339
Ascending reticular formation, 303
Asphalt plant noise, 86 ff.
Assessment of annoyance, 68
Atmospheric attenuation, 37
Auditory sensation, 39
Aural pain, 131, 133
Avalanche phenomenon, 304

## B

BSI committee, 354
Balance disturbance, 34, 97, 142
Band-pass filters, 20
Barbecue-spit rotation, 316
Binaural advantage, 49
Binaural threshold, 47 ff., 57
Biodynamic models, 123, 213, 237
Biological effects, 43
Blast furnace, 10, 81
Blast waves, 13
Blur, 273, 279
Blur level, 287
Boat vibration, 258, 260
Body posture, 203, 282
Body resonances, 123, 213, 237, 283
Boiler house, 10
Boiler rumble, 95
Bone conduction, 37
Bony labyrinth, 154
Buffeting, 74
Bus vibration, 258, 260

## C

Canal–otolith conflict, 313, 314, 316
Canal–otolith rearrangement, 311
Cardio-vascular behaviour, 217
Car vibration, 258, 260
Channel capacity test, 110
Chipping hammers, 203
Cinerama sickness, 311
Circular motion, 277
Collimated display, 243
Combined-axes vibrations, 202, 236 ff., 291
Combustion noise, 12
Commercial vehicles, 26, 73, 258, 260
Community reaction, 66
Comparator unit, 318
Compensatory eye movements, 270, 284
Compensatory tracking task, 237, 250 ff., 284

Complex balance test, 111
Complex object motions, 276
Complex subsidiary task, 111
Complex vibration, 291
Compressor noise, 11
Condenser microphone, 1, 3
Control-display ratio, 245
Control force, 245 ff.
Control force effects, 248
Coriolis adaptation test, 330
Coriolis sickness, 309
Coriolos vestibular reaction, 314
Corneo-retinal potential, 98
Counter rolling, 152, 168
Counter-rotation, 316
Criteria for passenger cars, 76 ff.
Cross-matching techniques, 193
Cross-modality matching, 193
Cupula, 156

## D

dB(A) scale, 65 ff.
Detection of infrasound, 1
Deterministic vibrations, 194
Dial reading errors, 270
Dieckman, 349
Diesel engine noise, 11
Discomfort (vibration), 189 ff.
Discomfort (visual), 281
Disturbance, 65
Diurnal fluctuations, 16
Double glazing, 9
Driving accidents, 35, 142, 269
Driving performance, 35
Drowsiness, 302, 303
Drugs (motion sickness), 336
Drum membrane retraction, 132
Dual-axis vibrations, 250, 255, 276, 278
Dual frequency motion, 277
Dynamic pressure chamber, 120, 121, 168, 181
Dynamic visual acuity, 267

## E

Eardrum, 132, 154
Eardrum rupture, 134
Earphones, 43
Eddy currents, 176 ff.

Electrodynamic loudspeaker, 42, 44, 53, 99
Electromyographic activity, 217
Electronics factory, 81
Endolymph, 154 ff.
Endolymphatic ducts, 157, 175
Endolymph displacement, 104
Engine noise, 31
Equalised binaural advantage, 49, 50
Equalised binaural threshold, 49
Equal loudness, 59 ff.
Equal loudness contours, 42
Equal sensation methods, 191
Equisection techniques, 194
Euphoria, 34
Eustachian tube, 180
Exposure limits, 146, 351
Exposure time, 279
Extractor fan, 82
Extraversion-introversion, 329
Eye, 263 ff.
Eye movements, 162, 265 ff.
Eye resonance, 286

## F

Factory boiler, 85, 86
Fatigue, 139
Fatigue decreased proficiency boundary, 288, 351, 352
Fear, 95
Ferry-boats, 33
Field dependence, 329
Field measurement of vibration, 257
Filters, infrasonic, 6, 20
Foot vibration, 204
Fractionation techniques, 194
Frequency-modulation microphone, 3
Frequency-modulation recorder, 4, 20, 67
Frequency response of headset, 45
Fume cupboard, 82, 84
Fusion frequency, 39

## G

Grindstones, 203
Growth of annoyance, 71, 78
Guinea pig, 158 ff.
Gun fire noise, 13
Gut reactions, 303

# H

Hair cells, 155, 174
Hand vibration, 203
Harmonic distortion, 39, 43, 47
Harness effects, 237, 245 ff.
Head movements, 340
Head reactions, 303
Head restraint, 308
Head-up display, 243
Head vibration, 207, 280, 282
Hearing acuity, 125
Hearing protection, 135
Hearing threshold, 37
Hearing tolerance limits, 135
Heave vibrations, 236 ff.
Helicopter, 33
Helicopter vibration, 258, 260
Helmholtz resonator, 21
Heterodyne analyser, 6
Home environment noise, 85
Homodyne analyser, 6
Hovercraft vibration, 258, 260
Human body analogues, 123, 213, 237
Human performance (visual), 268
Hydrofoil vibration, 258, 260

# I

IEC, 349
ISO, 349
ISO 2631, 240, 352
Illumination, 275
Impedance of the body, 213 ff., 282
Impulsive noise, 13
Incus, 175
Individual reaction, 66
Infrasound
  analysis, 6
  band-pass filter, 6, 20, 67
  commercial vehicles, 26
  detection, 1
  effects in transport, 33, 68 ff.
  energy, 25
  helicopters, 10, 33
  industry, 10
  measurements, 20, 67
  passenger cars, 21 ff.
  recording, 4
  ships, 9, 33
  sources (general), 67, 116

Infrasound—contd.
  sources in transport, 6, 31, 68 ff.
  subjective descriptions, 41, 106
  subjective effects, 102, 107, 122
  test facilities, 78, 119, 137
  trains, 9, 31, 79 ff.
International Electrotechnical Commission, 349
International Organisation for Standardisation, 349
Inter-vehicle comparisons, 76
Intoxication, 34

# J

Jet-edge mechanism, 21
Jet planes, 10, 42

# K

Kinaesthetic sensitivity, 188

# L

Labyrinth, 153
Landolt C, 241, 271, 274, 290
Latency of nystagmic response, 101
Lethargy, 34
Linear acceleration, 152
Long term monitoring, 15
Loudness, 37 ff.
Loudness and annoyance, 61 ff., 65 ff.
Low frequency annoyance, 66
Low frequency chamber, 53 ff.
Low frequency chamber (NPL), 53, 56
Low frequency headset, 44
Lung damage, 142

# M

Maculae, 188
Magnetic tape recording, 20
Magnitude estimation, 192
Mal de débarquement, 309, 318
Malleus, 175
Manual dexterity, 109
Measurement of infrasound, 20
Measurement of vibration, 225, 257
Membranous labyrinth, 154

Method of limits, 46
Microphone
  calibration, 4
  condenser, 1, 3
  frequency-modulation, 3
  moving coil, 2
  piezoelectric, 3
  Solion infrasonic, 2
  thermistor, 2
Middle ear, 132
Middle ear muscle displacement, 157
Mismatch signal, 319
Monaural threshold, 47 ff.
Monkey, 158 ff.
Motion sickness, 240, 258, 299 ff.
  drugs, 336
  frequency, 190
  screening, 334
  susceptibility, 326 ff., 334
Motivation, 239
Motorways, 7, 66
Moving coil microphone, 2
Multi-axis vibration, 202, 236 ff.
Multiple frequency motion, 277

N

Natural frequencies of body organs, 211
Neural mismatch theory, 301, 318, 339, 342
Neural storage unit, 318, 339
Nodal image, 241, 271, 274, 279, 285
Noise annoyance, 65 ff.
Noise assessment procedures, 66
Noise in transportation, 6 ff., 19 ff., 68 ff., 84
Noise rating number (NR), 65
Noise threshold, 51 ff.
Noisiness, 65
Non-stationary vibrations, 197
Non-vestibular proprioceptors, 299, 306 ff.
Number recognition test, 110
Nystagmus, 34, 98, 142, 153 ff.

O

Object and subject vibration, 293
Object illumination, 290

Object size, 275, 276, 290
Object vibration, 269
Oil-fired boilers, 66, 81
Open window, 25, 28, 74
Optical detector, 2
Ossicular chain, 157 ff.
Otoliths, 98, 188
Otolith overstimulation theory, 306 ff.
Oval window, 154, 177
Overtones, 38

P

Pain threshold, 1
Passenger cars, 21 ff., 68 ff., 76
Pensacola slow rotation room, 330
Perceived level (PLdB), 65 ff.
Perceived noise (PNdB), 65 ff.
Perception of vibration, 187
Perilymph, 154 ff.
Perilymphatic ducts, 157, 175
Perilymph displacement, 104
Perilymph pressure, 159 ff.
Peripheral visual acuity, 294
Phase response (eye), 271, 272
Physiological effects of vibration, 211
Piezoelectric microphone, 3
Pistonphone, 4, 39, 40, 67, 126
Pneumatic chisels, 203
Pointer following test, 34, 109
Positional nystgmaus, 180
Position feedback effects, 248
Postural equilibrium, 142
Power spectral density, 198
Proposed infrasound limits, 146
Protective adaptation, 313, 338
Pursuit eye movements, 270, 273

R

Radio-chemistry laboratory, 82
Rail test, 108, 143, 181
Random vibrations, 196, 291
Range of human hearing, 37
Raynaud's phenomenon, 203
Reaction time, 110
Reading, 269
  errors, 271 ff.
  time, 271, 273
Receptivity, 334

Receptivity and adaptability, 328
Recording of infrasound, 4
Reduced comfort boundary, 288, 355
Resonance (body), 123, 213, 237, 283
Respiratory effects, 140, 217
Retention of adaptation, 333 ff.
Retina, 264, 268
Ride
  railways, 224
  vehicles, 189, 209, 218, 220
Riveting hammers, 203
Road roughness, 19, 29, 218
Rocket noise, 42, 117
Rotary nystagmus, 165, 173
Round window, 177

**S**

Saccula, 155, 188
Seat
  characteristics, 209
  cushions, 242
Seated vibration, 205
Semi-circular canals, 88, 98, 153 ff., 285
Semi-supine condition, 291
Sensory conflict, 299, 309 ff., 310, 313
Sensory rearrangement, 299, 329
Sex, 328
Ships, 33
Shunt vibration, 236 ff.
Slope of noise spectra, 91 ff.
Social survey, 65
Solion infrasonic microphone, 2
Somaesthetic sensibility, 187
Somnolence, 302
Sonic bangs, 13, 128, 142
Sonic booms, 13, 128, 142
Sound level meter, 20, 67
Space flight, 314
Space sickness, 309
Speech intelligibility, 134
Sprung seats, 242
Standing vibration, 204, 291
Stapes displacement, 157 ff.
Stapes non-linearity, 171
Stationary vibrations, 197
Statistical definitions, 198
Statolith, 155 ff.
Steel works noise, 10
Streptomycin intoxication, 174

Strong and weak nervous systems, 329
Subject motivation, 239
Subject vibration, 187 ff., 235 ff., 280
Subjective descriptions (infrasound),
  41, 106
Subjective intrusiveness, 65
Subjective noisiness, 65
Supine position, 308, 341
Sway vibration, 236 ff.
Swing sickness, 313

**T**

Tactile sensitivity, 188
Tape recording, 20, 67
Task difficulty, 237, 238, 245
Task performance, 34, 139, 240 ff.
Temporary threshold shift, 109, 125
Test duration, 239
Thermistor microphone, 2
Threshold determining technique, 46
Threshold of hearing, 37 ff.
Time-course of adaptive effects, 318
Tolerance levels (infrasound), 144
Tolerance limits (vibration), 190, 352
Tracking task, 250, 267, 271
Traffic noise, 7
Trains, 31, 68, 79
Train vibration, 208, 258, 260
Transmissibility, 207 ff., 282
Transportation, 19
  noise, 6 ff., 19 ff., 68 ff.
Tremor (eye), 266
Tuning fork, 38
Turbulence, 7, 21, 31
Turnover frequency, 91 ff.
Tympanic membrane, 132, 154

**U**

Unease, 95
Unpleasantness of noise, 81
Urban traffic noise, 73
Utricle, 155, 188

**V**

Valsalva, 132
Vascular effects (vibration), 216
Vascular injection, 133

Vehicle ride, 189, 209, 218, 220 ff.
Vehicle vibrations, 259
Ventilation system noise, 12
Vertical nystagmus, 34
Vertical oscillation, 321
Vestibular
 apparatus, 188
 effects, 142
 ganglion neurons, 162
 nuclei, 303
 receptors, 177, 299
 stimulation, 311
 system, 151 ff., 305 ff., 310, 313, 326
Vestibulo-ocular reflex, 285
Vibration
 alleviation, 242
 amplitude (vision), 288
 and control manipulation, 244
 and performance, 199
 frequency (vision), 284
 greatness, 203
 greatness level, 194
 in aircraft, 258, 260
 in boats, 258, 260
 in buses, 258, 260
 in cars, 258, 260
 in helicopters, 258, 260
 in hovercraft, 258, 260
 in hydrofoils, 258, 260
 in trains, 208, 258, 260
 measurement techniques, 225, 257
 perception, 187 ff.
 test environment, 252
Viewing distance, 275, 289

Vigilance, 19, 35
Vision, 264 ff., 306
Visual
 acuity, 240 ff., 263 ff.
 blur, 273, 279, 289
 discomfort, 281
 feedback, 246
 —inertial conflict, 311, 312, 313
 —inertial rearrangement, 311
 nystagmus, 98, 142
 search, 294
Visually induced sickness, 308
Volume displacement, 176 ff.
Voluntary tolerance levels, 108

## W

Wesleyan University studies, 321
Whole-body infrasound, 53, 106, 136
Wind
 flutter, 21
 roar, 74
 -throb, 21
Work environment, 81

## Y

Y-axis vibration and performance, 201

## Z

Z-axis vibration and performance, 199
Zero-gravity flight, 314

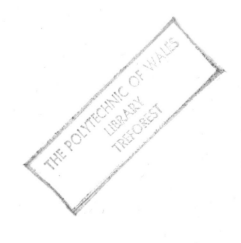